NURSING

A GUIDE TO

DIAGNOSIS

PLANNING CARE

HANDBOOK

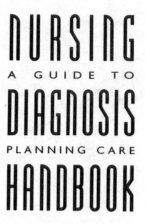

NURSING
A GUIDE TO
DIAGNOSIS
PLANNING CARE
HANDBOOK

Betty J. Ackley, MSN, Ed S RN
Professor of Nursing
Jackson Community College
Jackson, Michigan

Gail B. Ladwig, MSN, RN
Professor of Nursing
Jackson Community College
Jackson, Michigan

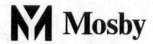
Mosby

St. Louis Baltimore Boston Chicago London Philadelphia Sydney Toronto

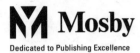

Mosby

Dedicated to Publishing Excellence

Publisher: Alison Miller
Editor: Terry Van Schaik
Developmental Editor: Janet Livingston
Project Manager: Mark Spann
Designer: David Zielinski

Printed in the United States of America

Mosby-Year Book, Inc.
11830 Westline Industrial Drive
St. Louis, Missouri 63146

ISBN 0-8016-7791-2

93 94 95 96 97   PC   9 8 7 6 5 4 3 2 1

Contributors

J. Keith Hampton, MSN, RN, CS
Nurse Manager, Dialysis Services,
University of Minnesota Hospital and Clinic,
Adjunct Faculty, School of Nursing,
University of Minnesota,
Minneapolis, Minnesota.

Mary Henrikson, MN, RNC, ARNP
Director of Nursing—Maternal Child Health
Services
Salem Hospital,
Salem, Oregon

Michelle Masta, RN, CCRN
Critical Care Educator,
Hillsdale Hospital,
Hillsdale, Michigan

Vicki McClurg, MN, RN
Assistant Professor of Nursing,
Seattle Pacific University,
Seattle, Washington

Cathy McLean, RN
Staff Nurse,
Home Health Services of Jackson,
Jackson, Michigan

Kathy A. Stimac O'Brien, MSN, RN
Pediatric Home Health Nurse,
Kids Club of Illinois,
Lombard, Illinois

Victoria L. Cole Schonlau, DNSc, MPA, RN
Nursing Faculty, Pediatrics,
California State University,
Los Angeles, California,
Nursing Supervisor,
Kenneth Norris Junior Cancer Hospital,
University of Southern California,
Los Angeles, California

Virginia Wall, MN, RN, IBCLC
Lactation Specialist,
University of Washington Medical Center,
Seattle, Washington

Peggy A. Wetsch, MSN, RN, CNA
Coordinator, Computer and Learning Resources,
School of Nursing, Los Angeles County Medical
Center
Los Angeles, California

Frances Wistrom, MSN, RN, CSW, CPN
Nurse Psychotherapist, Private Practice,
White Lake Counseling,
Whitehall, Michigan

Consultants

Constance Dellinger
Director, Adult and Community Education,
Jackson Public Schools, Tomlinson Center
Jackson, Michigan

Linda Williams, MSN, RN, C, CS
Associate Professor of Nursing,
Gerontological Clinical Nurse Specialist,
Jackson Community College,
Staff Nurse—Post Anesthesia Care Unit,
WA Foote Memorial Hospital,
Jackson, Michigan

Dedication

This book is dedicated:

- to Dale Ackley, the greatest guy in the world, without whose support this book would have never happened;

- to Dawn Ackley, who with Dale has been the joy of my life;

- to Jerry Ladwig, my husband, who is still supportive and patient after 28 years. I could not have done it without him.

- to my children and their spouses, Jerry and Kathy, Chrissy and John, Jenny and Jim and Amy—the greatest family anyone could ever hope for

- to our nursing faculty colleagues, especially Sharlene Shipley and Beverly Pickett. "Friends are one of life's most precious gifts."

Acknowledgements

We would like to acknowledge the help of the following people:

- Terry Van Schaik, Nursing Editor at Mosby, who championed this project with style and caring. We think she would make a great nurse!

- The nursing students and graduates of Jackson Community College who made us think and shared a very special time with us.

- The nurses at W.A. Foote Memorial Hospital and Doctors Hospital in Jackson, Michigan, who have helped us educate students and served as role models for excellence in nursing care.

- And each other, for perseverance, patience, and friendship.

Preface

The Nursing Diagnosis Handbook: A Guide to Planning Care is a convenient reference to help the practicing nurse or nursing student make a nursing diagnosis and write a plan of care with ease and confidence. The handbook helps the user correlate nursing diagnoses to what is known about the client based on assessment findings, established medical or psychiatric diagnoses, and the current treatment plan.

Making a nursing diagnosis and planning care are complex processes involving diagnostic reasoning and critical thinking skills. Nursing students and practicing nurses cannot possibly memorize over 1000 defining characteristics, related factors, and risk factors for the 110 diagnoses approved by the North American Nursing Diagnosis Association (NANDA). This book correlates suggested nursing diagnoses with what the nurse knows about the client and then offers a plan of care for each nursing diagnosis.

In Section II, Guide to Nursing Diagnoses, the reader can look up suggested nursing diagnoses for over 700 client symptoms, medical and psychiatric diagnoses, diagnostic procedures, surgical interventions, and clinical states. In Section III, Guide to Planning Care, the reader will find plans of care for all diagnoses suggested in Section II.

Nursing Diagnosis Handbook: A Guide to Planning Care includes medical diagnoses because nurses find them useful in suggesting appropriate nursing diagnoses. For example, under the medical diagnosis of AIDS, the reader will find the nursing diagnosis *Body Image Disturbance* related to (r/t) chronic contagious illness, cachexia. The nurse who is using this handbook will need to evaluate if this suggested nursing diagnosis is appropriate to the client.

Nursing Diagnosis Handbook: A Guide to Planning Care contains many features that contribute to its clinical utility:

- Suggested nursing diagnoses for over:

250	Signs and symptoms
200	Medical diagnoses
50	Surgeries
150	Maternal-child disorders
50	Mental health disorders
40	Geriatric disorders

- A format that facilitates a process nurses already use—analyzing signs and symptoms, which are defining characteristics of nursing diagnoses, to make a diagnosis.

- Use of NANDA terminology and approved diagnoses, including those approved at the Tenth NANDA Conference in 1992.

- Inclusion of two additional nursing diagnoses, *Grieving* and *Altered Comfort*, because of their usefulness when caring for many clients.

- Alphabetical formats for Section II, Guide to Nursing Diagnoses, and Section III, Guide to Planning Care, to allow for rapid access to information in the text.

- Nursing care plans for all nursing diagnoses that are listed in Section II.

- Specific geriatric and maternal-child interventions in appropriate plans of care.

- Specific client/family teaching interventions in each plan of care.

- Inclusion of commonly used abbreviations (for example, AIDS, MI, CHF) with cross-referencing to the complete term in the alphabetical listing of client data in Section II.

- Contributions by nurses who together represent all of the major nursing specialties and have extensive experience with nursing diagnosis and the nursing process.

The authors and contributors trust that readers will find *Nursing Diagnosis Handbook: A Guide to Planning Care* to be a valuable tool that will simplify the process of diagnosing clients and planning for their care and thus allow the nurse more time to provide care that will speed the client's recovery.

Contents

SECTION I

Nursing Diagnosis and the Nursing Process

NURSING DIAGNOSIS AND
THE NURSING PROCESS

The nursing process is an organizing framework for professional nursing practice. Components of the process include performing a nursing assessment, making nursing diagnoses, writing outcome/goal statements, determining appropriate nursing interventions, and then evaluating the nursing care that has been given. An essential part of this process is nursing diagnosis.

> A nursing diagnosis is a clinical judgment about individual, family, or community responses to actual or potential health problems/life processes. Nursing diagnoses provide the basis for selection of nursing interventions to achieve outcomes for which the nurse is accountable (NANDA, 1990).

ASSESSMENT

Before determining appropriate nursing diagnoses, the nurse must perform a thorough holistic nursing assessment of the client. The nurse may use the assessment format adopted by the facility in which he or she is practicing. Several organizational approaches to assessment are available, including Gordon's Functional Health Patterns and head-to-toe and body-systems approaches. Regardless of the approach used, the nurse will assess for client symptoms, which will help lead to the formation of a nursing diagnosis.

To elicit as many symptoms/problems as possible, the nurse uses open-ended, rather than yes/no, questions during the assessment. In addition to gathering data by questioning, the nurse obtains information via physical assessment and from diagnostic test results. If the client is critically ill or unable to respond verbally, the nurse will obtain most of the data from physical assessment and diagnostic test results and possibly from the client's significant others. The nurse can use data from each of these sources to formulate a nursing diagnosis.

NURSING DIAGNOSIS

The nurse makes a nursing diagnosis by categorizing symptoms, or defining characteristics, as common patterns of response to actual or potential health problems. After doing the assessment, the nurse lists all identified symptoms and clusters similar symptoms together. For example, the following symptoms may be identified in the assessment: shortness of breath, dyspnea, edema, hypotension. Of these, shortness of breath and dyspnea would be clustered because they are related. Both symptoms are defining characteristics listed under *Ineffective Breathing Pattern*. A diagnosis is made based on the client having the appropriate symptoms (defining characteristics) that correspond with a particular nursing diagnosis.

Nursing diagnosis statement

When using this book the reader may use one of two methods to develop the nursing diagnosis statement. The following is the first method:

A working nursing diagnosis statement has three parts:
    1.   The nursing diagnosis

2. "Etiology" or "related to" phrase
3. "Defining characteristics" phrase

The first part, called the *nursing diagnosis*, is taken from NANDA's list of approved nursing diagnoses. The authors have included two additional diagnoses, *Altered Comfort* and *Grieving*, because they have found these diagnoses to be useful in clinical practice. It is appropriate to develop new diagnoses when the NANDA-approved diagnoses do not adequately address the client's problem. Definitions, defining characteristics, risk factors, and related factors are provided in Section III for all NANDA-approved nursing diagnoses and for *Altered Comfort* and *Grieving*.

To determine a nursing diagnosis, use assessment data to make a list of tentative relevant nursing diagnoses for each client. Look up each chosen nursing diagnosis in Section III. To ensure that the diagnosis is appropriate for the client, read through the definition and defining characteristics. Many of the nursing diagnoses in Section III differentiate between major and minor defining characteristics or specify critical defining characteristics. For a diagnosis to be accurate, NANDA suggests that the client should have most of the major or critical defining characteristics. Research has shown that the major characteristics have appeared in most clients for whom the particular diagnosis has been made.

"Etiology" or "related to" phrase
The second part of the nursing diagnosis statement is the *etiology* or *related to (r/t)* phrase. This phrase states what may be causing or contributing to the nursing diagnosis. Pathophysiological and psychosocial changes, such as developmental age and cultural and environmental situations, may be causative factors. Ideally, the etiology, or cause, of the nursing diagnosis is something the nurse can treat. A carefully written, individualized "related to" statement enables the nurse to plan nursing interventions that will assist the client in accomplishing goals and returning to optimum health.

Refer to the common "related to" statements listed in this handbook, under the heading "Related Factors (r/t)," for each suggested nursing diagnosis. These "related to" statements may or may not be appropriate for the individual client. Readers may also refer to Section II to look for alternative "related to" statements as needed.

"Defining characteristics" phrase
The third part of the nursing diagnosis statement consists of defining characteristics (signs and symptoms) that the nurse gathered during the assessment phase. The phrase *as evidenced by (a.e.b.)* may be used to connect the etiology and defining characteristics.

The second method for using this book to develop a nursing diagnosis statement plus sample nursing diagnosis statements follow:

To write a nursing diagnosis statement using Section II of the *Nursing Diagnosis Handbook: A Guide to Planning Care* for a client with Addison's Disease, for example, look up the term *Addison's Disease*. Under the term you will find the following information:

Addison's Disease
Activity Intolerance (*Nursing Diagnosis*) r/t weakness, fatigue *(Etiology)*

To the information found in Section II, the "defining characteristics" phrase is added:
as evidenced by *generalized weakness* (*Defining Characteristic*—The defining characteristic is based on information the client shared or behavior the nurse observed during the assessment phase of the nursing process, such as "reports fatigue when walking length of hall" or "states weakness when standing more than 10 minutes")

With the above information, the nurse is able to make the following nursing diagnosis statement:
Activity Intolerance r/t weakness, fatigue a.e.b. generalized weakness.

To write a nursing diagnosis statement using Section II of *Nursing Diagnosis Handbook: A Guide to Planning Care* for a client with alopecia, look up the term *alopecia*. Under the term you will find the following information.

Alopecia
Body Image Disturbance (*Nursing Diagnosis*) r/t loss of hair, change in appearance *(Etiology)*

To the information found in Section II, the "defining characteristics" phrase is added:
a.e.b. verbalization of fear of rejection by others because of hair loss (*Defining Characteristic*).

With the above information, the nurse is able to make the following nursing diagnosis statement:
Body Image Disturbance r/t loss of hair, change in appearance a.e.b. verbalization of fear of rejection by others because of hair loss.

To use Section II of *Nursing Diagnosis Handbook: A Guide to Planning Care* to write a nursing diagnosis statement for a patient who has undergone leg amputation, look up the term *amputation*. Under the term, you will find the following information.

Amputation
Body Image Disturbance (*Nursing Diagnosis*) r/t negative effects of amputation *(Etiology)*

To the information in Section II, the "defining characteristics" phrase is added:
a.e.b. verbalization of change in lifestyle (*Defining Characteristic*).

With the above information, the nurse is able to make the following nursing diagnosis statement:
Body Image Disturbance r/t negative effects of amputation a.e.b. verbalization of change in lifestyle

PLANNING

Prioritizing
For most clients the nurse will make more than one nursing diagnosis. Therefore the next step in the nursing process is to determine the priority for care from the list of nursing diagnoses. The nurse can determine the highest priority nursing diagnoses by using Maslow's Hierarchy of Needs. In this hierarchy, highest priority is generally given to immediate problems that may be life threatening. For example, *Ineffective Airway Clearance* would have a higher priority than *Ineffective Individual Coping*. Refer to

Appendix A, "Nursing Diagnoses Arranged by Maslow's Hierarchy of Needs" for assistance in prioritizing nursing diagnoses.

Outcomes/Goals
After determining the appropriate priority of the nursing diagnoses, the nurse writes client outcome/goal statements. Suggested choices for outcomes/goals are listed in Section III for each nursing diagnosis. If at all possible, the nurse involves the client in determining appropriate outcomes/goals. Following discussion with the client, the nurse plans nursing care that will assist the client to accomplish the outcome/goal.

After the client outcomes/goals are selected, the nurse establishes a means to accomplish the outcomes/goals. The usual means are by nursing interventions.

Interventions
Interventions are like a road map directing nursing care and the best ways to provide it. The more clearly a nurse writes the intervention, the easier it will be to complete the journey and arrive at the destination of successful client outcomes/goals.

For each nursing diagnosis, Section III supplies choices for interventions. The reader may choose the ones appropriate for the client and individualize them accordingly or determine additional interventions.

Recording
The final planning phase is recording the nursing diagnoses, outcomes/goals, and interventions. Documentation is necessary for legal purposes and for financial reimbursement. Most commonly, this documentation is accomplished with the recording of the nursing care plan in an organized manner. Section III provides care plans that serve as models for documentation.

IMPLEMENTATION
The implementation phase of the nursing process is the actual initiation of the nursing care plan. Client outcomes/goals are achieved by the actual performance of the nursing interventions. During this phase the nurse continues to assess the client to determine the appropriateness of the selected interventions and to alter the interventions as necessary to achieve outcomes/goals. An important part of this phase is documentation. The nurse should use his or her facility's tool for documentation and accurately and carefully record all nursing interventions. Documentation is also necessary for legal reasons because in a dispute, "If it wasn't charted (or documented), it wasn't done,"

EVALUATION
Although evaluation is listed as the last phase of the nursing process, it is actually an integral part of each phase that the nurse does continuously, as is assessment. When evaluation is performed as the last phase, the nurse refers to the client's outcomes/goals and determines if they were met. If not met, the nurse begins again with assessment and determines why the outcomes/goals were not met. Were the goals not attainable? Was the wrong nursing diagnosis made? Should the interventions be changed? At this point, *Nursing Diagnosis Handbook: A Guide to Planning Care* will become useful again because the nurse can use it to look up any new symptoms or conditions that have been identified for the client and then adjust the care plan as needed.

SECTION II

Guide to Nursing Diagnoses

A

Abdominal Distention

Altered Nutrition: Less than Body Requirements r/t nausea/vomiting

Constipation r/t decreased activity, decreased fluid intake

Pain r/t retention of air and gastrointestinal secretions

Abdominal Hysterectomy

Refer to Hysterectomy

Abdominal Surgery

Altered Nutrition: Less than Body Requirements r/t high metabolic needs, decreased ability to digest food

Constipation r/t decreased activity, decreased fluid intake, anesthesia/narcotics

Knowledge Deficit r/t limited exposure to information

High Risk for Altered Tissue Perfusion: Peripheral r/t immobility and abdominal surgery resulting in stasis of blood flow

Pain r/t surgical procedure

High Risk for Infection r/t invasive procedure

Refer to Surgery

Abortion - Induced

Health Seeking Behaviors r/t desire to control fertility

High Risk for Infection r/t open uterine blood vessels, dilated cervix

Ineffective Family Coping: Compromised r/t unresolved feelings about decision

Knowledge Deficit r/t lack of exposure to situation

Self Esteem Disturbance r/t feelings of guilt

Spiritual Distress r/t perceived moral implications of decision

Abortion - Spontaneous

Altered Family Processes r/t unmet expectations for pregnancy/childbirth

Body Image Disturbance r/t perceived inability to carry pregnancy, produce child

Fear r/t implications for future pregnancies

High Risk for Fluid Volume Deficit r/t hemorrhage

High Risk for Dysfunctional Grieving r/t loss of fetus

High Risk for Infection r/t septic or incomplete abortion of products of conception, open uterine blood vessels, dilated cervix

Ineffective Family Coping: Disabling r/t unresolved feelings about loss

Ineffective Individual Coping r/t personal vulnerability

Knowledge Deficit r/t lack of exposure to situation

Pain r/t uterine contractions, surgical intervention

Self Esteem Disturbance r/t feelings of failure, guilt

Abruptio Placenta (>36 weeks)

Altered Family Processes r/t unmet expectations for pregnancy/childbirth

Anxiety r/t unknown outcome, change in birth plans

Fear r/t threat to well-being of self and fetus

High Risk for Altered Tissue Perfusion (Fetal) r/t uteroplacental insufficiency

High Risk for Fluid Volume Deficit r/t hemorrhage

High Risk for Infection r/t partial separation of the placenta

High Risk for Injury (Fetal) r/t hypoxia

High Risk for Injury (Maternal) r/t uterine rupture

Knowledge Deficit r/t limited exposure to situation

Pain r/t irritable uterus, hypertonic uterus

Abuse, Spouse, Parent, Significant Other or by Caregiver

Anxiety r/t to threat to self-concept or situational crisis of abuse

Caregiver Role Strain r/t chronic illness; self-care deficits; lack of respite care; extent of care-giving required

Defensive Coping r/t low self-esteem

Impaired Verbal Communication r/t psychological barriers of fear

Ineffective Family Coping: Compromised r/t abusive patterns

Post-Trauma Response r/t history of abuse

High Risk for Self-Directed Violence r/t history of abuse

Powerlessness r/t lifestyle of helplessness

Self-Esteem Disturbance r/t negative family interactions

Sleep Pattern Disturbance r/t psychological stress

Accessory Muscle Use (To Breath)

Ineffective Breathing Pattern r/t neuromuscular impairment, pain, musculoskeletal impairment, perception/cognitive impairment, anxiety, decreased energy/fatigue

Refer to COPD, Asthma, Bronchitis, Respiratory Infections, Acute Childhood

Achalasia

High Risk for Aspiration r/t nocturnal regurgitation

Impaired Swallowing r/t neuromuscular impairment

Ineffective Individual Coping r/t chronic disease

Pain r/t stasis of food in the esophagus

Acidosis, Metabolic

Altered Nutrition, Less than Body Requirements r/t inability to ingest, absorb nutrients

Altered Thought Processes r/t central nervous system depression

Decreased Cardiac Output r/t dysrhythmias from hyperkalemia

High Risk for Injury r/t disorientation, weakness, stupor

Pain: Headache r/t neuromuscular irritability, tetany

Acidosis, Respiratory

Activity Intolerance r/t imbalance between oxygen supply and demand

Altered Thought Processes r/t central nervous system depression

High Risk for Decreased Cardiac Output r/t arrhythmias associated with respiratory acidosis

Impaired Gas Exchange r/t ventilation perfusion imbalance

Acquired Immunodeficiency Syndrome
Refer to AIDS

Activity Intolerance

Activity Intolerance r/t bedrest/immobility; generalized weakness; sedentary life-style; imbalance between oxygen supply/demand; pain

Activity Intolerance, Potential to Develop

High Risk for Activity Intolerance r/t deconditioned status, presence of circulatory/respiratory problems, inexperience with the activity

Addison's Disease

Activity Intolerance r/t weakness, fatigue

Altered Nutrition: Less than Body Requirements r/t chronic illness

Fluid Volume Deficit r/t failure of regulatory mechanisms

High Risk for Injury r/t weakness

Knowledge Deficit r/t lack of informational sources

Adenoidectomy

Altered Comfort r/t effects of anesthesia: nausea and vomiting

High Risk for Altered Nutrition: Less than Body Requirements r/t hesitation/reluctance to swallow

High Risk for Aspiration/Suffocation r/t postoperative drainage and impaired swallowing

High Risk for Fluid Volume Deficit r/t decreased intake secondary to painful swallowing, effects of anesthesia

Ineffective Airway Clearance r/t hesitation/reluctance to cough secondary to pain

Knowledge Deficit r/t insufficient knowledge regarding postoperative nutrition and rest requirements, signs and symptoms of complications, positioning

Pain r/t surgical incision

Adjustment Disorder

Anxiety r/t inability to cope with psychosocial stressor

Impaired Adjustment r/t assault to self-esteem

Personal Identity Disturbance r/t psychosocial stressor (specific to individual)

Situational Low Self-Esteem r/t change in role function

Adjustment Impairment

Impaired Adjustment r/t disability requiring change in lifestyle, inadequate support systems, impaired cognition, sensory overload, assault to self-esteem, altered locus of control, incomplete grieving

Adolescent, Pregnant

Altered Family Processes r/t unmet expectations for adolescent, situational crisis

Altered Growth and Development r/t pregnancy

Altered Health Maintenance r/t denial of pregnancy, desire to keep pregnancy secret and fear

Altered Nutrition: Less than Body Requirements r/t lack of knowledge of nutritional needs during pregnancy and as a growing adolescent

Altered Role Performance r/t pregnancy

Anxiety r/t situational/maturational crisis—pregnancy

Body Image Disturbance r/t pregnancy superimposed on developing body

Decisional Conflict: Keeping child vs giving up child vs abortion r/t lack of experience with decision making, interference with decision making, multiple or divergent sources of information, lack of support system

Family Coping: Disabling r/t highly ambivalent family relationships, chronically unresolved feelings of guilt, anger, or despair

Fear r/t labor and delivery

Health Seeking Behaviors r/t desire for optimal maternal/fetal outcome

High Risk for Injury (Fetal and Maternal) r/t limitations of maturational age

Impaired Social Interaction r/t self-concept disturbance

Ineffective Denial r/t fear of consequences of pregnancy becoming known

Ineffective Individual Coping r/t situational/maturational crisis, personal vulnerability

Knowledge Deficit: Pregnancy, birth, parenting r/t lack of exposure to situation

Noncompliance r/t denial of pregnancy

Situational Low Self-Esteem r/t feelings of shame and guilt over becoming pregnant

Adult Respiratory Distress Syndrome
Refer to ARDS

Affective Disorders

Altered Health Maintenance r/t lack of ability to make good judgments regarding ways to obtain help

Chronic Low Self-Esteem r/t repeated unmet expectations

Colonic Constipation r/t inactivity, decreased fluid intake

Dysfunctional Grieving r/t lack of previous resolution of former grieving response

Fatigue r/t psychological demands

High Risk for Violence: Self-Directed r/t panic state

Hopelessness r/t feeling of abandonment, long-term stress

Ineffective Individual Coping r/t dysfunctional grieving

Knowledge Deficit r/t lack of motivation to learn new coping skills

Self Care Deficit: Specify r/t depression, cognitive impairment

Sexual Dysfucntion r/t loss of sexual desire

Sleep Pattern Disturbance r/t inactivity

Social Isolation r/t ineffective coping

Refer to specific disorder: Depression/major, Dysthymia, Mania

Aggressive Behavior

High Risk for Violence: Self Directed or Directed at Others r/t antisocial character, battered woman, catatonic excitement, child abuse, manic excitement, organic brain syndrome, panic states, rage reactions, suicidal behavior, temporal lobe epilepsy, toxic reactions to medication

Agoraphobia

Anxiety r/t real or perceived threat to physical integrity

Fear r/t leaving home and going out in public places

Ineffective Individual Coping r/t inadequate support systems

Impaired Social Interaction r/t disturbance in self-concept

Social Isolation r/t altered thought process

AIDS (Acquired Immunodeficiency Syndrome)

Altered Family Processes r/t distress over diagnosis of HIV infection

Altered Health Maintenance r/t knowledge deficit regarding transmission of infection, lack of exposure to information, misinterpretation of information

Altered Nutrition: Less than Body Requirements r/t decreased ability to eat and absorb nutrients secondary to anorexia, nausea, diarrhea

Altered Protection r/t high risk for infection secondary to inadequate immune system

Anticipatory Grieving: Family/Parental r/t potential/impending death of loved one

Anticipatory Grieving: Individual r/t loss of physiopsychosocial well-being

Body Image Disturbance r/t chronic contagious illness, cachexia

Caregiver Role Strain r/t unpredictable illness course; presence of situation stressors

Pain, Chronic r/t tissue inflammation/destruction

Diarrhea r/t inflammatory changes in bowel

Fatigue r/t disease process, stress, poor nutritional intake

Fear r/t powerlessness, threat to well-being

High Risk for Altered Oral Mucous Membranes r/t immunological deficit

High Risk for Altered Thought Processes r/t infection in brain

High Risk for Fluid Volume Deficit r/t diarrhea, vomiting, fever, bleeding

High Risk for Infection r/t inadequate immune system

High Risk for Impaired Skin Integrity r/t immunological deficit or diarrhea

Hopelessness r/t deteriorating physical condition

Situational Low Self Esteem r/t crisis of chronic contagious illness

Social Isolation r/t self-concept disturbance, therapeutic isolation

Spiritual Distress r/t challenged belief/moral system

Refer to Cancer; Pneumonia; AIDS in child

AIDS in Child

Altered Parenting r/t congenital acquisition of infection secondary to IV drug use, multiple sexual partners, history of tainted blood transfusion

Refer to AIDS; Hospitalized Child; Child With chronic condition; Terminally ill child/death of child

Airway Obstruction/Secretions

Ineffective Airway Clearance r/t decreased energy/fatigue, tracheobronchial infection, obstruction, secretions; perceptual/cognitive impairment, trauma, decreased force of cough from aging changes

Alcoholism

Altered Nutrition: Less than Body Requirements r/t anorexia

Altered Protection r/t malnutrition, sleep deprivation

Anxiety r/t loss of control

Compromised/Dysfunctional Family Coping r/t codependency issues

High Risk for Injury r/t alteration in sensory perceptual function

High Risk for Violence r/t reactions to substances used, impulsive behavior, disorientation, impaired judgment

Impaired Home Maintenance Management r/t memory deficits, fatigue

Ineffective Individual Coping r/t use of alcohol to cope with life events

Powerlessness r/t alcohol addiction

Self-Esteem Disturbance r/t failure at life events

Sleep Pattern Disturbance r/t irritability, nightmares, tremors

Social Isolation r/t unacceptable social behavior, values

Alcohol Withdrawal

Altered Nutrition: Less than Body Requirements r/t poor dietary habits

Altered Thought Processes r/t potential delirium tremors

Anxiety r/t situational crisis; withdrawal

Chronic Low Self Esteem r/t repeated unmet expectations

High Risk for Fluid Volume Deficit r/t excessive diaphoresis, agitation, decreased fluid intake

Ineffective Individual Coping r/t personal vulnerability

Knowledge Deficit r/t chronic illness or effects of alcohol consumption

High Risk for Violence r/t substance withdrawal

Sensory/Perceptual Alterations: Visual, Auditory, Kinesthetic, Tactile, Olfactory r/t neurochemical imbalance in brain

Sleep Pattern Disturbance r/t effect of depressants, alcohol withdrawal, anxiety

Alopecia

Body Image Disturbance r/t loss of hair, change in appearance

Alzheimer's Disease

Altered Thought Processes r/t chronic organic disorder

Anger r/t frustration secondary to memory deficits

Caregiver Role Strain r/t duration and extent of caregiving required

Fear r/t loss of self

High Risk for Injury r/t confusion

High Risk for Violence: Directed at Others r/t frustration, fear, anger

Hopelessness r/t deteriorating condition

Knowledge Deficit (Family) r/t limited exposure to information

Impaired Home Maintenance Management r/t impaired cognitive function, inadequate support systems

Impaired Physical Mobility r/t severe neurological dysfunction

Ineffective Family Coping: Compromised r/t altered family processes

Powerlessness r/t deteriorating condition

Self-Care Deficit: Specify r/t psychophysiological impairment

Sleep Pattern Disturbance r/t neurological impairment and naps during the day

Social Isolation r/t fear of disclosure of memory loss

Refer to Dementia

Refer to Maturational Issues, Adolescent

Anosmia—Loss of Smell

Sensory/Perceptual Alteration: Olfactory r/t altered sensory reception, transmission, or integration

Anticoagulant Therapy

Altered Protection r/t altered clotting function from anticoagulant

Anxiety r/t situational crisis

High Risk for Fluid Volume Deficit: Hemorrhage r/t altered clotting mechanism

Knowledge Deficit r/t lack of informational sources

Antisocial Personality Disorder

High Risk for Altered Parenting r/t inability to function as a parent or guardian; emotional instability

High Risk for Violence Directed at Others r/t history of violence

Impaired Social Interaction r/t sociocultural conflict; chemical dependence; inability to form relationships

Ineffective Individual Coping r/t frequently violating societies norms, rules

Anxiety

Anxiety r/t unconscious conflict about essential values/goals of life; threat to self-concept; threat of death threat to or change in health status; threat to or change in role functioning; threat to or change in environment; threat to or change in interaction patterns; situational/maturational crises; interpersonal transmission/contagion; unmet needs

Anxiety Disorder

Altered Thought Processes r/t anxiety

Anxiety r/t unmet security and safety needs

Decisional Conflict r/t low self esteem; fear of making a mistake

Ineffective Family Coping: Disabling r/t ritualistic behavior, actions*Ineffective Individual Coping* r/t not being able to express feelings appropriately

Powerlessness r/t lifestyle of helplessness

Self-Care Deficit r/t ritualistic behavior, activities

Sleep Pattern Disturbance r/t psychological impairment; emotional instability

Aortic Aneurysm Repair (Abdominal Surgery)

Refer to Aneurysm, Abdominal Surgery

Aortic Valvular Stenosis

Refer to Congenital Heart Disease/Cardiac Anomalies

Aphasia

Anxiety r/t situational crisis of aphasia

Impaired Verbal Communication r/t decrease in circulation to brain

Ineffective Individual Coping r/t loss of speech

Knowledge Deficit r/t lack of information on aphasia, alternative communication techniques

Apnea in Infancy

Refer to SIDS, Near Miss; Premature Infant

Apneustic Respirations

Impaired Breathing Pattern r/t perception/cognitive impairment, neuromuscular impairment

Refer to cause of Apneustic Respirations

Appendicitis

High Risk for Fluid Volume Deficit r/t anorexia, nausea and vomiting

High Risk for Infection r/t possible perforation of appendix

Pain r/t inflammation

Appendectomy

High Risk for Fluid Volume Deficit r/t fluid restriction; hypermetabolic state; nausea and vomiting

High Risk for Infection r/t perforation/rupture of appendix; surgical incision; peritonitis

Knowledge Deficit r/t unfamiliarity with information sources

Pain r/t surgical incision

Refer to Surgery, Hospitalized Child

ARDS (Adult Respiratory Distress Syndrome)

Impaired Gas Exchange r/t damage to alveolar-capillary membrane, change in lung compliance

Inability to Sustain Spontaneous Ventilation r/t damage to the alveolar capillary membrane

Ineffective Airway Clearance r/t excessive tracheobronchial secretions

Refer to Ventilator Client Care, Child with Chronic Condition

Arrhythmias

Refer to Dysrhythmias

Arthritis

Activity Intolerance r/t chronic pain, fatigue, weakness

Altered Family Process r/t disability of family member

Body Image Disturbance r/t ineffective coping with joint abnormalities

Pain, Chronic r/t progression of joint deterioration

Impaired Physical Mobility r/t musculoskeletal impairment

Knowledge Deficit r/t limited exposure to information

Self-Care Deficit: Specify r/t pain, musculoskeletal impairment

Refer to Rheumatoid Arthritis, Juvenile

Arthroplasty—Total Hip Replacement

Activity Intolerance r/t limitations from surgery

High Risk for Colonic Constipation r/t immobility

High Risk for Infection r/t invasive surgery, foreign object in body, anesthesia, immobility with stasis of respiratory secretions *High Risk for Injury* r/t interruption of arterial blood flow, dislocation of the prosthesis

High Risk for Peripheral Neurovascular Dysfunction r/t orthopedic surgery

Knowledge Deficit r/t lack of adequate information regarding potential postoperative complications and restrictions

Pain r/t tissue trauma associated with surgery

Refer to Surgery

Arthroscopy

Knowledge Deficit r/t unfamiliarity with procedure, postoperative restrictions

Ascites

Pain, Chronic r/t altered body function

High Risk for Altered Nutrition: Less Body Requirements r/t loss of appetite

Ineffective Breathing Pattern r/t increased abdominal girth

Knowledge Deficit r/t lack of informational sources, lack of interest in learning

Refer to cause of Cirrhosis or Cancer

Aspiration, Danger of

High Risk for Aspiration r/t reduced level of consciousness; depressed cough/gag reflexes; presence of tracheostomy or endotracheal tube; incomplete lower esophageal sphincter; presence of gastrointestinal tubes or tube feedings; medication administration; situations hindering elevation of upper body; increased intragastric pressure; increased gastric residual; decreased gastrointestinal motility; delayed gastric emptying; impaired swallowing;facial/oral/neck surgery or trauma; wired jaws

Assaultive Patient

Altered Thought Process r/t use of hallucinogenic substance, psychological disorder

17

High Risk for Violence r/t paranoid ideation

High Risk for Injury r/t confused thought process and impaired judgment

Ineffective Individual Coping r/t lack of control of impulsive actions

Asthma

Activity Intolerance r/t fatigue; energy shift to meet muscle needs for effective breathing and to overcome airway obstruction

Altered Health Maintenance r/t knowledge deficit regarding physical triggers, medications, treatment of early warning signs secondary to lack of exposure to information about asthma

Anxiety r/t inability to breathe effectively, fear of suffocation

Body Image Disturbance r/t decreased participation in physical activities at school

Impaired Home Maintenance Management r/t knowledge deficit regarding control of environmental triggers

Ineffective Airway Clearance r/t tracheobronchial narrowing, excessive secretions

Ineffective Breathing Pattern r/t anxiety

Ineffective Individual Coping r/t personal vulnerability to a situational crisis

Refer to Child with Chronic Condition; Hospitalized Child

Ataxia

Anxiety r/t change in health status

Body Image Disturbance r/t staggering gait

High Risk for Injury r/t gait alteration

Impaired Physical Mobility r/t neuromuscular impairment

Atelectasis

Impaired Gas Exchange r/t decreased alveolar-capillary surface

Ineffective Breathing Pattern r/t loss of functional lung tissue, depression of respiratory function or hypoventilation because of pain

Atrial Septal Defect

Refer to Congenital Heart Disease/Cardiac Anomalies

Autism

Altered Growth and Development r/t inability to develop relations with other human beings, inability to identify own body as separate from those of other people, inability to integrate concept of self

Altered Thought Processes r/t inability to perceive self or others, cognitive dissonance, perceptual dysfunction

High Risk for Self-Mutilation r/t autistic state

High Risk for Violence: Self and Other Directed r/t frequent destructive rages toward self or others, secondary to extreme response to changes in routine, fear of harmless things

Identity Disturbance r/t inability to distinguish between self and environment, inability to identify own body as separate from those of other people, inability to integrate concept of self

Impaired Social Interaction r/t communication barriers, inability to relate interpersonally to others

Impaired Verbal Communication r/t speech and language delays

Ineffective Family Coping: Compromised/Disabling r/t parental guilt over etiology of disease, inability to accept/adapt to child's condition, inability to help child and other family members seek treatment

Personal Identity Disturbance r/t inability to distinguish between self and environment, inability to identify own body as separate from those of other people, inability to integrate concept of self

Refer to Mental Retardation or Child With Chronic Condition

Autonomic Hyperreflexia

Dysreflexia r/t bladder distention, bowel distention, or other noxious stimuli

B

Back Pain

Anxiety r/t situational crisis; back injury

High Risk for Colonic Constipation r/t decreased activity

High Risk for Disuse Syndrome r/t severe pain

High Risk for Ineffective Individual Coping r/t situational crisis, back injury

Impaired Physical Mobility r/t pain

Knowledge Deficit r/t unfamiliarity with information resources, lack of information regarding prevention of further injury, body mechanics

Pain r/t back injury

Bathing/Hygiene Problems

Bathing/Hygiene Self-Care Deficit r/t intolerance to activity, decreased strength and endurance, pain, discomfort, perceptual or cognitive impairment, neuromuscular impairment, musculoskeletal impairment, depression, or severe anxiety

Battered Child Syndrome

Altered Growth and Development: Regression vs Delayed r/t diminished/absent environmental stimuli, inadequate caretaking, inconsistent responsiveness by caretaker

Altered Nutrition: Less than Body Requirements r/t inadequate caretaking

Anxiety/Fear (child) r/t threat of punishment for perceived wrongdoing

Chronic Low Self-Esteem r/t lack of positive feedback or excessive negative feedback

Diversional Activity Deficit r/t diminished/absent environmental or personal stimuli

High Risk for Poisoning r/t inadequate safeguards, lack of proper safety precautions, accessibility of illicit substances secondary to impaired home maintenance management

High Risk for Self Mutilation r/t feelings of rejection, dysfunctional family

High Risk for Suffocation/Aspiration r/t propped bottle, unattended child*High Risk for Trauma* r/t inadequate precautions, cognitive or emotional difficulties

Impaired Skin Integrity r/t altered nutritional state, physical abuse

Pain r/t physical injuries

Post-Trauma Response r/t physical abuse, incest/rape/molestation

Sleep Pattern Disturbance r/t hypervigilance, anxiety

Social Isolation, Family Imposed r/t fear of disclosure of family dysfunction and abuse

Battered Person

Refer to Abuse—Parent, Significant Other, Caregiver

Bedsores

Refer to Pressure Ulcers

Bedwetting

Refer to Enuresis

Benign Prostatic Hypertrophy

Refer to Prostatic Enlargement

Biliary Atresia

Altered Comfort r/t pruritis, nausea

Altered Nutrition: Less than Body Requirements r/t decreased absorption of fat and fat soluble vitamins; poor feeding

Anxiety/Fear r/t surgical intervention (Kasai procedure) and possible liver transplantation

High Risk for Ineffective Breathing Patterns r/t enlarged liver and development of ascites

High Risk for Injury: Bleeding r/t vitamin K deficiency and altered clotting mechanisms

High Risk for Impaired Skin Integrity r/t to pruritis
Refer to Hospitalized Child; Child With Chronic
Condition; Terminally Ill Child/Death of Child;
Cirrhosis as complication

Bipolar Disorder: Depression, Mania
Altered Health Maintenance r/t lack of ability to
make good judgments regarding ways to obtain
help
Chronic Low Self-Esteem r/t repeated unmet
expectations
Dysfunctional Grieving r/t lack of previous resolu-
tion of former grieving response
Fatigue r/t psychological demands
Ineffective Individual Coping r/t dysfunctional
grieving
Knowledge Deficit r/t lack of motivation to learn
new coping skills
Self Care Deficit: Specify r/t depression, cognitive
impairment
Social Isolation r/t ineffective coping
Refer to Depression or Mania

Bladder Distension
Urinary Retention r/t high urethral pressure caused
by weak detrusor; inhibition of reflex arc;
blockage; strong sphincter; fecal impaction

Bladder Training
Knowledge Deficit r/t protocol to follow for
bladder training
Stress Incontinence r/t degenerative change in
pelvic muscles and structural supports
Urge Incontinence r/t decreased bladder capacity,
increased urine concentration, overdistention of
bladder
Functional Incontinence r/t altered environment;
sensory, cognitive, or mobility deficit

Bladder Tumor
High Risk for Urinary Retention r/t clots obstruct-
ing urethra
Refer to TURP, Cancer

Blindness
Sensory Perceptual Alteration: Visual r/t altered
sensory reception, transmission, or integration

Blood Pressure Alteration
Refer to Hypertension, Hypotension

Body Image Change
Body Image Disturbance r/t chronic illness; loss of
body part; change in body appearance

Bone Marrow Biopsy
Fear r/t unkown outcome of results of aspiration
Knowledge Deficit r/t purpose and actual
procedure
Pain r/t bone marrow aspiration

Borderline Personality
Altered Thought Process r/t poor reality testing
Anxiety r/t perceived threat to self-concept
Defensive Coping r/t difficulty with relationships;
inability to accept blame for own behavior
Disturbance in Self Concept r/t unmet dependency
needs
High Risk for Caregiver Role Strain r/t care
receiver can not accept criticism or takes ad-
vantage of others to meet own needs; unreason-
able expectations of care receiver
High Risk for Self-Mutilation r/t ineffective
coping; feelings of self-hatred
High Risk for Violence: Self-Directed r/t feelings
of need to punish self/manipulative behavior
Ineffective Individual Coping r/t use of maladjust-
ed defense mechanisms, e.g., projection, denial
Powerlessness r/t lifestyle of helplessness
Social Isolation r/t immature interests

Boredom
Diversional Activity Deficit r/t environmental lack
of diversional activity

Bowel Incontinence
Bowel Incontinence r/t decreased awareness of need to defecate; loss of sphincter control; fecal impaction

Bowel Obstruction
Altered Nutrition: Less than Body Requirements r/t nausea, vomiting
Constipation r/t decreased motility; intestinal obstruction
Fluid volume Deficit r/t inadequate fluid volume intake; fluid loss in bowel
Pain r/t pressure from distended abdomen

Bowel Sounds, Absent or Diminished
Constipation r/t decreased or absent peristalsis
Fluid Volume Deficit r/t inability to ingest fluids; loss of fluids in bowel

Bowel Sounds, Hyperactive
Diarrhea r/t increased gastrointestinal motility

BPH (Benign Prostatic Hypertrophy)
High Risk for Infection r/t urinary residual postvoiding; bacterial invasion of bladder
Knowledge Deficit r/t unfamiliarity with information sources
Sleep Pattern Disturbance r/t nocturia
Urinary Retention r/t obstruction

Bradycardia
Altered Tissue Perfusion: Cerebral r/t decreased cardiac output secondary to bradycardia
Decreased Cardiac Output r/t slow heart rate supplying inadequate amount of blood for body function
High Risk for Injury r/t decreased cerebral tissue perfusion
Knowledge Deficit r/t cardiac medication effects

Bradypnea
Ineffective Breathing Pattern r/t neuromuscular impairment; pain; musculoskeletal impairment; perception/cognitive impairment; decreased energy/fatigue; drug effect
Refer to cause of Bradypnea

Brain Injury
Refer to Intracranial Pressure, Increased

Brain Surgery
Refer to Craniotomy/Craniectomy

Brain Tumor
Altered Thought Processes r/t altered circulation or destruction of brain tissue
Anticipatory Grieving r/t potential loss of physio-psychosocial well-being
Fear r/t threat to well-being
High Risk for Injury r/t sensory-perceptual alterations; weakness
Pain r/t neurologic injury
Sensory/Perceptual Alteration (Specify) r/t tumor growth compressing brain tissue
Refer to Craniotomy/Craniectomy; Cancer; Chemotherapy; Radiation Therapy; Hospitalized Child; Child with Chronic Condition; Terminally Ill Child

Breastfeeding, Effective
Effective Breastfeeding r/t basic breastfeeding knowledge; normal breast structure; normal infant oral structure; infant gestational age greater than 34 weeks; support sources or maternal confidence

Breastfeeding, Ineffective
Ineffective Breastfeeding r/t prematurity; infant anomaly; maternal breast anomaly; previous breast surgery; previous history of breastfeeding failure; infant receiving supplemental feedings with artificial nipple; poor infant sucking reflex; nonsupportive partner/family; knowledge

deficit; interruption in breastfeeding; maternal anxiety/ ambivalence

Refer to Painful Breasts-Engorgement; Painful Breasts-Cracked Nipples

Breastfeeding, Interrupted

Interrupted Breastfeeding r/t maternal or infant illness; prematurity; maternal employment; contraindications to breastfeeding (e.g., drugs, true breastmilk jaundice); need to abruptly wean infant

Breast Cancer

Disturbance in Self-Concept r/t surgery and possible side effects of chemotherapy and/or radiation

Fear r/t diagnosis of cancer

Ineffective Coping r/t treatment and prognosis

Sexual Dysfunction r/t loss of body part and partner's reaction to loss

Refer to Mastectomy

Breast Lumps

Knowledge Deficit r/t breast-self examination

Fear r/t potential for diagnosis of cancer

Breath Sounds, Decreased or Absent

Refer to Atelectasis, Pneumothorax

Breathing Pattern Alteration

Ineffective Breathing Pattern r/t neuromuscular impairment; pain; musculoskeletal impairment; perception/cognitive impairment; anxiety; decreased energy/fatigue

Bronchitis

Anxiety r/t potential chronic condition

Ineffective Airway Clearance r/t excessive thickened mucous secretion

Knowledge Deficit r/t lack of exposure to information; need for cessation of smoking

Bronchopulmonary Dysplasia (BPD)

Activity Intolerance r/t imbalance between oxygen supply and demand

Altered Nutrition: Less than Body Requirements r/t poor feeding; increased caloric needs secondary to increased work of breathing*Fluid Volume Excess* r/t sodium and water retention

Knowledge Deficit r/t lack of informational sources

Refer to Respiratory Conditions of the Neonate; Child With Chronic Condition; Hospitalized Child

Bruits, Carotid

Altered Tissue Perfusion: Cerebral r/t interruption of carotid blood flow

High Risk for Injury r/t loss of motor, sensory, or visual function

Bulimia

Altered Nutrition: Less than Body Requirements r/t induced vomiting

Altered Thought Processes r/t anorexia

Chronic Low Self-Esteem r/t lack of positive feedback

Defensive Coping r/t eating disorder

Disturbance in Body Image r/t misperception about actual appearance and body weight

Fear r/t food ingestion and weight gain

Ineffective Family Coping r/t chronically unresolved feelings: guilt, anger, and hostility

Noncompliance r/t negative feelings toward treatment regimen

Powerlessness r/t urge to purge self after eating

Refer to Maturational Issues, Adolescent

Burns

Altered Nutrition: Less than Body Requirements r/t increased metabolic needs; anorexia; protein and fluid loss

Altered Tissue Perfusion: Peripheral r/t circumferential burns; impaired arterial/venous circulation

Anticipatory Grieving r/t loss of bodily function; loss of future hopes and plans

Anxiety/Fear r/t pain from treatments; possible permanent disfigurement

Body Image Disturbance r/t altered physical appearance

Diversional Activity Deficit r/t long-term hospitalization

High Risk for Fluid Volume Deficit r/t loss from skin surface; fluid shift

High Risk for Hypothermia r/t impaired skin integrity

High Risk for Infection r/t loss of intact skin; trauma, invasive sites

High Risk for Ineffective Airway Clearance r/t potential tracheobronchial obstruction, edema

High Risk for Peripheral Neurovascular Dysfunction r/t eschar formation with circumferential burn

Impaired Physical Mobility r/t pain; musculoskeletal impairment; contracture formation

Impaired Skin Integrity r/t burn injury of skin

Pain r/t burn injury and treatments

Post-Trauma Response r/t life-threatening event

Refer to Safety, Childhood; Hospitalized Child

Bursitis

Impaired Physical Mobility r/t inflammation in joint

Pain r/t inflammation in joint

C

Cachexia
Altered Nutrition: Less than Body Requirements r/t inability to ingest food due to biological factors

Altered Protection r/t inadequate nutrition

Calcium Alteration
Refer to Hypocalcemia, Hypercalcemia

Cancer
Altered Nutrition: Less than Body Requirements r/t loss of appetite or difficulty swallowing; side effects of chemotherapy; obstruction by tumor

Altered Oral Mucous Membranes r/t chemotherapy; oral pH changes; decreased or altered oral flora

Altered Protection r/t cancer-suppressing immune system

Altered Role Performance r/t change in physical capacity; inability to resume prior role

Anticipatory Grieving r/t potential loss of significant others; high risk for infertility

Body Image Disturbance r/t side effects of treatment; cachexia

Pain, Chronic r/t metastatic cancer

Colonic Constipation r/t side effects of medication; altered nutrition; decreased activity

Decisional Conflict r/t selection of treatment choices; continuation/discontinuation of treatment; Do Not Resuscitate decision

Fear r/t serious threat to well-being

High Risk for Disuse Syndrome r/t severe pain; change in level of consciousness

High Risk for Infection r/t inadequate immune system

High Risk for Injury r/t bleeding secondary to bone marrow depression

High Risk for Impaired Home Maintenance Management r/t lack of familiarity with community resources

Hopelessness r/t loss of control; terminal illness

Impaired Physical Mobility r/t weakness; neuro-musculoskeletal impairment; pain

Impaired Skin Integrity r/t immunological deficit; immobility

Ineffective Denial r/t dysfunctional grieving process

Ineffective Family Coping: Compromised r/t prolonged disease or disability progression that exhausts the supportive ability of significant others functioning

Ineffective Individual Coping r/t personal vulnerability in situational crisis; terminal illness

Knowledge Deficit r/t limited exposure to prescribed treatment information

Powerlessness r/t treatment, progression of disease

Self-Care Deficit: Specify r/t pain; intolerance to activity; decreased strength

Sleep Pattern Disturbance r/t anxiety; pain

Social Isolation r/t hospitalization; lifestyle changes

Spiritual Distress r/t test of spiritual beliefs

Refer to Chemotherapy; Hospitalized Child; Child with Chronic Condition; Terminally Ill Child/Death of Child

Capillary Refill Time, Prolonged
Altered Tissue Perfusion: Peripheral r/t interruption of arterial/venous flow

High Risk for Peripheral Neurovascular Dysfunction r/t vascular obstruction

Impaired Gas Exchange r/t ventilation perfusion imbalance

Refer to Shock

Cardiac Catheterization
Altered Comfort r/t postprocedure restrictions, invasive procedure

Anxiety/Fear r/t invasive procedure, uncertainty of outcome of procedure

High Risk for Altered Tissue Perfusion r/t impaired arterial/venous circulation

High Risk for Decreased Cardiac Output r/t ventricular ischemia, arrhythmias

High Risk for Injury: Hematoma r/t invasive procedure

High Risk for Peripheral Neurovascular Dysfunction r/t vascular obstruction

Knowledge Deficit r/t limited exposure to information about the procedure and after procedure care

Cardiac Disorders in Pregnancy

Activity Intolerance r/t cardiac pathophysiology; increased demand secondary to pregnancy; weakness, fatigue

Altered Family Processes r/t changes in role; hospitalization; maternal incapacitation

Altered Role Performance r/t changes in lifestyle; expectations secondary to disease process with superimposed pregnancy

Anxiety r/t unknown outcomes of pregnancy and family well-being

Fatigue r/t metabolic demands; psychological-emotional demands

Fear r/t potential poor fetal/maternal outcome

High Risk for Altered Fetal Tissue Perfusion r/t poor maternal oxygenation

High Risk for Fluid Volume Excess r/t compromised regulatory mechanism with increased afterload, increased preload, increased circulating blood volume

High Risk for Impaired Gas Exchange r/t pulmonary edema

High Risk for Fetal Injury r/t hypoxia

High Risk for Maternal Injury r/t thromboembolic episode secondary to valvular defect

Ineffective Family Coping: Compromised r/t prolonged hospitalization or maternal incapacitation that exhausts supportive capacity of significant people

Ineffective Individual Coping r/t personal vulnerability

Knowledge Deficit r/t primiparity

Powerlessness r/t illness-related regime

Situational Low Self-Esteem r/t situational crisis of pregnancy

Social Isolation r/t limitations of activity; bedrest/hospitalization; separation from family and friends

Cardiac Dysrhythmias
Refer to Dysrhythmias

Cardiac Output Decrease
Decreased Cardiac Output r/t cardiac dysfunction

Caregiver Role Strain
Caregiver Role Strain r/t pathophysiological factors; developmental factors; psychosocial factors; situational factors

High Risk for Caregiver Role Strain r/t pathophysiological factors; developmental factors; psychosocial factors; or situational factors

Carious Teeth
Refer to Cavities in Teeth

Carotid Endarterectomy
Fear r/t surgery in vital area

High Risk for Altered Tissue Perfusion: Cerebral r/t hemorrhage, clot formation

High Risk for Injury r/t possible hematoma formation

High Risk for Ineffective Breathing Pattern r/t hematoma compressing trachea

Knowledge Deficit r/t unfamiliarity with information resources

Carpal Tunnel Syndrome
Impaired Physical Mobility r/t neuromuscular impairment

Pain r/t unrelieved pressure on median nerve

Carpopedal Spasm
Refer to Hypocalcemia

25

Casts

Diversional Activity Deficit r/t physical limitations from the cast

High Risk for Peripheral Neurovascular Dysfunction r/t mechanical compression from cast

High Risk for Impaired Skin Integrity r/t unrelieved pressure on skin

Impaired Physical Mobility r/t limb immobilization

Knowledge Deficit r/t cast management

Cataract Extraction

Anxiety r/t threat of permanent vision loss; surgical procedure

Sensory/Perceptual Alteration: Vision r/t adjustment to new lens or glasses

High Risk for Injury r/t increased intraocular pressure; accomodation to new visual field

Knowledge Deficit r/t postoperative restrictions

Catatonic Schizophrenia

Altered Nutrition: Less than Body Requirements r/t decrease in outside stimulation; no perception of hunger; resistance to instructions to eat

Impaired Physical Mobility r/t cognitive impairment; maintenance of rigid posture; inappropriate/ bizarre postures

Impaired Verbal Communication r/t mutism

Social Isolation r/t inability to communicate; immobility

Refer to Schizophrenia

Catheterization, Urinary

High Risk for infection r/t invasive procedure

Knowledge Deficit r/t care of catheter

Cavities in Teeth

Altered Health Maintenance r/t lack of knowledge regarding prevention of dental disease secondary to high sugar diet; giving infants/toddlers with erupted teeth bottles of milk at bedtime; lack of fluoride treatments; inadequate or improper brushing of teeth

Cellulitis

Altered Tissue Perfusion: Peripheral r/t edema

Impaired Skin Integrity r/t inflammatory process damaging skin

Pain r/t inflammatory changes in tissues from infection

Cellulitis, Periorbital

Impaired Skin Integrity r/t inflammation/infection of skin/tissues

Pain r/t edema and inflammation of skin/tissues

Sensory/Perceptual Alterations (visual) r/t decreased visual fields secondary to edema of eyelids

Hyperthermia r/t infectious process

Refer to Hospitalized Child

Central Line Insertion

High Risk for Infection r/t invasive procedure

Knowledge Deficit r/t precautions to take when central line in place

Cerebral Palsy

Impaired Physical Mobility r/t spasticity, neuromuscular impairment/weakness

Self Care Deficit (specify area and level) r/t neuromuscular impairments, sensory deficits

High Risk for Injury/Trauma r/t muscle weakness, inability to control spasticity

Impaired Verbal Communication r/t impaired ability to articulate/speak words secondary to facial muscle involvement

Diversional Activity Deficit r/t physical impairments; limitations on ability to participate in recreational activities

Impaired Social Interaction r/t impaired communication skills; limited physical activity; perceived differences from peers

High Risk for Altered Nutrition: Less than Body Requirements r/t spasticity, feeding/swallowing difficulties

Refer to Child With Chronic Condition

Cerebrovascular Accident
Refer to CVA

Cesarean Delivery
Altered Family Processes r/t unmet expectations for childbirth

Altered Role Performance r/t unmet expectations for childbirth

Alteration in Comfort: Nausea, Vomiting, Pruritis r/t side effects of systemic or epidural narcotics

Anxiety r/t unmet expectations for childbirth; unknown outcome of surgery

Body Image Disturbance r/t surgery, unmet expectations for childbirth

Fear r/t perceived threat to own well being

High Risk for Aspiration r/t positioning for general anesthesia

High Risk for Fluid Volume Deficit r/t increased blood loss secondary to surgery

High Risk for Infection r/t surgical incision; stasis of respiratory secretions secondary to general anesthesia

High Risk for Urinary Retention r/t regional anesthesia

Impaired Physical Mobility r/t pain

Knowledge Deficit r/t lack of exposure to situation

Pain r/t surgical incision; decreased or absent peristalsis secondary to anesthesia; manipulation of abdominal organs during surgery; immobilization; restricted diet

Situational Low Self-Esteem r/t inability to birth child vaginally

Chemical Dependency
Refer to Alcohol Abuse, Drug Abuse

Chemotherapy
Altered Comfort: Nausea and Vomiting r/t effects of chemotherapy

Altered Nutrition: Less than Body Requirements r/t side effects of chemotherapy

Altered Oral Mucous Membranes r/t effects of chemotherapy

Altered Protection r/t suppressed immune system; decreased platelets

Body Image Disturbance r/t loss of weight; loss of hair

Fatigue r/t disease process; anemia; drug effects

High Risk for Altered Tissue Perfusion r/t anemia

High Risk for Fluid Volume Deficit r/t vomiting, diarrhea

High Risk for Infection r/t immunosuppression

High Risk for Trauma/Injury r/t abnormal blood profile

Knowledge Deficit r/t action, side effects of chemotherapy

Refer to Cancer

Chest Pain
Fear r/t potential threat of death

High Risk for Decreased Cardiac Output r/t ventricular ischemia

Pain r/t myocardial injury, ischemia

Refer to Angina, MI

Chest Tubes
High Risk for Injury r/t presence of invasive chest tube

Impaired Gas Exchange r/t decreased functional lung tissue

Ineffective Breathing Pattern r/t asymmetrical lung expansion secondary to pain

Pain r/t presence of chest tubes, injury

Cheyne-Stokes Respirations
Ineffective Breathing Pattern r/t critical illness

Refer to cause of Cheyne-Stokes Respiration

CHF
Activity Intolerance r/t weakness, fatigue

Constipation r/t activity intolerance

Decreased Cardiac Output r/t impaired cardiac function

Fatigue r/t disease process

Fear r/t threat to well-being

Fluid Volume Excess r/t impaired excretion of sodium and water

High Risk for Impaired Gas Exchange r/t excessive fluid in interstitial space of lungs, alveoli

Knowledge Deficit r/t disease process and treatment

Refer to Congenital Heart Disease/Cardiac Anomalies, Hospitalized Child, Child with Chronic Condition

Chicken Pox
Refer to Communicable Diseases, Childhood

Child Abuse
Altered Growth and Development: Regression vs Delayed r/t diminished/absent environmental stimuli; inadequate caretaking; inconsistent responsiveness by caretaker

Altered Nutrition: Less than Body Requirements r/t inadequate caretaking

Altered Parenting r/t psychological impairment; physical, emotional abuse of parent; substance abuse; unrealistic expectations of child

Anxiety/Fear (child) r/t threat of punishment for perceived wrongdoing

Chronic Low Self-Esteem r/t lack of positive feedback or excessive negative feedback

Diversional Activity Deficit r/t diminished/absent environmental/personal stimuli

High Risk for Poisoning r/t inadequate safeguards; lack of proper safety precautions; accessibility of illicit substances secondary to impaired home maintenance management

High Risk for Suffocation/Aspiration r/t propped bottle; unattended child

High Risk for Trauma r/t inadequate precautions; cognitive or emotional difficulties

Impaired Skin Integrity r/t altered nutritional state; physical abuse

Pain r/t physical injuries

Post Trauma Response r/t physical abuse; incest/rape/molestation

Sleep Pattern Disturbance r/t hypervigilance; anxiety

Social Isolation, Family Imposed r/t fear of disclosure of family dysfunction and abuse

Child With Chronic Condition
Activity Intolerance r/t fatigue associated with chronic illness

Altered Family Processes r/t intermittent situational crisis of illness/disease and hospitalization

Altered Growth and Development r/t regression or lack of progression toward developmental milestones secondary to frequent/prolonged hospitalization; inadequate/inappropriate stimulation; cerebral insult; chronic illness; effects of physical disability; prescribed dependence

Altered Health Maintenance r/t exhausting family resources (financial, physical energy, support systems)

Altered Nutrition: Less than Body Requirements r/t anorexia; fatigue secondary to physical exertion

Altered Nutrition: More than Body Requirements r/t effects of steroid medications on appetite

Altered Sexuality Patterns (Parental) r/t disrupted relationship with sexual partner

Chronic Low Self-Esteem r/t actual or perceived differences and/or peer acceptance; decreased ability to participate in physical/school/social activities

Chronic Pain r/t physical, biological, chemical, psychological factors

Decisional Conflict r/t treatment options and conflicting values

Diversional Activity Deficit r/t immobility; monotonous environment; frequent/lengthy treatments; reluctance to participate; self-imposed social isolation

Family Coping: Potential for Growth r/t impact of crisis on family values, priorities, goals, or relationships; changes in family choices to optimize wellness

High Risk Altered Parenting r/t impaired/disrupted bonding; child with perceived overwhelming care needs

High Risk for Infection r/t debilitating physical condition

High Risk for Noncompliance r/t complex, prolonged, home care regimens; expressed intent to not comply secondary to value systems, health beliefs, and cultural/religious practices

Hopelessness (Child) r/t prolonged activity restriction; long-term stress; lack of involvement in care/passively allowing care secondary to parental overprotection

Impaired Home Maintenance Management r/t over-taxed family members, e.g., exhausted, anxious

Impaired Social Interaction r/t developmental lag/delay; perceived differences

Ineffective Family Coping: Compromised r/t prolonged disease or disability progression that exhausts supportive capacity of significant people

Ineffective Family Coping: Disabling r/t prolonged over-concern for child; distortion of reality regarding child's health problem, including extreme denial about its existence or severity

Ineffective Individual Coping (Child) r/t situational or maturational crises

Knowledge Deficit: Potential for Enhanced Health Maintenance r/t knowledge/skill acquisition regarding health practices; acceptance of limitations; promotion of maximum potential of child; self-actualization of rest of family

Parental Role Conflict r/t separation from child due to chronic illness; home care of child with special needs; interruptions of family life due to home care regimen

Powerlessness (Child) r/t health care environment; illness-related regimen; lifestyle of learned helplessness

Sleep Pattern Disturbance (Child or Parent) r/t time intensive treatments; exacerbation of condition; 24-hour care needs

Social Isolation: Family: Self-Imposed r/t actual or perceived social stigmatization; complex care requirements

Chills
Hyperthermia r/t infectious process
Altered Comfort r/t discomfort of chills

Chlamydia Infection
Refer to Sexually Transmitted Disease

Choking/Coughing with Feeding
High Risk for Aspiration r/t depressed cough and gag reflexes
Impaired Swallowing r/t neuromuscular impairment

Cholecystectomy
Altered Nutrition: Less than Body Requirements r/t high metabolic needs; decreased ability to digest fatty foods
High Risk for Fluid Volume Deficit r/t restricted intake; nausea and vomiting
High Risk for Ineffective Breathing Pattern r/t proximity of incision to lungs resulting in pain with deep breathing
Knowledge Deficit r/t lack of exposure to information
Pain r/t recent surgery
Refer to Abdominal Surgery

Cholelithiasis
Altered Nutrition: Less than Body Requirements r/t anorexia, nausea and vomiting
Knowledge Deficit r/t lack of information about treatment plan
Pain r/t obstruction of bile flow, inflammation in gallbladder

Chovstek's Sign
Refer to Hypocalcemia

29

Chronic Obstructive Pulmonary Disease
Refer to COPD

Chronic Pain
Refer to Pain, Chronic

Circumcision
High Risk for Fluid Volume Deficit r/t hemorrhage
High Risk for Infection r/t surgical wound
Knowledge Deficit: Parental r/t lack of exposure
   to situation
Pain r/t surgical intervention

Cirrhosis
Altered Nutrition: Less than Body Requirements r/t
   loss of appetite, nausea, vomiting
Chronic Low Self-Esteem r/t chronic illness
Chronic Pain r/t liver enlargement
Diarrhea r/t dietary changes, medications
Fatigue r/t malnutrition
High Risk for Altered Oral Mucous Membranes r/t
   altered nutrition
High Risk for Altered Thought Processes r/t chron-
   ic organic disorder with increased ammonia
   levels/substance abuse
High Risk for Fluid Volume Deficit: Hemorrhage
   r/t abnormal bleeding from esophagus
High Risk for Injury r/t substance intoxication,
   potential delirium tremors
Knowledge Deficit r/t lack of information about
   correlation between lifestyle habits and disease
   process
Ineffective Management of Therapeutic Regimen
   r/t denial of seriousness of illness
Noncomplinace r/t denial of illness

Cleft Lip/Cleft Palate
Altered Health Maintenance r/t lack of parental
   knowledge regarding feeding techniques, wound
   care, use of elbow restraints
Altered Nutrition: Less than Body Requirements r/t
   inability to feed with normal techniques

Altered oral Mucous Membranes r/t surgical
   correction
Fear: (Parental) r/t special care needs, surgery
Grieving r/t (loss of perfect child) birth of child
   with congenital defect
High Risk for Aspiration r/t common feeding/
   breathing passage
High Risk for Body Image Disturbance r/t disfigurement and speech impediment
High Risk for Infection r/t invasive procedure; disruption of eustachian tube development; aspiration
Impaired Physical Mobility r/t imposed restricted
   activity and use of elbow restraints
Impaired Skin Integrity r/t incomplete joining of
   lip/palate ridges
Impaired Verbal Communication r/t inadequate
   palate function and possible hearing loss from
   infected eustachian tubes
Ineffective Airway Clearance r/t common feeding/
   breathing passage; postoperative laryngeal or
   incisional edema
Ineffective Infant Feeding Pattern r/t cleft lip/cleft
   palate
Ineffective Breastfeeding r/t infant anomaly
Pain r/t surgical correction and elbow restraints

Clotting Disorder
Altered Protection r/t clotting disorder
Anxiety/Fear r/t threat to well-being
High Risk for Fluid Volume Deficit r/t
   uncontrolled bleeding
Knowledge Deficit r/t treatment of disease
Refer to Hemophilia, Anticoagulant Therapy, DIC

Coarctation of the Aorta
Refer to Congenital Heart Disease/Cardiac
   Anomalies

Cocaine Abuse
Altered Thought Processes r/t excessive stimulation of nervous system by cocaine

30

Ineffective Breathing Pattern r/t drug effect on respiratory center

Ineffective Individual Coping r/t inability to deal with life stresses

Co-Dependency

Caregiver Role Strain r/t codependency

Decisional Conflict r/t support system deficit

Denial r/t unmet self-needs

Impaired Verbal Communication r/t psychological barriers

Ineffective Individual Coping r/t inadequate support systems

Powerlessness r/t lifestyle of helplessness

Cognitive Deficit

Altered Thought Processes r/t neurological impairment

Colectomy

Altered Nutrition: Less than Body Requirements r/t high metabolic needs; decreased ability to ingest/digest food

Constipation r/t decreased activity; decreased fluid intake

High Risk for Infection r/t invasive procedure

Knowledge Deficit r/t limited exposure to information

Pain r/t recent surgery

Refer to abdominal surgery

Colitis

Diarrhea r/t inflammation in colon

Pain r/t inflammation in colon

Refer to Ulcerative Colitis, Crohn's Disease, or Irritable Bowel Syndrome

Colostomy

Body Image Disturbance r/t presence of stoma; daily care of fecal material

High Risk for Altered Sexuality Pattern r/t altered body image, self concept

High Risk for Constipation/Diarrhea r/t inappropriate diet

High Risk for Impaired Skin Integrity r/t irritation from bowel contents

High Risk for Social Isolation r/t anxiety over appearance of stoma and possible leakage

Knowledge Deficit r/t self-care, treatment needs

Coma

Altered Family Processes r/t illness/disability of family member

Altered Thought Processes r/t neurophysiological changes

High Risk for Altered Oral Mucous Membranes r/t dry mouth

High Risk for Aspiration r/t impaired swallowing, loss of cough/gag reflex

High Risk for Disuse Syndrome r/t altered level of consciousness impairing mobility

High Risk for Impaired Skin Integrity r/t immobility

High Risk for Injury r/t potential seizure activity

Self-Care Deficit: Specify r/t neuromuscular impairment

Total Incontinence r/t neurological dysfunction

Refer to the cause of client's comatose state

Comfort, Loss of

Altered Comfort r/t injury agent

Communicable Diseases, Childhood (Measles, Mumps, Rubella, Chicken Pox, Scabies, Lice, Impetigo)

Altered Comfort r/t Hyperthermia secondary to infectious disease process

Altered Comfort r/t pruritus secondary to skin rash or subdermal organisms

Altered Health Maintenance r/t nonadherence with appropriate immunization schedules; lack of prevention of transmission of infection

Diversional Activity Deficit r/t imposed isolation from peers; disruption in usual play activities; fatigue/activity intolerance

31

High Risk for Infection: Transmission to Others r/t contagious organisms

Knowledge Deficit: Potential for Enhanced Health Maintenance r/t knowledge acquisition regarding appropriate, preventive health practices

Pain r/t impaired skin integrity, edema

Refer to Respiratory Infections, Acute Childhood; Meningitis/Encephalitis; Reye Syndrome

Communication Problems

Impaired Verbal Communication r/t decrease in circulation to brain; brain tumor; physical barrier (tracheostomy, intubation); anatomical defect, cleft palate; psychological barriers; cultural difference; developmental or age related

Compulsion

Refer to Obsessive Compulsive Personality Disorder

Conduction Disorders (Cardiac)

Refer to Dysrhythmias

Confusion

Altered Thought Processes r/t organic mental disorder; disruption of cerebral arterial blood flow; chemical imbalance/intoxication

High Risk for Injury r/t confusion

Sensory/Perceptual Alteration r/t disruption of cerebral arterial blood flow; electrolyte imbalance; neurological dysfunction

Congenital Heart Disease/Cardiac Anomalies

Acyanotic: Patent ductus arteriosus (PDA); Atrial/Ventricular septal defect (ASD/VSD); Pulmonary Stenosis; Endocardial Cushion Defect; Aortic Valvular Stenosis; Coarctation of the Aorta

Cyanotic: Tetralogy of Fallot; Tricuspid Atresia; Transposition of the Great Vessels; Truncus Arteriosus; Total Anomalous Pulmonary Venous Return (TAPVR); Hypoplastic Left Lung

Activity Intolerance r/t fatigue; generalized weakness; lack of adequate oxygenation

Altered Family Processes r/t to ill child

Altered Growth and Development r/t inadequate oxygen and nutrients to tissues

Altered Nutrition: Less than Body Requirements r/t fatigue, generalized weakness; inability of infant to suck and feed; increased caloric requirements

Decreased Cardiac Output r/t cardiac dysfunction

Fluid Volume Excess r/t cardiac defect, side effects of medication

High Risk for Fluid Volume Deficit r/t side effects of diuretics

High Risk for Ineffective Thermoregulation r/t neonatal age

High Risk for Poisoning r/t potential toxicity of cardiac medications

Impaired Gas Exchange r/t cardiac defect; pulmonary congestion

Ineffective Breathing Patterns r/t pulmonary vascular disease

Refer to Hospitalized Child; Child With Chronic Illness

Congestive Heart Failure

Refer to CHF

Conjunctivitis

High Risk for Injury r/t change in visual acuity

Pain r/t inflammatory process

Sensory/Perceptual Alteration r/t change in visual acuity from inflammation

Constipation

Constipation r/t decreased fluid intake; decreased intake of foods containing bulk; inactivity, immobility; knowledge deficit of appropriate bowel routine; lack of privacy for defecation

Constipation, Colonic with Hard, Dry Stool

Colonic Constipation r/t less than adequate fluid intake; less than adequate dietary intake

Constipation, Perceived

Perceived Constipation r/t cultural/family health beliefs; faulty appraisal; impaired thought processes

Conversion Reaction

Altered Role Performance r/t physical conversion symptom

Anxiety r/t unresolved conflict

High Risk for Injury r/t physical conversion symptom

Hopelessness r/t long-term stress

Impaired Physical Mobility r/t physical conversion symptom

Impaired Social Interaction r/t altered thought process

Ineffective Individual Coping r/t personal vulnerability

Powerlessness r/t lifestyle of helplessness

Self-Esteem Disturbance r/t unsatisfactory or inadequate interpersonal relationships

Convulsions

Anxiety r/t concern over controlling convulsions

High Risk for Altered Thought Processes r/t seizure activity

High Risk for Aspiration r/t impaired swallowing

High Risk for Injury r/t seizure activity

Knowledge Deficit r/t need for medication and care during seizure activity

Refer to Seizure Disorders, Childhood

COPD

Activity Intolerance r/t imbalance between oxygen supply and demand

Altered Family Process r/t role changes

Altered Nutrition: Less than Body Requirements r/t decreased intake because of dyspnea, unpleasant taste in mouth left by medications

Anxiety r/t breathlessness, change in health status

Chronic Low Self-Esteem r/t chronic illness

High Risk for Infection r/t stasis of respiratory secretions

Impaired Gas Exchange r/t ventilation-perfusion inequality

Impaired Social Interaction r/t social isolation secondary to oxygen use, activity intolerance

Ineffective Airway Clearance r/t bronchoconstriction, increased mucous, ineffective cough, and infection

Knowledge Deficit r/t lack of information/ motivation

Noncompliance r/t reluctance to accept responsibility for changing detrimental health practices

Powerlessness r/t progressive nature of the disease

Self-Care Deficit: Specify r/t fatigue secondary to increased work of breathing

Sleep Pattern Disturbance r/t dyspnea; side effect of medications

Coping Problems

Ineffective Individual Coping r/t situational crises; maturational crises; personal vulnerability

Defensive Coping r/t superior attitude toward others; difficulty establishing/maintaining relationships; hostile laughter or ridicule of others; difficulty in reality testing perceptions; lack of follow through or participation in treatment or therapy

Refer to Family Problems

Coronary Artery Bypass Grafting

Decreased Cardiac Output r/t dysrhythmias, depressed cardiac function; increased systemic vascular resistance

Fear r/t outcome of surgical procedure

Fluid Volume Deficit r/t intraoperative fluid loss; use of diuretics in surgery

Knowledge Deficit r/t lifestyle adjustment after surgery

Pain r/t traumatic surgery

Corneal Reflex, Absent

High Risk for Injury r/t accidental corneal abrasion, drying of cornea

33

Costovertebral Angle Tenderness
Refer to Nephrolithiasis, Pyelonephritis

Cough, Effective/Ineffective
Ineffective Airway Clearance r/t decreased energy/ fatigue; normal aging changes
Refer to COPD, Bronchitis, Pulmonary Edema

Crack Abuse
Refer to Cocaine Abuse

Crack Baby
Altered Growth and Development r/t effects of maternal use of drugs; neurological impairment; decreased attentiveness to environmental stimuli
Altered Nutrition: Less than Body Requirements r/t feeding problems; uncoordinated/ineffective suck and swallow; effects of diarrhea, vomiting, colic
Altered Parenting r/t impaired or lack of attachment behaviors; inadequate support systems
Altered Protection r/t effects of maternal substance abuse
Diarrhea r/t effects of withdrawal; increased peristalsis secondary to hyperirritability
High Risk for Infection (Skin, Meningeal, Respiratory) r/t effects of withdrawal
Ineffective Airway Clearance r/t pooling of secretions secondary to lack of adequate cough reflex
Ineffective Infant Feeding r/t prematurity; neurological impairment
Sensory-Perceptual Alteration r/t hypersensitivity to environmental stimuli
Sleep Pattern Disturbance r/t hyperirritability, hypersensitivity to environmental stimuli

Crackles in Lungs, Fine
Ineffective Breathing Pattern r/t decreased energy; fatigue; surgery.
If crackles cardiac in origin, refer to CHF; if from pulmonary infection refer to Bronchitis or Pneumonia

Crackles in Lungs, Coarse
Ineffective Airway Clearance r/t excessive secretions in airways; ineffective cough
Refer to cause of coarse crackles

Craniectomy
Altered Tissue perfusion: Cerebral r/t cerebral edema; decreased cerebral perfusion; increased intracranial pressure
Fear r/t threat to well-being
High Risk for Altered Thought Processes r/t neurophysiological changes
High Risk for Injury r/t potential confusion
Pain r/t recent surgery, headache
Refer to Coma, if relevant

Crepitation, Subcutaneous
Refer to Pneumothorax

Crisis
Anticipatory Grieving r/t potential significant loss
Anxiety r/t threat to or change in environment, health status, interaction patterns, situation, self-concept, role-functioning; threat of death, self/significant other
Fear r/t crisis situation
Ineffective Family Coping: Compromised r/t situational or developmental crisis
Ineffective Individual Coping r/t situational or maturational crisis
Situational Low Self-Esteem r/t perception of inability to handle crisis
Spiritual Distress r/t intense suffering

Crohn's Disease
Altered Nutrition: Less than Body Requirements r/t diarrhea; altered ability to digest and absorb food
Anxiety r/t change in health status
Diarrhea r/t inflammatory process
High Risk for Fluid Volume Deficit r/t abnormal fluid loss with diarrhea

Ineffective Individual Coping r/t repeated episodes of diarrhea
Knowledge Deficit r/t management of the disease
Pain r/t increased peristalsis
Powerlessness r/t chronic disease

Croup
Refer to Respiratory Infections, Acute Childhood

Cushing's Syndrome
Activity Intolerance r/t fatigue, weakness
Body Image Disturbance r/t change in appearance from disease process
Fluid Volume Excess r/t failure of regulatory mechanisms
High Risk for Infection r/t suppression of the immune system secondary to increased coritisol
High Risk for Injury r/t decreased muscle strength, osteoporosis
Knowledge Deficit r/t treatment of the disease
Sexual Dysfucntion r/t loss of libido

CVA (Cerebrovascular Accident)
Altered Family Process r/t illness, disability of family member
Altered Thought Processes r/t neurophysiological changes
Anxiety r/t situational crisis; change in physical/ emotional condition
Body Image Disturbance r/t chronic illness, paralysis
Constipation r/t decreased activity
Dysfunctional Grieving r/t loss of health
High Risk for Caregiver Role Strain r/t cognitive problems of care receiver; need for significant home care
High Risk for Disuse Syndrome r/t paralysis
High Risk for Aspiration r/t impaired swallowing, loss of gag reflex
High Risk for Injury r/t sensory-perceptual alteration
High Risk for Impaired Skin Integrity r/t immobility

High Risk for Unilateral Neglect r/t disturbed perception from loss of half of the visual field, loss of sensation on affected side
Impaired Physical Mobility r/t loss of balance and coordination
Impaired Social Interaction r/t limited physical mobility, limited ability to communicate
Impaired Swallowing r/t neuromuscular dysfunction
Impaired Verbal Communication r/t pressure damage/decreased circulation to the speech center of the brain
Ineffective Individual Coping r/t disability
Knowledge Deficit r/t lack of informational sources
Reflex Incontinence r/t loss of feeling to void
Self-Care Deficit r/t decreased strength and endurance; paralysis
Sensory/Perceptual Alteration: Visual, Tactile, Kinesthetic r/t neurological deficit
Total Incontinence r/t neurological dysfunction

Cyanosis, Central with Cyanosis of Oral Mucous Membranes
Impaired Gas Exchange r/t alveolar-capillary membrane changes

Cyanosis, Peripheral with Cyanosis of Nailbeds
Altered Tissue Perfusion r/t interruption of arterial flow; severe vasoconstriction; cold
High Risk for Peripheral Neurovascular Dysfunction r/t condition causing a disruption in circulation

Cystic Fibrosis
Activity Intolerance r/t imbalance between oxygen supply and demand
Altered Nutrition: Less than Body Requirements r/t anorexia; decreased absorption of nutrients/fat; increased work of breathing
Anxiety r/t dyspnea and oxygen deprivation

35

Body Image Disturbance r/t changes in physical appearance and treatment of chronic lung disease (clubbing, barrel chest, home oxygen therapy)

High Risk for Caregiver Role Strain r/t illness severity of the care receiver; unpredictable illness course

High Risk for Fluid Volume Deficit r/t decreased fluid intake and increased work of breathing

High Risk for Infection r/t thick, tenacious mucous; harboring bacterial organisms; debilitated state

Impaired Gas Exchange r/t ventilation perfusion imbalance

Impaired Home Maintenance Management r/t extensive daily treatment, medications necessary for health, mist/oxygen tents

Ineffective Airway Clearance r/t increased production of thick mucus

Refer to Hospitalized Child; Child With Chronic Condition; Terminally Ill Child/Death of Child

Cystitis

Altered Pattern of Urinary Elimination: Frequency r/t urinary tract infection

Knowledge Deficit r/t methods to treat and prevent UTIs

Pain: *Dysuria* r/t inflammatory process in bladder

Refer to Pyelonephritis

Cystoscopy

High Risk for Infection r/t invasive procedure

Knowledge Deficit r/t post-operative care

Urinary Retention r/t edema in urethra obstructing flow of urine

D

Deafness
Sensory Perceptual Alteration: Auditory r/t alteration in sensory reception, transmission, or integration

Death, Oncoming
Anticipatory Grieving r/t loss of significant other
Fear r/t threat of death
Ineffective Individual Coping r/t personal vulnerability
Ineffective Family Coping: Compromised r/t client's inability to provide support to the family
Powerlessness r/t effects of illness, oncoming death
Social Isolation r/t altered state of wellness
Spiritual Distress r/t intense suffering
Refer to Terminally Ill Child; Death of Child

Decisions, Difficulty Making
Decisional Conflict r/t unclear personal values/beliefs; perceived threat to value system; lack of experience or interference with decision making; lack of relevant information; support system deficit; multiple or divergent sources of information

Decubitus Ulcer
Refer to Pressure Ulcer

Deep Vein Thrombosis
Refer to DVT

Defensive Behavior
Defensive Coping r/t nonacceptance of blame; denial of problems/weakness

Dehiscence, Abdominal
Fear r/t threat of death, severe dysfunction
High Risk for Infection r/t loss of skin integrity
Impaired Skin Integrity r/t altered circulation; malnutrition; opening in incision

Impaired Tissue Integrity r/t exposure of abdominal contents to external environment
Pain r/t stretching of abdominal wall

Dehydration
Altered oral Mucous Membranes r/t decreased salivation and fluid deficit
Fluid Volume Deficit r/t active fluid volume loss
Knowledge Deficit r/t treatment and prevention of dehydration

Delerium Tremens
Refer to Alcohol Withdrawal

Delusions
Anxiety r/t content of intrusive thoughts
High Risk for Violence: Self-Directed or Directed at Others r/t delusional thinking
Impaired Verbal Communication r/t psychological impairment; delusional thinking
Ineffective Individual Coping r/t distortion and insecurity of life events

Dementia
Altered Family Process r/t disability of family member
Altered Nutrition: Less than Body Requirements r/t psychological impairment
Altered Thought Processes r/t organic mental disorder
High Risk for Caregiver Role Strain r/t amount of caregiving tasks; duration of caregiving required
High Risk for Injury r/t confusion, decreased muscle coordination
High Risk for Impaired Skin Integrity r/t altered nutritional status, immobility
Impaired Home Maintenance Management r/t inadequate support system
Impaired Physical Mobility r/t neuromuscular impairment

Self-Care Deficit: Specify r/t psychological/
neuromuscular impairment
Sleep Pattern Disturbance r/t neurological impairment; naps during the day
Total Incontinence r/t neuromuscular impairment

Denial of Health Status
Ineffective Denial r/t lack of perception about
health status effects of illness
Ineffective Management of Therapeutic Regimen
r/t denial of seriousness of health situation

Dental Caries
Altered Health Maintenance r/t lack of knowledge
regarding prevention of dental disease secondary to high sugar diet; giving infants/toddlers
with erupted teeth bottles of milk at bedtime;
lack of fluoride treatments; inadequate or improper brushing of teeth

Depression, Major
Altered Health Maintenance r/t lack of ability to
make good judgments regarding ways to obtain
help
Chronic Low Self-Esteem r/t repeated unmet
expectations
Colonic Constipation r/t inactivity; decreased fluid
intake
Dysfunctional Grieving r/t lack of previous resolu-
tion of former grieving response
Fatigue r/t psychological demands
High Risk for Violence: Self-Directed r/t panic
state
Hopelessness r/t feeling of abandonment; long-
term stress
Ineffective Individual Coping r/t dysfunctional
grieving
Knowledge Deficit r/t lack of motivation to learn
new coping skills
Powerlessness r/t pattern of helplessness
Self Care Deficit: *Specify* r/t depression; cognitive
impairment
Sexual Dysfucntion r/t loss of sexual desire

Sleep Pattern Disturbance r/t inactivity
Social Isolation r/t ineffective coping

Dermatitis
Altered Comfort: *Pruritus* r/t inflammation of skin
Anxiety r/t situational crisis imposed by illness
Knowledge Deficit r/t methods to decrease inflam-
mation
Impaired Skin Integrity r/t side effect of medica-
tion; allergic reaction

Despondency
Hopelessness r/t long-term stress
Refer to Depression

Diabetes Mellitus
Altered Nutrition: Less than Body Requirements r/t
inability to utilize glucose (Type I Diabetes)
Altered Nutrition: More than Body Requirements
r/t excessive intake of nutrients (Type II Diabetes)
Altered Tissue Perfusion: Peripheral r/t impaired
arterial circulation
High Risk for Altered Thought Processes r/t hypo-
glycemia/hyperglycemia
High Risk for Infection r/t hyperglycemia,
impaired healing, circulatory changes
High Risk for Injury:
Hypoglycemia/Hyperglycemia
r/t failure to consume adequate calories or failure to take insulin
High Risk for Impaired Skin Integrity r/t loss of
pain perception in extremities
Ineffective Management of Therapeutic Regimen
r/t complexity of therapeutic regimen
Knowledge Deficit r/t limited exposure to information
Noncompliance r/t restrictive lifestyle; changes in
diet, medication, and exercise
Powerlessness r/t perceived lack of personal
control

Sexual Dysfucntion r/t neuropathy associated with disease

Diabetes Mellitus, Juvenile (IDDM Type I)

Altered Health Maintenance r/t parental/child knowledge deficit regarding dietary management, medication administration, physical activity, and interaction between the three; daily changes in diet, medication, and activity related to child growth spurts and needs; r/t need to instruct other caregivers and teachers regarding signs and symptoms of hyperglycemia/hypoglycemia and treatment

Altered Nutrition: Less than Body Requirements r/t inability of body to adequately metabolize and utilize glucose and nutrients; increased caloric needs of child to promote growth; physical activity participation with peers

Body Image Disturbance r/t to imposed deviations from biophysical and psychosocial norm; perceived differences from peers

High Risk for Noncompliance r/t body image disturbance; impaired adjustment secondary to adolescent maturational crises

Impaired Adjustment r/t inability to participate in normal childhood activities

Pain r/t insulin injections; peripheral blood glucose testing

Refer to Diabetes Mellitus; Child With Chronic Illness; Hospitalized Child

Dialysis

Refer to Hemodialysis, Peritoneal Dialysis

Diaphragmatic Hernia

Refer to Respiratory Conditions of the Neonate

Diaphoresis

Altered Comfort r/t excessive sweating

Diarrhea

Diarrhea r/t infection; change in diet/food; gastrointestinal disorders; stress; medication effect; impaction

DIC (Disseminated Intravascular Coagulation)

Fear r/t threat to well-being

Fluid Volume Deficit: Hemorrhage r/t depletion of clotting factors

High Risk for Altered Tissue Perfusion: Peripheral r/t hypovolemia from profuse bleeding; formation of microemboli in vascular system

D & C (Dilatation and Curretage)

High Risk for Altered Sexuality Patterns r/t painful coitus; fear associated with surgery on genital area

High Risk for Fluid Volume Deficit: Hemorrhage r/t excessive blood loss during or after the procedure

High Risk for Infection r/t surgical procedure

Knowledge Deficit r/t postoperative self-care

Pain r/t uterine contractions

Digitalis Toxicity

Decreased Cardiac Output r/t drug toxicity affecting cardiac rhythm, rate

Knowledge Deficit r/t action of medication, need for potassium, side effects of digitalis

Discharge Planning

Altered Health Maintenance r/t lack of material sources

Knowledge Deficit r/t lack of exposure to information for home care

Impaired Home Maintenance Management r/t family members disease or injury interfering with home maintenance

Discomforts of Pregnancy

Alteration in Comfort r/t pityalism secondary to increased estrogen; nausea secondary to hormonal changes; shortness of breath secondary

39

to limited diaphragm expansion; nasal stuffiness secondary to increased vascularization; leukorrhea secondary to hormone stimulation, abdominal distention secondary to enlarging uterus; pruritus secondary to increased excretory function of skin and stretching of skin; urinary frequency secondary to vascular engorgement and altered bladder function; reduced bladder capacity reduced by enlarging uterus and fetal presenting part

Body Image Disturbance r/t physiological edema; pityalism; body shape changes secondary to enlarging uterus and breasts; spider nevi; palmar erythema; varicose veins; striae gravidarum, chloasma; acne

Constipation r/t decreased GI tract motility; compression of intestines secondary to enlarging uterus; supplementary iron; hemorrhoids

Fatigue r/t increased levels of hormones; elevated basal body temperature; sleep pattern disturbance

High Risk for Injury r/t faintness or syncope secondary to vasomotor lability or postural hypotension; venous stasis in lower extremities

Pain: *Indigestion-Heart Burn* r/t decreased GI tract motility; reverse peristalsis; relaxed cardiac sphincter; Braxton Hicks' contractions; Hemorrhoids r/t constipation, enlarging uterus and pelvic venous stasis, bearing down for bowel movement, decreased GI motility; *Joint and Backache* r/t relaxation of symphyses and sacroiliac joints secondary to hormones, exaggerated lumbar and cervicothoracic curves secondary to change in center of gravity from enlarging abdomen; *Leg Cramps* r/t compression of nerves supplying lower extremities by gravid uterus, reduced level of diffusible calcium or elevation of serum phosphorus; *Headache* r/t vascular engorgement and congestion of sinuses from hormone stimulation

Sleep Pattern Disturbance r/t fetal movement; muscular cramping; urinary frequency; shortness of breath

Stress Incontinence r/t high intraabdominal pressure secondary to gravid uterus, fetal movement

Disseminated Intravascular Coagulation
Refer to DIC

Dissociative Disorder
Alteration in Thought Processes r/t repressed anxiety

Anxiety r/t psychosocial stress

Disturbance in Self-Concept r/t childhood trauma; childhood abuse

Ineffective Individual Coping r/t personal vulnerability in crisis of accurate self-perception

Personal Identify Disturbance r/t inability to distinguish self caused by multiple personality disorder, depersonalization or disturbance in memory

Sensory/Perceptual Alteration: Kinesthetic r/t underdeveloped ego

Disuse Syndrome, Potential to Develop
High Risk for Disuse Syndrome r/t paralysis; mechanical immobilization; prescribed immobilization; severe pain; altered level of consciousness

Diversional Activity, Lack of
Diversional Activity Deficit r/t environmental lack of diversional activity

Diverticulitis
Altered Nutrition: Less than Body Requirements r/t loss of appetite

Constipation r/t dietary deficiency of fiber and roughage

Diarrhea r/t increased intestinal motility secondary to inflammation

High Risk for Fluid Volume Deficit r/t diarrhea

Knowledge Deficit r/t diet needed to control disease, medication regime

Pain r/t inflammation of bowel

Dizziness
Altered Tissue Perfusion: Cerebral r/t interruption of cerebral arterial blood flow
Decreased Cardiac Output r/t dysfunctional electrical conduction
High Risk for Injury r/t difficulty maintaining balance
Impaired Physical Mobility r/t dizziness

Down Syndrome
Refer to Mental Retardation; Child With Chronic Illness

Dressing Self, Inability to Do
Dressing/Grooming Self Care Deficit r/t intolerance to activity; decreased strength and endurance; pain, discomfort; perceptual or cognitive impairment; neuromuscular impairment; musculoskeletal impairment; depression; severe anxiety

Dribbling of Urine
Stress Incontinence r/t degenerative changes in pelvic muscles and structural supports

Drooling
Impaired Swallowing r/t neuromuscular impairment; mechanical obstruction

Drug Abuse
Altered Nutrition: Less than Body Requirements r/t poor eating habits
Anxiety r/t threat to self concept; lack of control of drug use
Ineffective Individual Coping r/t situational crisis
High Risk for Injury r/t hallucinations, drug effects
High Risk for Violence r/t poor impulse control
Noncompliance r/t denial of illness
Sensory/Perceptual Alterations: Specify r/t substance intoxication
Sleep Pattern Disturbance r/t effects of drugs or medications

Drug Withdrawal
Altered Nutrition: Less than Body Requirements r/t poor eating habits
Anxiety r/t physiological withdrawal
Ineffective Individual Coping r/t situational crisis, withdrawal
High Risk for Injury r/t hallucinations
High Risk for Violence r/t poor impulse control
Noncompliance r/t denial of illness
Sensory/Perceptual Alterations: Specify r/t substance intoxication
Sleep Pattern Disturbance r/t effects of drugs or medications

DTs (Delerium Tremens)
Refer to Alcohol Withdrawal

DVT (Deep Vein Thrombosis)
Altered Tissue Perfusion: Peripheral r/t interruption of venous blood flow
Colonic Constipation r/t inactivity; bedrest
Impaired Physical Mobility r/t pain in extremity; forced bedrest
Knowledge Deficit r/t self-care needs; treatment regimen, outcome
Pain r/t vascular inflammation; edema
Refer to Anticoagulant Therapy

Dysfunctional Eating Pattern
High Risk for Altered Nutrition: More than Body Requirements r/t observed use of food as a reward or comfort measure
Refer to Anorexia Nervosa, Bulimia

Dysfunctional Grieving
Dysfunctional Grieving r/t actual or perceived loss

Dysfunctional Family Unit
Refer to Family Problems

Dysmenorrhea
Knowledge Deficit r/t prevention and treatment of painful menstruation

Pain r/t cramping from hormonal effects

Dyspareunia
Sexual Dysfunction r/t lack of lubrication during intercourse; alteration in reproductive organ function

Dyspepsia
Anxiety r/t pressures of personal role
Knowledge Deficit r/t treatment/prevention of dyspepsia
Pain r/t gastrointestinal disease; consumption of irritating foods

Dysphagia
High Risk for Aspiration r/t loss of gag, cough reflex
Impaired Swallowing r/t neuromuscular impairment

Dysphasia
Impaired Social Interaction r/t difficulty in communicating
Impaired Verbal Communication r/t decrease in circulation to the brain

Dyspnea
Activity Intolerance r/t imbalance between oxygen supply and demand
Fear r/t threat to state of well-being, potential death
Impaired Gas Exchange r/t alveolar-capillary damage
Ineffective Airway Clearance r/t decreased energy, fatigue
Ineffective Breathing Pattern r/t decreased lung expansion; neurological impairment affecting respiratory center; extreme anxiety
Sleep Pattern Disturbance r/t difficulty breathing; positioning required for effective breathing

Dysreflexia
Dysreflexia r/t bladder distention; bowel distention; noxious stimuli

Dysrhythmia
Activity Intolerance r/t decreased cardiac output
Altered Tissue Perfusion: Cerebral r/t interruption of cerebral arterial flow secondary to decreased cardiac output
Anxiety/Fear r/t threat of death; change in health status
Decreased Cardiac Output r/t altered electrical conduction
Knowledge Deficit r/t unfamiliarity with information resources

Dysthmia
Altered Health Maintenance r/t lack of ability to make good judgments regarding ways to obtain help
Altered Sexual Pattern r/t loss of sexual desire chronic
Chronic Low Self-Esteem r/t repeated unmet expectations
Ineffective Individual Coping r/t impaired social interaction
Knowledge Deficit r/t lack of motivation to learn new coping skills
Sleep Pattern Disturbance r/t anxious thoughts
Social Isolation r/t ineffective coping

Dysuria
Altered Urinary Elimination r/t urinary tract infection

E

Earache

Pain r/t trauma; edema

Sensory Perceptual Alteration: Auditory r/t altered sensory reception, transmission or integration

Ear Surgery

High Risk for Injury r/t dizziness from excessive stimuli to vestibular apparatus

Knowledge Deficit r/t postoperative care

Pain r/t edema in ears from surgery

Sensory/Perceptual Alteration: Auditory r/t invasive surgery of ears; dressings

Refer to Hospitalized Child

Eclampsia

Altered Family Processes r/t unmet expectations for pregnancy/childbirth

Fear r/t threat of well-being to self and fetus

High Risk for Altered Fetal Tissue Perfusion r/t uteroplacental insufficiency

High Risk for Aspiration r/t seizure activity

High Risk for Fluid Volume Excess r/t decreased urine output secondary to renal dysfunction

High Risk for Injury: Maternal r/t seizure activity

High Risk for Injury: Fetal r/t hypoxia

Ectopic Pregnancy

Altered Role Performance r/t loss of pregnancy

Body Image Disturbance r/t negative feelings about the body and reproductive functioning

Fear r/t threat to self, surgery, implications for future pregnancy

Fluid Volume Deficit r/t loss of blood

High Risk for Altered Family Processes r/t situational crisis

High Risk for Infection r/t traumatized tissue and blood loss

High Risk for Ineffective Individual Coping r/t loss of pregnancy

High Risk for Spiritual Distress r/t grief process

Pain r/t stretching or rupture of implantation site

Situational Low Self-Esteem r/t loss of pregnancy and inability to carry pregnancy to term

Eczema

Body Image Disturbance r/t change in appearance from inflamed skin

Knowledge Deficit r/t methods to decrease inflammation

Impaired Skin Integrity r/t side-effect of medication, allergic reaction

Pain: Pruritus r/t inflammation of skin

Edema

Fluid Volume Excess r/t excessive fluid intake; cardiac dysfunction; renal dysfunction; loss of plasma proteins

High Risk for Impaired Skin Integrity r/t impaired circulation; fragility of skin

Knowledge Deficit r/t treatment of edema

Elderly Abuse

Refer to Battered Person

Emaciated Person

Altered Nutrition: Less than Body Requirements r/t inability to ingest or digest food or absorb nutrients due to biological, psychological, or economic factors

Emesis

Refer to Vomiting

Emotional Problems

Refer to Coping Problems

Emphysema

Refer to COPD

Encephalitis

Refer to Meningitis/Encephalitis

Endocardial Cushion Defect

Refer to Congenital Heart Disease/Cardiac Anomalies

Endocarditis

Altered Tissue Perfusion:
Cardiopulmonary/Peripheral r/t high risk for development of emboli

High Risk for Activity Intolerance r/t reduced cardiac reserve and prescribed bedrest

High Risk for Alteration in Nutrition: Less than Body Requirements r/t fever, hypermetabolic state associated with fever

High Risk for Decreased Cardiac Output r/t inflammation of lining of heart and change in structure in valve leaflets, increased myocardial workload

High Risk for Impaired Gas Exchange r/t high risk for congestive heart failure

Knowledge Deficit r/t preventive measures against initial and recurring attacks of rheumatic fever

Pain r/t biological injury and inflammation

Endometriosis

Anticipatory Grieving r/t possible infertility

Knowledge Deficit r/t disease condition, medications and other treatments

Pain r/t onset of menses with distention of endometrial tissue

Sexual Dysfunction r/t painful coitus

Endometritis

Anxiety r/t prolonged hospitalization and fear of the unknown

Hyperthermia r/t infectious process

Knowledge Deficit r/t limited experience with condition, treatment, and antibiotic regime

Pain r/t infectious process in reproductive tract

Enuresis

Altered Health Maintenance r/t unachieved developmental task; neuromuscular immaturity; diseases of the urinary system, infections, or ill-nesses, such as diabetes mellitus or insipidus; regression in developmental stage secondary to hospitalization or stress; parental knowledge deficit regarding involuntary urination at night after age 6; fluid intake at bedtime; lack of control during sound sleep; male gender

Refer to Toilet Training

Epididymitis

Altered Pattern of Sexuality r/t edema of epididymis and testes

Anxiety r/t situational crisis, pain, threat to future fertility

Knowledge Deficit r/t treatment for pain and infection

Pain r/t inflammation in scrotal sac

Epiglotitis

Refer to Respiratory Infections, Acute Childhood

Epilepsy

Anxiety r/t threat to role functioning

High Risk for Altered Thought Processes r/t excessive, uncontrolled neurological stimuli

High Risk for Aspiration r/t impaired swallowing, excessive secretions

High Risk for Injury r/t environmental factors during seizure

Knowledge Deficit r/t seizures and seizure control

Refer to Seizure Disorders, Childhood

Episiotomy

Anxiety r/t fear of pain

Body Image Disturbance r/t fear of resuming sexual relations

High Risk for Infection r/t tissue trauma

Impaired Physical Mobility r/t pain, swelling, and tissue trauma

Impaired Skin Integrity r/t perineal incision

Pain r/t tissue trauma

Sexual Dysfunction r/t altered body structure and tissue trauma

Epistaxis

Fear r/t large amount of blood loss

High Risk for Fluid Volume Deficit r/t excessive
fluid loss

Esophageal Varices

Fear r/t threat of death

Fluid Volume Deficit: Hemorrhage r/t portal
hypertension, distended variceal vessels that can
easily rupture

Refer to Cirrhosis

Esophagitis

Knowledge Deficit r/t treatment regimen

Pain r/t inflammation/infection

Evisceration

Refer to Dehisence

Exposure to Hot or Cold Environment

High Risk for Altered Body Temperature r/t exposure

Eye Surgery

Anxiety r/t possible loss of vision

High Risk for Injury r/t impaired vision

Knowledge Deficit r/t postoperative activity, medication and eye care

Self-Care Deficit r/t impaired vision

Sensory/Perceptual Alteration: Visual r/t surgical
procedure

Refer to Hospitalized Child

Frequency of Urination

Altered Urinary Elimination r/t anatomical
   obstruction; sensory motor impairment; urinary
   tract infection

Stress Incontinence r/t degenerative change in
   pelvic muscles and structural supports

Urge Incontinence r/t decreased bladder capacity;
   irritation of bladder stretch receptors causing
   spasm; alcohol; caffeine; increased fluids;
   increased urine concentration; overdistention of
   bladder

Urinary Retention r/t high urethral pressure caused
   by weak detrusor; inhibition of reflex arc;
   strong sphincter; blockage

Frostbite

Impaired Skin Integrity r/t freezing of skin

Pain r/t decreased circulation from prolonged
   exposure to cold

Refer to Hypothermia

Fusion, Lumbar

Anxiety r/t fear of surgical procedure and possible
   recurring problems

High Risk for Injury r/t improper body mechanics

Impaired Physical Mobility r/t limitations related
   to the surgical procedure; presence of brace

Knowledge Deficit r/t postoperative mobility
   restrictions, body mechanics

Pain r/t discomfort at bone donor site

G

Gag Reflex, Depressed or Absent

High Risk for Aspiration r/t depressed cough/gag reflex

Impaired Swallowing r/t neuromuscular impairment

Gallop Rhythm

Decreased Cardiac Output r/t decreased contractility of heart

Gallstones

Refer to Cholelithiasis

Gangrene

Altered Tissue Perfusion: Peripheral r/t obstruction of arterial flow

Fear r/t possible loss of extremity

Gas Exchange, Impaired

Impaired Gas Exchange r/t ventilation perfusion imbalance

Gastritis

Refer to Gastroenteritis

Gastroenteritis

Altered Nutrition:Less than Body Requirements r/t vomiting; inadequate intestinal absorption of nutrients; restricted dietary regimen intake

Diarrhea r/t infectious process involving intestinal tract

Fluid Volume Deficit r/t excessive loss from gastrointestinal tract secondary to diarrhea, vomiting

Pain r/t increased peristalsis causing cramping

Refer to Gastroenteritis - Child

Gastroenteritis - Child

Altered Health Maintenance r/t lack of parental knowledge regarding fluid and dietary changes

Impaired Skin Integrity (diaper rash) r/t acidic excretions on perineal tissues

Refer to Gastroenteritis; Hospitalized Child

Gastroesophageal Reflux

Altered Nutrition: Less than Body Requirements r/t poor feeding and vomiting

Anxiety/Fear, Parental r/t possible need for surgical intervention (Nissen fundoplication/gastrostomy tube)

Fluid Volume Deficit r/t persistent vomiting

High Risk for Altered Parenting r/t disruption in bonding secondary to irritable, inconsolable infant

High Risk for Aspiration r/t entry of gastric contents in tracheal/bronchial tree

Ineffective Airway Clearance r/t reflux of gastric contents into esophagus and tracheal/bronchial tree

Knowledge Deficit: Potential for Enhanced Health Maintenance r/t knowledge/skill acquisition regarding anti-reflux regime, e.g., positioning, oral/enteral feeding techniques, medications; possible home apnea monitoring

Pain r/t irritation of esophagus from gastric acids

Refer to Hospitalized Child; Child With Chronic Condition

Gastrointestinal Hemorrhage

Refer to GI Bleed

Gastroschisis/Omphalocele

Altered Bowel Elimination Pattern r/t effects of congenital herniated abdominal contents

Anticipatory Grieving r/t threatened loss of infant, loss of "perfect birth/infant" secondary to serious medical condition

High Risk for Fluid Volume Deficit r/t inability to feed secondary to condition and subsequent electrolyte imbalance

High Risk for Infection r/t disrupted skin integrity with exposure of abdominal contents

High Risk for Injury r/t disrupted skin integrity and altered protection

Impaired Gas Exchange r/t effects of anesthesia and subsequent atelectasis

Ineffective Airway Clearance r/t complications of anesthetic effects

Refer to Hospitalized Child; Premature Infant

Gestational Diabetes (Diabetes in Pregnancy)

Altered Maternal Nutrition: Less than Body Requirements r/t decreased insulin production and glucose uptake into cells

Altered Fetal Nutrition: More than Body Requirements r/t excessive glucose uptake

Anxiety r/t threat to self or fetus

High Risk for Fetal Injury r/t macrosomia; congenital defects; maternal hypoglycemic or hyperglycemic incidents

High Risk for Maternal Injury r/t delivery of large infant; hypoglycemic or hyperglycemia incidents

Knowledge Deficit r/t maternal learning needs about diabetes in pregnancy

Powerlessness r/t lack of control over outcome of pregnancy

GI Bleed

Altered Nutrition: Less than Body Requirements r/t nausea, vomiting

Fatigue r/t loss of circulating blood volume, decreased ability to transport oxygen

Fear r/t threat to well-being, potential death

Fluid Volume Deficit r/t gastrointestinal bleeding

High Risk for Ineffective Individual Coping r/t personal vulnerability in a crisis, bleeding and hospitalization

Pain r/t irritated mucosa from acid secretion

Gingivitis

Altered Oral Mucous Membranes r/t ineffective oral hygiene

Glaucoma

Sensory/Perceptual Alteration: Visual r/t increased intraocular pressure

Glomerulonephritis

Altered Nutrition: Less than Body Requirements r/t anorexia, restrictive diet

Fluid Volume Excess r/t renal impairment

Knowledge Deficit r/t treatment of disease

Pain r/t edema of kidney

Gonorrhea

High Risk for Infection r/t spread of organism throughout reproductive organs

Knowledge Deficit r/t treatment and prevention of disease

Pain r/t inflammation of reproductive organs

Gout

Impaired Physical Mobility r/t musculoskeletal impairment

Knowledge Deficit r/t medications and home care

Pain r/t inflammation of affected joint

Grandiosity

Defensive Coping r/t inaccurate perception of self and abilities

Grieving

Anticipatory Grieving r/t anticipated significant loss

Dysfunctional Grieving r/t actual or perceived significant loss

Grieving r/t actual significant loss; change in life status, lifestyle or function

Grooming, Inability to Groom Self

Dressing/Grooming Self-Care Deficit r/t intolerance to activity; decreased strength and endurance; pain, discomfort; perceptual or cognitive impairment; neuromuscular impairment; musculoskeletal impairment; depression; severe anxiety

Growth and Development Lag

Altered Growth and Development r/t inadequate caretaking; indifference, inconsistent responsiveness, multiple caretakers; separation from significant others; environmental and stimulation deficiencies; effects of physical disability; prescribed dependence

Guilt

Self-Esteem Disturbance r/t unmet expectations of self

Anticipatory Grieving r/t potential loss of significant person, animal, or prized material possession

Dysfunctional Grieving r/t actual loss of significant person, animal, or prized material possession

H

Hair Loss
Altered Nutrition: Less than Body Requirements r/t inability to ingest food due to biological, psychological, or economic factors
Body Image Disturbance r/t psychological reaction to loss of hair

Halitosis
Altered Oral Mucous Membranes r/t ineffective oral hygiene

Hallucinations
Altered Thought Processes r/t inability to control bizarre thoughts
Anxiety r/t threat to self-concept
High Risk for Self-Mutilation r/t command hallucinations
High Risk for Violence: Self-Directed or Directed at Others r/t catatonic excitment; manic excitement; rage/panic reactions; response to violent internal stimuli

Head Injury
Refer to Intracranial Pressure, Increased

Headache
Pain: Headache r/t lack of knowledge of pain control techniques or methods to prevent headaches

Health Maintenance Problems
Altered Health Maintenance r/t significant alteration in communication skills; lack of ability to make deliberate and thoughtful judgments; perceptual/cognitive impairment; ineffective individual coping; dysfunctional grieving; unachieved developmental tasks; ineffective family coping; disabling spiritual distress; lack of material resources

Health Seeking Person
Health Seeking Behavior r/t expressed desire for increased control of own personal health

Hearing Impairment
Impaired Verbal Communication r/t inability to hear own voice
Sensory/Perceptual Alteration: Auditory r/t altered state of auditory system
Social Isolation r/t difficulty with communication

Heartburn
High Risk for Altered Nutrition: Less than Body Requirements r/t pain after eating
Knowledge Deficit r/t information about factors that cause esophageal reflex
Pain: Heartburn r/t gastroesophageal reflux

Heart Failure
Refer to CHF

Heart Surgery
Refer to Coronary Artery Bypass Grafting

Heat Stroke
Altered Thought Processes r/t hyperthermia, increased oxygen needs
Fluid Volume Deficit r/t profuse diaphoresis
Hyperthermia r/t vigorous activity, hot environment

Hematemesis
Refer to GI Bleed

Hematuria
High Risk for Fluid Volume Deficit r/t excessive loss of blood through urinary system
Refer to cause of Hematuria

Hemianopsia
Anxiety r/t change in vision

Sensory/Perceptual Alteration: Visual r/t altered sensory reception, transmission, or integration

Unilateral Neglect r/t effects of disturbed perceptual abilities

Hemiplegia

Anxiety r/t change in health status

Body Image Disturbance r/t functional loss of one side of the body

High Risk for Impaired Skin Integrity r/t alteration in sensation, immobility

High Risk for Injury r/t impaired mobility

Impaired Physical Mobility r/t loss of neurological control of involved extremities

Self-Care Deficit: Specify r/t neuromuscular impairment

Unilateral Neglect r/t r/t neurological impairment, loss of sensation, vision, or movement

Refer to CVA

Hemodialysis

Altered Family Processes r/t changes in role responsibilities due to therapy regimen

Caregiver Role Strain r/t complexity of care receiver treatment

High Risk for Fluid Volume Deficit r/t excessive removal of fluid during dialysis

High Risk for Infection r/t exposure to blood products and risk for developing hepatitis B/C

High Risk for Injury: Clotting of Blood Access r/t abnormal surface for blood flow

Ineffective Individual Coping r/t situational crisis

Knowledge Deficit r/t hemodialysis procedure, restrictions, blood access care

Noncompliance: Dietary Restrictions r/t denial of chronic illness

Powerlessness r/t treatment regimen

Refer to Renal Failure, Oliguric; Renal Failure—Acute/Chronic, Childhood

Hemodynamic Monitoring

High Risk for Infection r/t invasive procedure

High Risk for Injury r/t inadvertent wedging of catheter; dislodgement of catheter; disconnections of catheter; embolism

Hemolytic Uremic Syndrome

Altered Comfort: Nausea/Vomiting r/t effects of uremia

Fluid Volume Deficit r/t vomiting and diarrhea

High Risk for Impaired Skin Integrity r/t diarrhea

High Risk for Injury r/t decreased platelet count, seizure activity

Refer to Renal Failure, Acute/Chronic, Child; Hospitalized Child

Hemophilia

Altered Protection r/t deficient clotting factors

Fear r/t high risk for AIDS secondary to contaminated blood products

High Risk for Injury r/t deficient clotting factors and child's developmental level; age-appropriate play; inappropriate use of toys, sports equipment

Impaired Physical Mobility r/t pain from acute bleeds and imposed activity restrictions

Pain r/t bleeding into body tissues

Potential for Enhanced Health Maintenance r/t knowledge/ skill acquisition regarding home administration of IV clotting factors, protection from injury

Refer to Hospitalized Child; Child With Chronic Condition; Maturational Issues, Adolescence

Hemoptysis

Fear r/t serious threat to wellbeing

High Risk for Fluid Volume Deficit r/t excessive loss of blood

High Risk for Ineffective Airway Clearance r/t obstruction of airway with blood and mucous

Hemorrhage

Fear r/t threat to well-being

Fluid Volume Deficit r/t massive blood loss

Refer to cause of Hemorrhage; Hypovolemic Shock

53

Hemorrhoidectomy

Anxiety r/t embarrassment, need for privacy

Colonic Constipation r/t fear of defecation

High Risk for Fluid Volume Deficit: Hemorrhage r/t surgical wound

High Risk for Urinary Retention r/t pain, anesthesia effect

Knowledge Deficit r/t pain relief, use of stool softeners, dietary changes

Pain r/t surgical procedure

Hemorrhoids

Constipation r/t painful defecation, poor bowel habits

Knowledge Deficit r/t lack of information sources

Pain: Pruritus r/t inflammation of hemorrhoids

Hepatitis

Activity Intolerance r/t weakness or fatigue secondary to infection

Altered Nutrition: Less than Body Requirements r/t anorexia, impaired utilization of proteins and carbohydrates

Diversional Activity Deficit r/t isolation

Fatigue r/t infectious process, altered body chemistry

High Risk for Fluid Volume Deficit r/t excessive loss of fluids via vomiting and diarrhea

Knowledge Deficit r/t disease process and home management

Pain r/t edema of liver, bile irritating skin

Social Isolation r/t treatment-imposed isolation

Hernia

Refer to Inguinal Hernia Repair, Hiatal Hernia

Herniorrhapy

Refer to Inguinal Hernia Repair

Herpes Simplex I

Altered Oral Mucous Membranes r/t inflammatory changes in mouth

Herpes Simplex II

Altered Urinary Elimination r/t pain with urination

Impaired Tissue Integrity r/t active herpes lesion

Knowledge Deficit r/t lack of exposure to situation

Pain r/t active herpes lesion

Situational Low Self-Esteem r/t expressions of shame/guilt

Herpes in Pregnancy

Altered Urinary Elimination r/t pain with urination

Fear r/t threat to fetus and impending surgery

High Risk for Fetal Injury r/t herpes virus

Impaired Tissue Integrity r/t active herpes lesion

Knowledge Deficit r/t lack of exposure to situation

Pain r/t active herpes lesion

Situational Low Self-Esteem r/t threat to fetus secondary to disease process

Hiatal Hernia

High Risk for Altered Nutrition: Less than Body Requirements r/t pain after eating

Knowledge Deficit r/t information about factors that cause esophageal reflex

Pain: Heartburn r/t gastroesophageal reflux

Hip Fracture

Colonic Constipation r/t immobility, narcotics, anesthesia

Fear r/t outcome of treatment, future mobility, and present helplessness

High Risk for Altered Thought Processes r/t change in environment, stress of surgery, sensory deprivation

High Risk for Fluid Volume Deficit Hemorrhage r/t postoperative complication, surgical blood loss

High Risk for Impaired Skin Integrity r/t immobility

High Risk for Infection r/t invasive procedure

High Risk for Injury r/t dislodged prosthesis; unsteadiness when ambulating

Impaired Physical Mobility r/t surgical incision and temporary absence of weight bearing

Pain r/t injury, surgical procedure
Powerlessness r/t health care environment
Self-Care Deficit: Specify r/t musculoskeletal
impairment

Hirschsprung's Disease
Altered Health Maintenance r/t parental knowledge deficit regarding temporary stoma care, dietary management, treatment for constipation/diarrhea
Altered Nutrition: Less than Body Requirements r/t anorexia; pain from distended colon
Constipation (bowel obstruction) r/t inhibited peristalsis secondary to congenital absence of parasympathetic ganglion cells in the distal colon
Grieving r/t to loss of perfect child, birth of child with congenital defect, even though child expected to be normal within 2 years
Impaired Skin Integrity r/t stoma; potential skin care problems associated with stoma
Pain r/t distended colon; incisional pain postoperative
Refer to Hospitalized Child

Hirsutism
Body Image Disturbance r/t excessive hair

HIV (Human Immunodeficiency Virus)
Altered Protection r/t depressed immune system
Fear r/t possible death
Refer to AIDS

Hodgkin's Disease
Refer to Cancer and Anemia

Home Maintenance Problems
Impaired Home Maintenance Management r/t individual/family member disease or injury; insufficient family organization or planning; insufficient finances; unfamiliarity with neighborhood resources; impaired cognitive or emotional functioning; lack of knowledge; lack of role modeling; inadequate support systems

Hopelessness
Hopelessness r/t prolonged activity restriction creating isolation; failing or deteriorating physiological condition; long-term stress; abandonment; lost belief in transcendent values/God

Hospitalized Child
Activity Intolerance r/t fatigue associated with acute illness
Altered Family Processes r/t situational crisis of illness/disease and hospitalization
Altered Growth and Development r/t regression or lack of progression toward developmental milestones secondary to frequent/prolonged hospitalization; inadequate/inappropriate stimulation; cerebral insult; chronic illness; effects of physical disability; prescribed dependence
Anxiety: Separation (child) r/t familiar surroundings and separation from family/friends
Diversional Activity Deficit r/t immobility; monotonous environment; frequent/lengthy treatments; reluctance to participate; therapeutic isolation; separation from peers
Family Coping: Potential for Growth r/t impact of crisis on family values, priorities, goals, or relationships in family
Fear r/t knowledge deficit or maturational level with fear of unknown, mutilation, painful procedures, surgery
High Risk for Altered Growth and Development:
Regression r/t disruption of normal routine, unfamiliar environment/caregivers; developmental vulnerability of young children
High Risk for Altered Nutrition: Less than Body Requirements r/t anorexia; absence of familiar foods; cultural preferences

High Risk for Ineffective Family Coping: Compromised r/t possible prolonged hospitalization that exhausts supportive capacity of significant people

High Risk for Injury r/t unfamiliar environment, developmental age or lack of parental knowledge regarding safety, e.g., side rails, IV site/pole

Hopelessness (child) r/t prolonged activity restriction and/or uncertain prognosis

Ineffective Individual Coping (parent) r/t possible guilt regarding hospitalization of child; parental inadequacies

Sleep Pattern Disturbance (child or parent) r/t 24-hour care needs of hospitalization

Pain r/t treatments, diagnostic or therapeutic procedures

Powerlessness (child) r/t health care environment; illness-related regimen

Hostile Behavior

High Risk for Violence: Self-Directed or Directed at Others r/t antisocial personality disorder

Hydrocephalus

Altered Family Processes r/t situational crisis

Altered Growth and Development r/t sequelae of increased intracranial pressure

Altered Nutrition: Less than Body Requirements r/t inadequate intake secondary to anorexia, nausea and/or vomiting, feeding difficulties

Altered Tissue Perfusion: Cerebral r/t interrupted flow and/or hypervolemia of cerebral ventricles

Decisional Conflict: Parental regarding selection of treatment modality r/t unclear or conflicting values

Fluid Volume Excess: Cerebral Ventricles r/t compromised regulatory mechanism

High Risk for Infection r/t sequelae of invasive procedure (shunt placement)

Impaired Skin (Tissue) Integrity r/t impaired physical mobility/mechanical irritation

Refer to Premature Infant; Child With Chronic Condition; Hospitalized Child; Mental Retardation, if appropriate

Hygiene, Inability to Provide Own Hygiene

Bathing/Hygiene Self-Care Deficit r/t intolerance to activity, decreased strength and endurance; pain, discomfort; perceptual or cognitive impairment; neuromuscular impairment; musculoskeletal impairment; depression, severe anxiety

Hyperactive Syndrome

Altered Role Performance: Parent(s) r/t stressors associated with dealing with hyperactive child; perceived or projected blame for causes of child's behavior; unmet needs for support/care, and lack of energy to provide for those needs

Decisional Conflict regarding education programs, nutrition regimens, medication regimens r/t multiple or divergent sources of information; willingness to change own food habits; limited resources

High Risk for Altered Parenting r/t disruptive, uncontrollable behaviors of child

High Risk for Violence: Parent or Child r/t frustration with disruptive behavior, anger, unsuccessful relationship(s)

Impaired Social Interaction r/t impulsive, overactive behaviors; concomitant emotional difficulties; distractibility and excitability

Ineffective Family Coping: Compromised r/t unsuccessful strategies to control excessive activity/behaviors, frustration and anger

Parental Role Conflict (when siblings present) r/t increased attention towards hyperactive child

Self-Esteem Disturbance or Chronic Low Self-Esteem r/t inability to achieve socially acceptable behaviors, frustration; frequent reprimands, punishment, scoldings secondary to uncontrolled activity/behaviors; mood fluctuations and restlessness; inability to succeed academically; lack of peer support

Hyperalimentation
Refer to TPN

Hyperbilirubinemia
Altered Nutrition: Less than Body Requirements r/t disinterest in feeding due to jaundice related lethargy

Anxiety r/t threat to infant and unknown future

High Risk for Altered Body Temperature r/t phototherapy

High Risk for Injury r/t kernicterus, phototherapy lights

Knowledge Deficit: Parental r/t lack of exposure to situation

Parental Role Conflict r/t interruption of family life due to home care regimen

Sensory/Perceptual Alteration: Visual r/t use of eye patches for protection of eyes during phototherapy

Hypercalcemia
Altered Thought Processes r/t elevated calcium levels causing paranoia

Altered Nutrition: Less than Body Requirements r/t gastrointestinal manifestations of hypercalcemia, nausea, anorexia, ileus

High Risk for Decreased Cardiac Output r/t bradydysrhythmias

Impaired Physical Mobility r/t decreased tone in smooth and striated muscle

Hypercapnea
Fear r/t difficulty breathing

Impaired Gas Exchange r/t ventilation perfusion imbalance

Hyperemesis Gravidarum
Altered Nutrition: Less than Body Requirements r/t vomiting

Anxiety r/t threat to self and infant, hospitalization

Fluid Volume Deficit r/t vomiting

Impaired Home Maintenance Management r/t chronic nausea and inability to function

Powerlessness r/t illness-related regimen

Social Isolation r/t hospitalization

Hyperglycemia
Refer to Diabetes Mellitus

Hyperkalemia
High Risk for Impaired Intolerance r/t muscle weakness

High Risk for Decreased Cardiac Output r/t possible dysrhythmias

High Risk for Fluid Volume Excess r/t untreated renal failure

Hypernatremia
High Risk for Fluid Volume Deficit r/t abnormal water loss, inadequate water intake

Hyperosmolar Hyperglycemic Nonketotic Coma
Altered Thought Processes r/t dehydration, electrolyte imbalance

Fluid Volume Deficit r/t polyuria, inadequate fluid intake

High Risk for Injury: Seizures r/t hyperosmolar state, electrolyte imbalance

Refer to Diabetes

Hypertension
Altered Nutrition: More than Body Requirements r/t lack of knowledge of relationship between diet and the disease process

High Risk for Decreased Cardiac Output r/t increased afterload

High Risk for Noncompliance r/t side effects of treatment

Knowledge Deficit r/t treatment and control of disease process

Pain: Headache r/t cerebral vascular changes

Hyperthermia

Hyperthermia r/t exposure to hot environment; vigorous activity; medications/anesthesia; inappropriate clothing; increased metabolic rate; illness or trauma; dehydration; inability or decreased ability to perspire

Hyperthyroidism

Activity Intolerance r/t increased oxygen demands from increased metabolic rate

Altered Nutrition: Less than Body Requirements r/t increased metabolic rate, increased gastrointestinal activity

Anxiety r/t increased stimulation, loss of control

Diarrhea r/t increased gastric motility

High Risk for Injury: Eye damage r/t exophthalmos

Knowledge Deficit r/t medications, methods of coping with stress

Sleep Pattern Disturbance r/t anxiety, excessive sympathetic discharge

Hyperventilation

Ineffective Breathing Pattern r/t anxiety; acid-base imbalance

Hypocalcemia

Altered Nutrition: Less than Body Requirements r/t effects of vitamin D deficiency; renal failure; malabsorption; laxative use

High Risk for Activity Intolerance r/t neuromuscular irritability

High Risk for Ineffective Breathing Pattern r/t laryngospasm

Hypoglycemia

Altered Nutrition: Less than Body Requirements r/t imbalance of glucose/insulin level

Altered Thought Processes r/t insufficient blood glucose to brain

Knowledge Deficit r/t disease process, home and self-care

Refer to Diabetes

Hypokalemia

Activity Intolerance r/t muscle weakness

Decreased Cardiac Output r/t possible dysrhythmias

Hyponatremia

Altered Thought Processes r/t electrolyte imbalance

Fluid Volume Excess r/t excessive intake of hypotonic fluids

Hypoplastic Left Lung

Refer to Congenital Heart Disease/Cardiac Anomalies

Hypotension

Altered Thought Processes r/t decreased oxygen supply to brain

Altered Tissue Perfusion:

Cardiopulmonary/Peripheral r/t hypovolemia; decreased contractility; decreased afterload

Decreased Cardiac Output r/t decreased preload

High Risk for Fluid Volume Deficit r/t excessive fluid loss

Refer to cause of Hypotension

Hypothermia

Hypothermia r/t exposure to cold environment; illness or trauma; damage to hypothalmus; malnutrition; aging

Hypothyroidism

Activity Intolerance r/t muscular stiffness, shortness of breath on exertion

Altered Nutrition: More than Body Requirements r/t decreased metabolic process

Colonic Constipation r/t decreased gastric motility

High Risk for Altered Thought Processes r/t altered metabolic process

Impaired Gas Exchange r/t possible respiratory depression

Impaired Skin Integrity r/t edema, dry scaly skin

Knowledge Deficit r/t disease process and self-care

Hypoxia
Altered Thought Processes r/t decreased oxygen supply to brain
Fear r/t breathlessness
Impaired Gas Exchange r/t altered oxygen supply, inability to transport oxygen
Ineffective Airway Clearance r/t decreased energy and fatigue; increased secretions

Hysterectomy
Anticipatory Grieving r/t change in body image, loss of reproductive status
Constipation r/t narcotics, anesthesia, bowel manipulation during surgery
High Risk for Altered Tissue Perfusion r/t thromboembolism
High Risk for Fluid Volume Deficit r/t abnormal blood loss, hemorrhage
High Risk for Ineffective Individual Coping r/t situational crisis of surgery
High Risk for Sexual Dysfunction r/t disturbance in self-concept
High Risk for Urinary Retention r/t edema in area, anesthesia/narcotics, pain
Knowledge Deficit r/t home care restrictions and needs
Pain r/t surgical injury
Refer to Surgery

I

Irritable Bowel Syndrome (IBS)

Constipation r/t low residue diet, stress

Diarrhea r/t increased motility of intestines associated with stress

Knowledge Deficit r/t treatment of disease

Ineffective Management of Therapeutic Regimen r/t knowledge deficit, powerlessness

Pain r/t spasms and increased motility of bowel

Idiopathic Thrombocytopenia (ITP)

Altered Protection r/t decreased platelet count

Diversional Activity Deficit r/t activity restrictions and safety precautions

High Risk for Injury r/t decreased platelet count and developmental level; age-appropriate play

Impaired Home Health Maintenance r/t parental lack of ability to follow through with safety precautions secondary to child's developmental stage (active toddler)

Refer to Hospitalized Child

Ileal Conduit

Body Image Disturbance r/t presence of stoma

High Risk for Altered Sexuality Pattern r/t altered body function and structure

High Risk for Impaired Skin Integrity r/t difficulty obtaining good seal of appliance

High Risk for Social Isolation r/t alteration in physical appearance, fear of accidental spill of ostomy contents

Ineffective Management of Therapeutic Regimen r/t new skills required to care for appliance and self

Knowledge Deficit r/t routines of care of stoma

Ileostomy

Body Image Disturbance r/t presence of stoma

High Risk for Altered Sexuality Pattern r/t altered body function and structure

High Risk for Constipation/Diarrhea r/t dietary changes, change in intestinal motility

High Risk for Impaired Skin Integrity r/t difficulty obtaining good seal of appliance, caustic drainage

High Risk for Social Isolation r/t alteration in physical appearance, fear of accidental spill of ostomy contents

Ineffective Management of Therapeutic Regimen r/t new skills required to care for appliance and self

Knowledge Deficit r/t limited practice of stoma care, dietary modifications

Ileus

Constipation r/t decreased gastric motility

Fluid Volume Deficit r/t loss of fluids from vomiting

Pain r/t pressure and abdominal distention

Immobility

Altered Thought Process r/t sensory deprivation from immobility

Altered Tissue Perfusion: Peripheral r/t interruption of venous flow

Constipation r/t immobility

High Risk for Disuse Syndrome r/t immobilization

High Risk for Impaired Skin Integrity r/t pressure on immobile parts, shearing forces when moving

Impaired Physical Mobility r/t medically imposed bedrest

Ineffective Breathing Pattern r/t inability to deep breathe in prone position

Powerlessness r/t forced immobility from health care environment

Immunosuppression

Altered Protection r/t medications/treatments suppressing immune system function

High Risk for Infection r/t immunosuppression

Impaction of Stool

Colonic Constipation r/t decreased fluid intake; less than adequate amounts of fiber and bulk-forming foods in diet; immobility

Impetigo

Inpaired Skin Integrity r/t pruritis
Refer to Communicable Diseases, Childhood

Impotence

Self-Esteem Disturbance r/t physiological crisis, inability to practice usual sexual activity
Sexual Dysfunction r/t altered body function

Incompetent Cervix

Refer to Premature Dilation of the Cervix

Incontinence of Stool

Bowel Incontinence r/t decreased awareness of need to defecate, loss of sphincter control
High Risk for Impaired Skin Integrity r/t incontinence of stool
Knowledge Deficit r/t lack of information on normal bowel elimination
Self-Care Deficit r/t toileting needs
Situational Low Self-Esteem r/t inability to control the elimination of stool

Incontinence of Urine

Functional Incontinence r/t altered environment; sensory, cognitive, or mobility deficits
High Risk for Impaired Skin Integrity r/t presence of urine
Reflex Incontinence r/t neurological impairment
Self-Care Deficit: Toileting r/t neurological dysfunction
Situational Low Self-Esteem r/t inability to control passage of urine
Stress Incontinence r/t degenerative change in pelvic muscles and structural supports associated with increased age; high intraabdominal pressure (e.g., obesity, gravid uterus); incompetent bladder outlet; overdistention between voidings; weak pelvic muscles and structural supports
Total Incontinence r/t neuropathy preventing transmission of reflex indicating bladder fullness; neurological dysfunction causing triggering of micturition at unpredictable times; independent contraction of detrusor reflex due to surgery; trauma or disease affecting spinal cord nerves; anatomical (fistula)
Urge Incontinence r/t decreased bladder capacity (e.g., history of PID, abdominal surgeries, indwelling urinary catheter); irritation of bladder stretch receptors causing spasm (e.g., bladder infection); alcohol, caffeine, increased fluids, increased urine concentration; overdistention of bladder

Indigestion

Altered Comfort r/t unpleasant sensations experienced when eating: "burning, bloating, heaviness"
Altered Nutrition, Less than Body Requirements r/t discomfort when eating

Induction of Labor

Anxiety r/t medical interventions
Decisional Conflict r/t perceived threat to idealized birth
Ineffective Individual Coping r/t situational crisis of medical intervention in birthing process
Self-Esteem Disturbance r/t inability to carry out normal labor

Infant Apnea

Refer to Premature Infant; Respiratory Conditions of the Neonate; Sudden Infant Death Syndrome

Infant Feeding Pattern, Ineffective

Ineffective Infant Feeding Pattern r/t prematurity; neurological impairment/delay; oral hypersensitivity; prolonged NPO

Infant of Diabetic Mother

Altered Nutrition: Less than Body Requirements r/t hypotonia, lethargy, and poor sucking; postnatal metabolic changes from hyperglycemia to hypoglycemia and hyperinsulinism

Fluid Volume Deficit r/t increased urinary excretion and osmotic diuresis

High Risk for Decreased Cardiac Output r/t increased incidence of cardiomegaly

High Risk for Impaired Gas Exchange r/t increased incidence of cardiomegaly; prematurity

High Risk for Altered Growth and Development r/t prolonged and severe postnatal hypoglycemia

Refer to Premature Infant; Respiratory Conditions of the Neonate

Infant of Substance Abusing Mother (Fetal Alcohol Syndrome, Crack Baby, other drug withdrawal infants)

Altered Growth and Development r/t effects of maternal use of drugs, effects of neurological impairment, decreased attentiveness to environmental stimuli or inadequate stimuli

Altered Nutrition: Less than Body Requirements r/t feeding problems, uncoordinated/ineffective suck and swallow; effects of diarrhea, vomiting, colic associated with maternal substance abuse

Altered Parenting r/t impaired or lack of attachment behaviors, inadequate support systems

Altered Protection r/t effects of maternal substance abuse

Diarrhea r/t effects of withdrawal, increased peristalsis secondary to hyperirritability

High Risk for Infection (skin, meningeal, respiratory) r/t effects of withdrawal

Ineffective Airway Clearance r/t pooling of secretions secondary to lack of adequate cough reflex; effects of viral or bacterial lower airway infection secondary to altered protective state

Ineffective Infant Feeding Pattern r/t uncoordinated/ineffective sucking reflex

Interrupted Breastfeeding r/t use of drugs, alcohol by mother

Sensory-Perceptual Alteration r/t hypersensitivity to environmental stimuli

Sleep Pattern Disturbance r/t hyperirritability, hypersensitivity to environmental stimuli

Refer to Failure to Thrive; Sudden Infant Death Syndrome; Hospitalized Child; Cerebral Palsy; Hyperactive Syndrome

Infantile Spasms

Refer to Seizure Disorders, Childhood

Infection

High Risk for Infection r/t inadequate primary defenses: broken skin, traumatized tissue, decrease in ciliary action, stasis of body fluids, change in ph secretions, altered peristalsis; inadequate secondary defenses (e.g., decreased hemoglobin, leukopenia, suppressed inflammatory response) and immunosuppression inadequate acquired immunity; tissue destruction and increased environmental exposure; chronic disease; invasive procedures; malnutrition; pharmaceutical agents; trauma; rupture of amniotic membranes; insufficient knowledge to avoid exposure to pathogens

Inflammatory Bowel Disease, Child and Adult

Altered Nutrition: Less than Body Requirements r/t anorexia, decreased absorption of nutrients from GI tract

Diarrhea r/t effects of inflammatory changes of the bowel

Fluid Volume Deficit r/t frequent, loose stools

Inpaired Skin Integrity r/t frequent stools and development of anal fissures

Ineffective Individual Coping r/t repeated episodes of diarrhea

Pain r/t abdominal cramping and anal irritation

Social Isolation r/t diarrhea

Refer to Crohn's Disease; Hospitalized Child; Child With Chronic Condition; Maturational Issues— Adolescent

Influenza
Fluid Volume Deficit r/t inadequate fluid intake
Hyperthermia r/t infectious process
Ineffective Management of Therapeutic Regimen r/t lack of knowledge regarding preventive immunizations
Knowledge Deficit r/t treatment of disease
Pain r/t inflammatory changes in joints

Inguinal Hernia Repair
High Risk for Infection r/t surgical procedure
Impaired Physical Mobility r/t pain at surgical site and fear of causing hernia to "break open"
Pain r/t surgical procedure
Urinary Retention r/t possible edema at surgical site

Injury
High Risk for Injury r/t environmental conditions interacting with the individual's adaptive and defensive resources

Insomnia
Anxiety r/t actual or perceived lose of sleep
Sleep Pattern Disturbance r/t sensory alterations; internal factors; external factors

Insulin Shock
Refer to Hypoglycemia

Intermittent Claudication
Altered Tissue Perfusion: Peripheral r/t interruption of arterial flow
High Risk for Peripheral Neurovascular Dysfunction r/t disruption in arterial flow
Knowledge Deficit r/t lack of knowledge of cause and treatment of peripheral vascular diseases
High Risk for Injury r/t tissue hypoxia

Pain r/t decreased circulation to extremities with activity
Refer to Peripheral Vascular Disease

Intervertebral Disc Excision
Refer to Laminectomy

Intoxication
Altered Thought Process r/t effect of substance on central nervous system
Anxiety r/t loss of control of actions
Ineffective Individual Coping r/t use of mind altering substances as a means of coping
High Risk for Violence r/t inability to control thoughts and actions
Sensory/Perceptual Alterations: Visual, Auditory, Kinesthetic, Tactile, Olfactory r/t neurochemical imbalance in the brain

Intracranial Pressure, Increased
Altered Thought Processes r/t pressure damage to brain
Altered Tissue Perfusion: Cerebral r/t the effects of increased intracranial pressure
Ineffective Breathing Patterns r/t pressure damage to breathing center in brainstem
Sensory/Perceptual Alteration r/t pressure damage to sensory centers in brain
Refer to Cause of Increased Intracranial Pressure

Intra-aortic Balloon Counterpulsation
Anxiety/Fear r/t device providing cardiovascular assistance
Decreased Cardiac Output r/t failing heart needing counterpulsation
High Risk for Peripheral Neurovascular Dysfunction r/t vascular obstruction in balloon catheter; thrombus formation; emboli; edema
Impaired Physical Mobility r/t restriction of movement because of mechanical device

Irregular Pulse
Refer to Dysrhythmias

Irritable Bowel Syndrome
Refer to IBS

Itching
Altered Comfort r/t irritation of the skin
High Risk for Infection r/t potential break in skin

J

Jaundice

High Risk for Altered Thought Processes r/t possible toxic blood metabolites

High Risk for Impaired Skin Integrity r/t pruritus, itching

Pain: Pruritus r/t toxic metabolites excreted in the skin

Refer to Cirrhosis

Jaw Surgery

Altered Nutrition: Less than Bodily Requirements r/t liquid diet

High Risk for Aspiration r/t wired jaws

Impaired Swallowing r/t possible edema from surgery

Knowledge Deficit r/t emergency care for wired jaw (cutting bands/wires) and oral care

Pain r/t surgical procedure

Joint Replacement

High Risk for Peripheral Neurovascular Dysfunction r/t orthopedic surgery

Refer to Total Joint Replacement

K

Kawasaki Disease (formerly called Mucocutaneous Lymph Node Syndrome)

Altered Nutrition: Less than Body Requirements r/t altered oral mucous membranes

Altered Oral Mucous Membranes r/t inflamed mouth and pharynx; swollen lips that progress to dry, cracked, and fissured

Anxiety, Parental r/t progression of disease and complications of arthritis and cardiac involvement

Hyperthermia r/t inflammatory disease process

Impaired Skin Integrity r/t inflammatory skin changes

Pain r/t enlarged lymph nodes; erythematous skin rash that progresses to desquamation, peeling and denuding of skin

Refer to Hospitalized Child

Kegel Exercise

Health Seeking Behavior r/t desire for information to relieve incontinence

Stress Incontinence r/t degenerative change in pelvic muscles

Urge Incontinence r/t decreased bladder capacity

Ketoacidosis

Altered Nutrition: Less than Body Requirements r/t body's inability to use nutrients

Fluid Volume Deficit r/t excess excretion of urine, nausea, vomiting and increased respiration

High Risk for Noncompliance (with Diabetic Regime) r/t ineffective coping with chronic disease

Ineffective Management of Therapeutic Regimen r/t denial of illness, lack of understanding of preventive measures and adequate blood sugar control

Refer to Diabetes

Kidney Failure

Refer to Renal Failure

Kidney Stones

Altered Patterns of Urinary Elimination: Frequency, Urgency r/t anatomical obstruction, irritation caused by stone

High Risk for Fluid Volume Deficit r/t nausea, vomiting

High Risk for Infection r/t obstruction of urinary tract with stasis of urine

Knowledge Deficit r/t fluid requirements and dietary restrictions

Pain r/t obstruction from renal calculi

Knowledge Deficit

Altered Health Maintenance r/t lack of or significant alteration in communication skills (written, verbal, and/or gestural)

Knowledge Deficit r/t lack of exposure; lack of recall; information misinterpretation; cognitive limitation; lack of interest in learning; unfamiliarity with information resources

Korsakoff's Syndrome

Altered Thought Process r/t impairment of short-term memory

High Risk for Altered Nutrition r/t lack of adequate balanced intake

High Risk for Injury r/t sensory dysfunction; lack of coordination when ambulating

L

Labor, Induction of
Refer to Induction of Labor

Labor—Normal
Anxiety r/t fear of the unknown and situational crisis
Fatigue r/t childbirth
Health Seeking Behaviors r/t healthy outcome of pregnancy, prenatal care, and childbirth eduction
High Risk for Fluid Volume Deficit r/t excessive loss of blood
High Risk for Infection r/t multiple vaginal examinations, tissue trauma, and prolonged rupture of membranes
High Risk for Injury (Fetal) r/t hypoxia
Knowledge Deficit r/t lack of preparation for labor
Impaired Skin Integrity r/t passage of infant through birth canal, episiotomy
Pain r/t uterine contractions and stretching of cervix and birth canal

Laminectomy
Anxiety r/t change in health status, surgical procedure
High Risk for Impaired Tissue Perfusion r/t edema, hemorrhage and/or embolism
High Risk for Urinary Retention r/t competing sensory impulses, narcotics, anesthesia
Impaired Physical Mobility r/t neuromuscular impairment
Knowledge Deficit r/t appropriate postoperative activites and after discharge
Pain r/t localized inflammation and edema
Sensory/Perceptual Alteration: Tactile r/t possible edema or nerve injury
Refer to Surgery, Scoliosis

Laproscopic Laser Cholecystectomy
Refer to Cholecystectomy; Laser Surgery

Laryngectomy
Alteration in Family Process r/t surgery, serious condition of family member, difficulty communicating
Alteration in Nutrition: Less than Body Requirements r/t absence of oral feeding, difficulty swallowing, increased need for fluids
Alteration in Oral Mucous Membranes r/t absence of oral feeding
Anticipatory Grieving r/t loss of voice, fear of death
Body Image Disturbance r/t change in body structure and function
High Risk for Infection r/t invasive procedure, surgery
Impaired Verbal Communication r/t removal of the larynx
Impaired Swallowing r/t edema, laryngectomy tube
Ineffective Airway Clearance r/t surgical removal of the glottis, decreased humidification of air
Knowledge Deficit r/t self-care needs

Laser Surgery
Knowledge Deficit r/t preoperative and postoperative care associated with laser procedure
Pain r/t heat from action of the laser
High Risk for Infection r/t delayed heating reaction of tissue exposed to laser
High Risk for Injury r/t accidental exposure to laser beam
Constipation r/t laser intervention in vulva and perianal areas

Laxative Abuse
Perceived Constipation r/t health belief, faulty appraisal, impaired thought processes

Lethargic/Listless
Altered Tissue Perfusion: Cerebral r/t lack of oxygen supply to brain
Fatigue r/t decreased metabolic energy production

67

Sleep Pattern Disturbance r/t internal/external stressors
Refer to cause of Lethargy

Leukemia
Altered Protection r/t abnormal blood profile
High Risk for Infection r/t ineffective immune system
High Risk for Fluid Volume Deficit r/t side effects of treatment: nausea, vomiting, bleeding
Refer to Chemotherapy, Cancer

Leukopenia
High Risk for Infection r/t low white blood count

Level of Consciousness, Decreased
Refer to Confusion

Lice
Refer to Communicable Diseases, Childhood

Limb Reattachment Procedures
Anticipatory Grieving r/t unknown outcome of reattachment procedure
Body Image Disturbance r/t unpredictability of function and appearance of reattached body part
Anxiety r/t unknown outcome of reattachment procedure; use of limb, appearance of limb
High Risk for Fluid Volume Deficit: *Hemorrhage* r/t severed vessels
High Risk for Peripheral Neurovascular Dysfunction r/t trauma, orthopedic, neurovascular surgery; compression of nerves, blood vessels
Refer to Surgery Postoperative Procedures

Loneliness
Social Isolation r/t delay in accomplishing developmental tasks; immature interests; alterations in physical appearance; alterations in mental status; unacceptable social behavior; unacceptable social values; altered state of wellness; inadequate personal resources; inability to engage in satisfying personal relationships

Loose Stools
Diarrhea r/t increased gastric motility
Refer to Cause of Diarrhea

Low Back Pain
Chronic Pain r/t degenerative processes; musculotendinous strain; injury; inflammation; congenital deformities
Impaired Physical Mobility r/t back pain
Ineffective Management of Therapeutic Regimen r/t knowledge deficit regarding proper posture, lifting techniques, and conditioning exercises
Urinary Retention r/t possible spinal cord compression

Lupus Erythromatosus
Body Image Disturbance r/t change in skin: rash, lesions, ulcers, mottled erythema
Fatigue r/t increased metabolic requirements
High Risk for Impaired Skin Integrity r/t chronic inflammation, edema, and altered circulation
Knowledge Deficit r/t medication, diet, and activity
Pain r/t inflammatory process
Powerlessness r/t unpredictability of course of the disease
Spiritual Distress r/t chronicity of disease; unknown etiology

Lyme Disease
Fatigue r/t increased energy requirements
High Risk for Decreased Cardiac Output r/t dysrhythmias
Pain r/t inflammation of joints, urticaria, and rash

M

Major Depression
Refer to Depression

Maladaptive Behavior
Refer to Crisis; Suicide

Malnutrition
Altered Nutrition: Less than Body Requirements r/t inability to ingest or digest food or absorb nutrients due to biological, psychological, economic factors, institutionalization, i.e., lack of menu choices

Altered Protection r/t inadequate nutrition

Ineffective Management of Therapeutic Regimen r/t economic difficulties

Knowledge Deficit r/t misinformation about normal nutrition, social isolation, lack of food preparation facilities

Mania
Altered Family Porcesses r/t family members illness

Altered Nutrition: Less than Body Requirements r/t lack of time and motivation to eat, constant movement

Altered Role Performance r/t impaired social interactions

Altered Thought Processes r/t mania

Anxiety r/t change in role function

Fluid Volume Deficit r/t decreased intake

High Risk for Caregiver Role Strain r/t unpredictability of the condition; mood swings

High Risk for Violence: Self-Directed or Directed at Others r/t bizarre hallucinations, delusions

Impaired Home Maintenance Management r/t altered psychological state, inability to concentrate

Ineffective Denial r/t fear of inability to control behavior

Ineffective Individual Coping r/t situational crisis

Ineffective Management of Therapeutic Regimen r/t lack of social supports

Noncompliance r/t denial of illness

Sleep Pattern Disturbance r/t constant anxious thoughts

Manipulative Behavior
Defensive Coping r/t superior attitude towards others

High Risk for Self-Mutilation r/t inability to cope with increased psychological/physiological tension in a healthy manner

Impaired Social Interaction r/t self-concept disturbance

Ineffective Individual Coping r/t inappropriate use of defense mechanisms

Mastectomy
Body Image Disturbance r/t loss of sexually significant body part

Fear r/t change in body image and prognosis

High Risk for Disuse Syndrome of arm on affected side r/t pain; lack of knowledge concerning need for range of motion

High Risk for Impaired Physical Mobility r/t nerve, muscle damage, pain

High Risk for Sexual Dysfunction r/t change in body image, fear of loss of feminism

Knowledge Deficit r/t self-care activities

Pain r/t surgical procedure

Refer to Cancer; Surgery

Mastitis
Altered Role Performance r/t change in capacity to function in expected role

Anxiety r/t threat to self and concern over safety of milk for infant

High Risk for Ineffective Breastfeeding r/t breast pain and conflicting advice from health care providers

69

Knowledge Deficit r/t antibiotic regimen and comfort measures

Pain r/t infectious disease process and swelling of breast tissue

Maturational Issues, Adolescent

Altered Family Porcesses r/t developmental crises of adolescence secondary to challenge of parental authority and values; situational crises secondary to change in parental marital status

High Risk for Impaired Social Interaction r/t ineffective/ unsuccessful/dysfunctional interaction with peers

High Risk for Injury/Trauma r/t thrill-seeking behaviors

Ineffective Individual Coping r/t maturational crises

Knowledge Deficit: Potential for Enhanced Health Maintenance r/t information misinterpretation; lack of education regarding age related factors

Social Isolation r/t perceived alteration in physical appearance, social values not accepted by dominant peer group

Refer to Sexuality—Adolescent; Substance Abuse—Adolescent

Measles (Rubeola)

Refer to Communicable Diseases, Childhood

Meconium Aspiration

Refer to Respiratory Conditions of the Neonate

Melena

Fear r/t presence of blood in feces

High Risk for Fluid Volume Deficit r/t hemorrhage

Refer to Gastrointestinal Bleeding

Memory Deficit

Anxiety r/t memory loss

Altered Thought Process r/t psychosocial or physiological stress; neurological deficit

High Risk for Injury r/t memory loss

Knowledge Deficit r/t techniques to improve memory

Meningitis/Encephalitis

Altered Comfort: Nausea and Vomiting r/t CNS inflammation

Altered Comfort: Photophobia r/t increased sensitivity to external stimuli secondary to CNS inflammation

Altered Thought Processes r/t inflammation of brain, fever

Altered Tissue Perfusion: Cerebral r/t inflamed cerebral tissues and meninges; increased intracranial pressure

Fluid Volume Excess r/t increased intracranial pressure; inappropriate secretion of antidiuretic hormone (SIADH)

High Risk for Altered Growth and Development r/t brain damage secondary to infectious process, increased intracranial pressure

High Risk for Aspiration r/t seizure activity

High Risk for Ineffective Airway Clearance r/t seizure activity

Pain r/t neck (nuchal) rigidity, inflammation of meninges, headache, kinesthetic sensory-perceptual alteration (skin is painful to touch), fever, earache

High Risk for Injury r/t seizure activity

Impaired Mobility r/t neuromuscular/CNS insult

Sensory-Perceptual Alteration: Hearing r/t CNS infection, ear infection

Sensory-Perceptual Alteration: Kinesthetic r/t CNS infection

Sensory-Perceptual Alteration: Visual r/t photophobia secondary to CNS infection

Refer to Hospitalized Child

Meningocele

Refer to Neurotube Defects

Menopause

Altered Sexuality Patterns r/t altered body structure; lack of physiological lubrication and lack of knowledge of artificial lubrication

Health Seeking Behavior r/t menopause and therapies associated with change in hormonal levels

High Risk for Altered Nutrition: More than Body Requirements r/t change in metabolic rate caused by fluctuating hormone levels

Ineffective Thermoregulation r/t changes in hormonal levels

Menorrhagia

Fear r/t loss of large amounts of blood

High Risk for Fluid Volume Deficit r/t excessive loss of menstrual blood

Mental Retardation

Altered Family Porcesses r/t crisis of diagnosis and situational transition

Altered Growth and Development r/t cognitive/perceptual impairment and developmental delay

Chronic Low Self-Esteem r/t perceived differences

Grieving r/t loss of perfect child; birth of child with congenital defect or subsequent head injury

Family Coping: Potential for Growth r/t adaptation and acceptance of child's condition and needs

High Risk for Self-Mutilation r/t separation anxiety; depersonalization

Impaired Home Maintenance Management r/t insufficient support systems

Impaired Social Interaction r/t developmental lag/delay, perceived differences

Impaired Swallowing r/t neuromuscular impairment

Impaired Verbal Communication r/t developmental delay

Parental Role Conflict r/t home care of child with special needs

Self-Care Deficit: Bathing/Hygiene;
Dressing/Grooming; Feeding; Toileting r/t perceptual or cognitive impairment

Refer to Safety—Childhood; Child With Chronic Condition

Midlife Crisis

Ineffective Individual Coping r/t inability to deal with changes associated with aging

Powerlessness r/t lack of control over life situation

Spiritual Distress r/t questioning belief/value system

Migraine Headache

Knowledge Deficit r/t prevention and treatment of headaches

Pain: Headache r/t vasodilatation of cerebral and extracerebral vessels

Miscarriage

Refer to Pregnancy Loss

Mitral Stenosis

Anxiety r/t possible worsening of symptoms; activity intolerance; fatigue

Activity Intolerance r/t imbalance between oxygen supply and demand

Decreased Cardiac Output r/t incompetent heart valves; abnormal forward or backward blood flow; flow into a dilated chamber; flow through an abnormal passage between chambers

Fatigue r/t reduced cardiac output

Mitral Valve Prolapse

Altered Tissue Perfusion: Cerebral r/t postural hypotension

Anxiety r/t symptoms of condition: palpitations, chest pain

Fatigue r/t abnormal catecholamine regulation and decreased intravascular volume

Fear r/t lack of knowledge about mitral valve prolapse; feelings of having a heart attack

High Risk for Infection r/t invasive procedures

Knowledge Deficit r/t methods to relieve pain, treatment of dysrhythmias and shortness of breath, need prophylactic antibiotics before invasive procedures

Pain r/t mitral valve regurgitation

Mobility, Impaired Physical

Impaired Physical Mobility r/t intolerance to activity; decreased strength and endurance; pain/discomfort/ perceptual/cognitive impairment; neuromuscular impairment; musculoskeletal impairment; depression/severe anxiety

Mononucleosis

Activity Intolerance r/t generalized weakness

High Risk for Injury r/t possible rupture of spleen

Hyperthermia r/t infectious process

Impaired Swallowing r/t irritation of oropharyngeal cavity

Ineffective Management of Therapeutic Regimen r/t knowledge deficit concerning transmission and treatment of disease

Pain r/t enlargement of lymph nodes, irritation of oropharyngeal cavity

Mottling of Peripheral Skin

Altered Tissue Perfusion: Peripheral r/t interruption of arterial flow; decreased circulating blood volume

Mouth Lesions

Refer to Mucous Membranes, Impaired

Mucocutaneous Lymph Node Syndrome

Refer to Kawasaki Disease

Mucous Membranes, Altered Oral

Altered Oral Mucous Membranes r/t pathological conditions—oral cavity (radiation to head or neck); dehydration; trauma (chemical, e.g., acidic foods, drugs, noxious agents, alcohol; mechanical, e.g., ill-fitting dentures, braces, tubes (endotracheal/nasogastric), surgery in oral cavity); NPO for more than 24 hours; ineffective oral hygiene; mouth breathing; malnutrition; infection; lack of or decreased salivation; medication

Multiple Gestation

Altered Nutrition: Less than Body Requirements r/t physiological demands of a multifetal pregnancy

Anxiety r/t uncertain outcome of pregnancy

Fatigue r/t physiologic demands of a multifetal pregnancy and/or care of more than one infant

High Risk for Ineffective Breastfeeding r/t lack of support, physical demands of feeding more than one infant

Impaired Home Maintenance Management r/t fatigue

Impaired Physical Mobility r/t increased uterine size

Knowledge Deficit r/t caring for more than one infant

Sleep Pattern Disturbance r/t discomforts of multiple gestation or care of infants

Stress Incontinence r/t increased pelvic pressure

Multiple Personality

Anxiety r/t loss of control of behavior and feelings

Body-Image Disturbance r/t feelings of powerlessness with personality changes

Chronic Low Self-Esteem r/t inability to deal with life events; history of abuse

Defensive Coping r/t unresolved past traumatic events; severe anxiety

High Risk for Self-Mutilation r/t need to act out to relieve stress

Ineffective Individual Coping r/t history of abuse

Hopelessness r/t long-term stress

Personal Identity Disturbance r/t severe child abuse

Refer to Dissociative Disorder

Multiple Sclerosis

Anticipatory Grieving r/t high risk for loss of normal body functioning

High Risk for Altered Nutrition: Less than Body Requirements r/t impaired swallowing, depression

High Risk for Disuse Syndrome r/t physical immobility

High Risk for Ineffective Airway Clearnace r/t decreased energy/fatigue

High Risk for Injury r/t altered mobility, sensory dysfunction

High Risk for Urinary Retention r/t inhibition of the reflex arc

Impaired Physical Mobility r/t neuromuscular impairment

Powerlessness r/t progressive nature of disease

Self-Care Deficit: Specify r/t neuromuscular impairment

Sensory/Perceptual alteration: Specify r/t pathology in sensory tracts

Sexual Dysfucntion r/t biopsychosocial alteration of sexuality

Spiritual Distress r/t perceived hopelessness of diagnosis

Refer to Nervous System Disorders

Mumps

Refer to Communicable Diseases, Childhood

Murmurs

Decreased Cardiac Output r/t incompetent heart valves; abnormal forward or backward blood flow; flow into a dilated chamber; flow through an abnormal passage between chambers

Muscular Atrophy/Weakness

Disuse Syndrome r/t impaired physical mobility

Muscular Dystrophy

Activity Intolerance r/t fatigue

Altered Nutrition: Less than Body Requirements r/t impaired swallowing/chewing

Altered Nutrition: More than Body Requirements r/t inactivity

Decreased Cardiac Output r/t effects of congestive heart failure

High Risk for Aspiration r/t impaired swallowing

High Risk for Constipation r/t immobility

High Risk for Disuse Syndrome r/t complications of immobility

High Risk for Fatigue r/t increased energy requirements to perform activities of daily living

High Risk for Impaired Gas Exchange r/t ineffective airway clearance and ineffective breathing patterns secondary to muscle weakness

High Risk for Impaired Skin Integrity r/t immobility and braces/adaptive devices

High Risk for Ineffective Breathing Patterns r/t muscle weakness

High Risk for Infection r/t pooling of pulmonary secretions secondary to immobility and muscle weakness

High Risk for Injury r/t muscle weakness and unsteady gait

Impaired Mobility r/t muscle weakness and development of contractures

Ineffective Airway Clearance r/t muscle weakness and decreased cough

Self-Care Deficits: Feeding, Bathing, Dressing, Toileting r/t muscle weakness and fatigue

Refer to Hospitalized Child; Child With Chronic Condition; Terminally Ill Child/Death of Child

Myasthenia Gravis

Altered Family Process r/t crisis of dealing with diagnosis

Altered Nutrition r/t difficulty eating and swallowing

High Risk for Caregiver Role Strain r/t severity of illness of client

Fatigue r/t paresthesia and aching muscles

Impaired Physical Mobility r/t defective transmission of nerve impulses at the neuromuscular junction

73

Impaired Swallowing r/t neuromuscular impairment

Ineffective Airway Clearance r/t decreased ability to cough and swallow

Ineffective Management of Therapeutic Regimen r/t lack of knowledge of treatment and uncertainty of outcome

Myelocele
Refer to Neurotube Defects

Myelogram, Contrast
High Risk for Altered Tissue Perfusion: Cerebral r/t hypotension; loss of cerebral spinal fluid

High Risk for Fluid Volume Deficit r/t possible dehydration; loss of cerebral spinal fluid

Pain r/t irritation of nerve roots

Urinary Retention r/t pressure on spinal nerve roots

Myelomeningocele
Refer to Neurotube Defects

Myocardial Infarction
Altered Family Porcesses r/t crisis, role change

Anxiety r/t threat of death; possible change in role status

Colonic Constipation r/t decreased peristalsis from decreased physical activity, medication effect, change in diet

Decreased Cardiac Output r/t ventricular damage, ischemia; dysrhythmias

Fear r/t threat to well-being

High Risk for Altered Sexuality Pattern r/t fear of chest pain, possibility of heart damage

High Risk for Ineffective Denial r/t fear or knowledge deficit about heart disease

High Risk for Situational Low Self-Esteem r/t crisis of myocardial infarction

Ineffective Family Coping r/t spouse/significant other fear of partner loss

Knowledge Deficit r/t self-care program

Pain r/t myocardial tissue damage from inadequate blood supply

Myocarditis
Activity Intolerance r/t reduced cardiac reserve and prescribed bedrest

Decreased Cardiac Output r/t impaired contractility of ventricles

Knowledge Deficit r/t treatment of disease

Refer to Congestive Heart Failure, if appropriate

Myxedema
Refer to Hypothyroidism

N

Nasogastric Suction
High Risk for Fluid Volume Deficit r/t loss of gastrointestinal fluids without adequate replacement

Altered Comfort r/t presence of nasogastric tube

Nausea
High Risk for Altered Nutrition: Less than Body Requirements r/t nausea (specify cause)

High Risk for Fluid Volume Deficit r/t inadequate fluid intake secondary to nausea

Near Drowning
Altered Health Maintenance r/t parental knowledge deficit regarding safety measures appropriate for age

Anticipatory/Dysfucntional Grieving r/t potential death of child; unknown sequelae; guilt over accident

Aspiration r/t aspiration of fluid into the lungs

Fear, Parental r/t possible death of child; possible permanent, debilitating sequelae

High Risk for Altered Growth and Development r/t hypoxemia; cerebral anoxia

High Risk for Infection r/t aspiration, invasive monitoring

Hypothermia r/t CNS injury, prolonged submersion in cold water

Impaired Gas Exchange r/t laryngospasm, breath holding, aspiration

Ineffective Airway Clearance/Ineffective Breathing Pattern r/t aspiration and impaired gas exchange

Refer to Safety—Childhood; Hospitalized Child; Child With Chronic Condition; Terminally Ill Child/Death of Child

Neck Vein Distention
Fluid Volume Excess r/t excess fluid intake or compromised regulatory mechanisms

Refer to Congestive Heart Failure

Necrotizing Enterocolitis (NEC)
Altered Nutrition: Less than Body Requirements r/t decreased ability to absorb nutrients; decreased perfusion to GI tract

Altered Tissue Perfusion: Gastrointestinal r/t shunting of blood away from mesenteric circulation, toward vital organs secondary to perinatal stress, hypoxia

Fluid Volume Deficit r/t vomiting; GI bleed

High Risk for Infection r/t bacterial invasion of GI tract; invasive procedures

Ineffective Breathing Pattern r/t abdominal distention, hypoxia

Refer to Premature Infant; Hospitalized Child

Negative Feelings About Self
Chronic Low Self-Esteem r/t long-standing negative self-evaluation

Self-Esteem Disturbance r/t inappropriate learned negative feelings about self

Neglectful Care of Family Member
Caregiver Role Strain r/t care demands of family member and lack of social/financial support

Ineffective Family Coping: Disabling r/t highly ambivalent family relationships, lack of respite care

Knowledge Deficit r/t care needs

Nephrectomy
Anxiety r/t surgical recovery; prognosis

Alteration in Urinary Elimination r/t loss of kidney

Constipation r/t lack of return of peristalsis

High Risk for Infection r/t invasive procedure, lack of deep breathing due to location of surgical incision

High Risk for Fluid Volume Deficit r/t vascular losses, decreased intake

Ineffective Breathing Pattern r/t location of surgical incision

Pain r/t incisional discomfort

Nephrotic Syndrome
Activity Intolerance r/t generalized edema
Altered Confort r/t edema
Altered Nutrition: Less than Body Requirements r/t anorexia and protein loss
Altered Nutrition: More than Body Requirements r/t increased appetite secondary to steroid therapy
Body Image Disturbance r/t edematous appearance and side effects of steroid therapy
Fluid Volume Excess r/t edema secondary to oncotic fluid shift from serum protein loss and renal retention of salt and water
High Risk for Impaired Skin Integrity r/t edema
High Risk for Infection r/t altered immune mechanisms secondary to disease itself and effects of steroids
High Risk for Noncompliance r/t side effects encountered with home steroid therapy
Social Isolation r/t edematous appearance
Refer to Hospitalized Child; Child With Chronic Condition

Nervous System Disorders
Altered Family Porcesses r/t situational crisis, illness/disability of family member
Anticipatory Grieving r/t loss of usual body functioning
Altered Nutrition, Less than Body Requirements r/t impaired swallowing, depression, difficulty feeding self
High Risk for Disuse Syndrome r/t physical immobility, neuromuscular dysfunction
High Risk for Impaired Skin Integrity r/t altered sensation, altered mental status, paralysis
High Risk for Ineffective Airway Clearnace r/t perceptual/cognitive impairment, decreased energy/fatigue
High Risk for Injury r/t altered mobility, sensory dysfunction, cognitive impairment

Impaired Home Maintenance Management r/t individual/family members disease
Impaired Physical Mobility r/t neuromuscular impairment
Ineffective Individual Coping r/t disability requiring change in lifestyle
Powerlessness r/t progressive nature of disease
Self-Care Deficit: Specify r/t neuromuscular dysfunction
Sexual Dysfunction r/t biopsychosocial alteration of sexuality
Social Isolation r/t altered state of wellness

Neuritis
Activity Intolerance r/t pain with movement
Knowledge Deficit r/t treatment of disease
Pain r/t stimulation of affected nerve endings; inflammation of sensory nerves

Neurogenic Bladder
Reflex Incontinence r/t neurological impairment
Urinary Retention r/t interruption in the lateral spinal tracts

Neurotube Defects (Meningocele, Myelomeningocele, Spina Bifida, Anencephaly)
Altered Growth and Development r/t physical impairments, possible cognitive impairment
Chronic Low Self-Esteem r/t perceived differences; decreased ability to participate in physical and social activities at school
Colonic Constipation r/t immobility or less than adequate mobility
Family Coping: Potential for Growth r/t effective adaptive response by family members
Grieving r/t (loss of perfect child) birth of child with congenital defect
High Risk for Altered Nutrition: More than Body Requirements r/t diminished/limited/impaired physical activity
High Risk for Impaired Skin Integrity (Lower Extremities) r/t decreased sensory perception
Impaired Mobility r/t neuromuscular impairment

Impaired Skin Integrity r/t incontinence

Sensory/Perceptual Alteration: Visual r/t altered reception secondary to strabismus

Urge Incontinence vs Reflex Incontinence r/t neurogenic impairment vs Total Incontinence r/t neurological dysfunction

Refer to Premature Infant; Child With Chronic Condition

Newborn, Normal

Altered Protection r/t immature immune system

Effective Breastfeeding r/t normal oral structure and gestational age greater than 34 weeks

High Risk for Infection r/t open umbilical stump

High Risk for Injury r/t immaturity and need for caretaking

Ineffective Thermoregulation r/t immaturity of neuroendocrine system

Newborn, Postmature

High Risk for Aspiration r/t meconium aspiration

High Risk for Injury r/t hypoglycemia secondary to depleted glycogen stores

Hypothermia r/t depleted stores of subcutaneous fat

Impaired Skin Integrity r/t cracked and peeling skin secondary to decreased vernix

Newborn, Small for Gestational Age (SGA)

Altered Nutrition: Less than Body Requirements r/t inadequate sucking reflex

Ineffective Thermoregulation r/t immaturity of neuroendocrine system; decreased brown fat and subcutaneous fat

Nicotine Addiction

Altered Health Maintenance r/t lack of ability to make a judgement about smoking cessation

Powerlessness r/t perceived lack of control over ability to give up nicotine

Nightmares

Post-Trauma Response r/t disasters, wars, epidemics rape, assault, torture, catastrophic illness or accident

Rape-Trauma Syndrome, Rape-Trauma Syndrome: Compound Reaction, Rape-Trauma Syndrome Silent Reaction r/t forced violent sexual penetration against the victim's will and consent

Nocturia

Altered Urinary Elimination r/t sensory motor impairment, urinary tract infection

Total Incontinence r/t neuropathy preventing transmission of reflex indicating bladder fullness; neurological dysfunction causing triggering of micturition at unpredictable times; independent contraction of detrusor reflex due to surgery; trauma or disease affecting spinal cord nerves; anatomic (fistula)

Urge Incontinence r/t decreased bladder capacity; irritation bladder stretch receptors causing spasm; alcohol; caffeine; increased fluids; increased urine concentration; overdistention of bladder

Noncompliance r/t patient value system; health beliefs, cultural influences, spiritual values; client-provider relationships, knowledge deficit

Altered Nutrition: Less than Body Requirements r/t inability to ingest or digest food or absorb nutrients due to biological, psychological, or economic factors

Altered Nutrition: More than Body Requirements r/t excessive intake in relation to metabolic need

O

Obesity

Altered Nutrition: More than Body Requirements r/t caloric intake exceeding energy expenditure

Body Image Disturbance r/t eating disorder, excess weight

Chronic Low Self-Esteem r/t ineffective individual coping, overeating

Obsessive Compulsive Disorder

Altered Thought Process r/t persistent thoughts, ideas, and impulses that will not relent and seem irrelevant

Anxiety r/t threat to self-concept; unmet needs

Decisional Conflict r/t inability to make a decision for fear of reprisal

Ineffective Family Coping: Disabling r/t family process being disrupted by client's ritualistic activities

Ineffective Individual Coping r/t expression of feelings in an unacceptable way; ritualistic behavior

Powerlessness r/t unrelenting repetitive thoughts to perform irrational activities

Obstruction, Bowel

Refer to Bowel Obstruction

Oliguria

Fluid Volume Deficit r/t active fluid loss; failure of regulatory mechanism

Refer to Renal Failure; Shock; Decreased Cardiac Output

Oophorectomy

High Risk for Altered Sexuality Patterns r/t altered body function

Refer to Surgery

Open Reduction of Fracture with Internal Fixation (Femur)

Anxiety r/t outcome of corrective procedure

High Risk for Peripheral Neurovascular Dysfunction r/t mechanical compression, orthopedic surgery, immobilization

Impaired Physical Mobility r/t position required post-operatively; abduction of leg and avoidance of acute flexion

Powerlessness r/t loss of control; unanticipated change in lifestyle

Refer to Surgery Post-Operative

Oral Mucous Membrane, Altered

Altered Oral Mucous Membrane r/t pathological conditions—oral cavity (radiation to head or neck): dehydration; trauma (chemical, e.g., acidic foods, drugs, noxious agents, alcohol; mechanical, e.g., ill-fitting dentures, braces, tubes (endotracheal/nasogastric, surgery in oral cavity); NPO for more than 24 hours; ineffective oral hygiene; mouth breathing; malnutrition; infection; lack of or decreased salivating; medication

Organic Mental Syndromes

High Risk for Injury r/t disorientation to time, place and person

Impaired Social Interaction r/t altered thought processes

Refer to Dementia

Orthopnea

Ineffective Breathing Pattern r/t inability to breathe with the head of the bed flat

Decreased Cardiac Output r/t inability of heart to meet demands of body

Orthostatic Hypotension

Refer to Dizziness

Osteomylitis

Altered Health Maintenance r/t continued immobility at home, possible extensive casts, continued antibiotics

Diversional Activity Deficit r/t prolonged immobilization and hospitalization

Fear: Parental r/t concern regarding possible growth plate damage secondary to infection or concern that infection may become chronic

High Risk for Colonic Constipation r/t immobility

High Risk for Impaired Skin Integrity r/t irritation from splint/cast

High Risk for (Spread of) Infection r/t inadequate primary defenses, secondary defenses

Hyperthermia r/t infectious process

Impaired Physical Mobility r/t imposed immobility secondary to infected area

Pain r/t inflammation in affected extremity

Refer to Hospitalized Child

Osteoporosis

Altered Nutrition: Less than Body Requirements r/t inadequate intake of calcium and vitamin D

High Risk for Injury: Fractures r/t lack of activity; risk of falling from environmental hazards; neuromuscular disorders; diminished senses; cardiovascular responses; responses to drugs

Impaired Physical Mobility r/t pain, skeletal changes

Knowledge Deficit r/t diet, exercise, and need to abstain from alcohol and nicotine

Pain r/t fracture and muscle spasm

Ostomy

Refer to Colostomy; Ileostomy; Ileal Conduit; Child with Chronic Condition

Otitis Media

High Risk for Infection r/t eustachian tube obstruction, traumatic eardrum perforation, or following infectious disease process

Pain r/t inflammation, infectious process

Sensory/Perceptual Alteration: Auditory r/t incomplete resolution of otitis media, presence of excess drainage in the middle ear

Pacemaker

Anxiety r/t change in health status; presence of pacemaker

High Risk for Decreased Cardiac Output r/t malfunction of pacemaker

High Risk for Infection r/t invasive procedure, presence of foreign body: catheter and generator

Knowledge Deficit r/t self-care program; when to seek medical attention

Pain r/t surgical procedure

Pain

Pain r/t injury agents (biological, chemical, physical, psychological)

Pain, Chronic

Chronic Pain r/t chronic physical/psychosocial disability

Painful Breasts—Cracked Nipples

Altered Role Performance r/t change in physical capacity to assume the role of breastfeeding mother

High Risk for Infection r/t break in skin

Impaired Skin Integrity r/t mechanical factors involved in suckling and breastfeeding management

Ineffective Breastfeeding r/t pain

Pain r/t cracked nipples

Painful Breasts—Engorgement

Altered Role Performance r/t change in physical capacity to assume the role of breastfeeding mother

High Risk for Ineffective Breastfeeding r/t pain and infant's inability to latch-on to engorged breast

Impaired Tissue Integrity r/t excessive fluid in breast tissues

Pain r/t distension of breast tissue

Pallor of Extremities

Altered Tissue Perfusion: Peripheral r/t interruption of vascular flow

Pancreatitis

Altered Nutrition: Less than Body Requirements r/t inadequate dietary intake, increased nutritional needs secondary to acute illness, increased metabolic needs caused by increased body temperature

Diarrhea r/t decrease in pancreatic secretions resulting in steatorrhea

Fluid Volume Deficit r/t vomiting, decreased fluid intake, fever with diaphoresis and fluid shifts

High Risk for Ineffective Breathing Pattern r/t splinting from severe pain

High Risk for Ineffective Denial r/t ineffective coping (alcohol use)

Knowledge Deficit r/t lack of knowledge concerning diet, alcohol use and medication

Pain r/t irritation and edema of the inflamed pancreas

Panic Attacks

Anxiety r/t situational crisis

Ineffective Individual Coping r/t personal vulnerability

Post-Trauma Response r/t previous catastrophic event

Social Isolation r/t fear of lack of control

Paralysis

Body Image Disturbance r/t biophysical changes, loss of movement, mobility

Colonic Constipation r/t effects of spinal cord disruption; diet inadequate in fiber

High Risk for Disuse Syndrome r/t paralysis

High Risk for Impaired Skin Integrity r/t altered circulation, altered sensation, and immobility

High Risk for Injury r/t altered mobility, sensory dysfunction

Impaired Physical Mobility r/t neuromuscular impairment

Knowledge Deficit r/t impaired home maintenance management

Pain r/t prolonged immobility

Powerlessness r/t illness-related regimen

Reflex Incontinence r/t neurological impairment

Self-Care Deficit: Specify r/t neuromuscular impairment

Sexual Dysfucntion r/t loss of sensation; biopsychosocial alteration

Refer to Child with Chronic Condition; Hospitalized Child; Neurotube Defects; Hemiplegia, Spinal Cord Injury

Paralytic Ileus

Constipation r/t decreased gastric motility

Fluid Volume Deficit r/t loss of fluids from vomiting

Pain r/t pressure and abdominal distention

Paranoid Disorder

Altered Thought Processes r/t psychological conflicts

Anxiety r/t uncontrollable intrusive, suspicious thoughts

Chronic Low Self-Esteem r/t inability to trust others

High Risk for Violence: Directed at Others r/t suspicious of others and others actions

Sensory/Perceptual Alteration: Specify r/t psychological dysfunction; suspicious thoughts

Social Isolation r/t inappropriate social skills

Paraplegia

Refer to Spinal Cord Injury

Parental Role Conflict

Parental Role Conflict r/t separation from child due to chronic illness; intimidation with invasive or restrictive modalities (e.g., isolation, intubation) specialized care center, policies; home care of a child with special need (e.g. apnea monitoring, postural drainage, hyperalimentation); change in marital status; interruptions of family life due to home care regimen (treatments, caregivers lack of respite)

Parenthood, Adjustment to New

Refer to Adjustment to Parenthood

Parenting, Altered

Altered Parenting r/t lack of available role model; ineffective role model; physical and psychosocial abuse of nurturing figure; lack of support between/from significant other(s); unmet social/emotional maturation needs of parenting figures; interruption in bonding process, i.e., maternal, paternal, other; unrealistic expectation for self, infant, partner; physical illness; presence of stress (financial, legal, recent crisis, cultural move); lack of knowledge; limited cognitive functioning; lack of role identity; lack of appropriate response of child to relationship; multiple pregnancies

Parenting, High Risk for Altered

High Risk for Altered Parenting r/t lack of available role model; ineffective role model; physical and psychosocial abuse of nurturing figure; lack of support between/from significant other(s); unmet social/emotional maturation needs of parenting figures; interruption in bonding process, i.e., maternal, paternal, other; unrealistic expectation for self, infant, partner; physical illness; presence of stress (financial, legal, recent crisis, cultural move); lack of knowledge; limited cognitive functioning; lack of role identity; lack or inappropriate response of child to relationship; multiple pregnancies

Paresthesia

Sensory/Perceptual Alteration: Tactile r/t altered sensory reception, transmission, or integration

Parkinson's Disease

Alteration in Nutrition: Less than Body Requirements r/t tremor, slowness in eating, difficulty in chewing and swallowing

High Risk for Colonic Constipation r/t weakness of defecation muscles; lack of exercise; inadequate fluid intake; decreased autonomic nervous system activity

High Risk for Injury r/t tremors, slow reactions, altered gait

Impaired Verbal Communication r/t decreased speech volume, slowness of speech, impaired facial muscles

Refer to Nervous System Disorders

Paroxsysmal Nocturnal Dyspnea

Decreased Cardiac Output r/t failure of the left ventricle

Ineffective Breathing Pattern r/t increase in carbon dioxide levels decrease in oxygen levels

Patent Ductus Arteriosus (PDA)

Refer to Congenital Heart Disease/Cardiac Anomalies

Patient-Controlled Analgesia (see PCA)

Patient Education

Health Seeking Behaviors r/t expressed or observed desire to seek a higher level of wellness or control of health practices

Knowledge Deficit r/t lack of exposure to information; information misinterpretation; unfamiliarity with information resources

PCA

Altered Comfort r/t medication side effects: pruritus, nausea or vomiting

Knowledge Deficit r/t self-care of pain control

High Risk for Injury r/t possible complications associated with PCA

Pelvic Inflammatory Disease

Refer to PID

Pericardial Friction Rub

Decreased Cardiac Output r/t inflammation in pericardial sac, fluid accumulation compressing heart

Pain r/t inflammation, effusion

Pericarditis

Activity Intolerance r/t reduced cardiac reserve and prescribed bedrest

Altered Tissue Perfusion: Cardiopulmonary/Peripheral r/t high risk for development of emboli

High Risk for Alteration in Nutrition: Less than body Requirements r/t fever, hypermetabolic state associated with fever

High Risk for Decreased Cardiac Output r/t inflammation in pericardial sac, fluid accumulation compressing heart function

Knowledge Deficit r/t unfamiliarity with information sources

Pain r/t biological injury and inflammation

Peripheral Neurovascular Dysfunction, High Risk For

High Risk for Peripheral Neurovascular Dysfunction r/t fractures; mechanical compression; orthopedic surgery; trauma; immobilization; burns; vascular obstruction

Peripheral Vascular Disease

Activity Intolerance r/t imbalance between peripheral oxygen supply and demand

Altered Tissue Perfusion: Peripheral r/t interruption of vascular flow

Chronic Pain: Intermittent Claudication r/t ischemia

High Risk for Impaired Skin Integrity r/t altered circulation, sensation

High Risk for Injury r/t tissue hypoxia, altered mobility, altered sensation

High Risk for Peripheral Neurovascular Dysfunction r/t possible vascular obstruction

Knowledge Deficit r/t prevention of circulatory complications

Peritoneal Dialysis

High Risk for Fluid Volume Excess r/t retention of dialysate

High Risk for Ineffective Breathing Pattern r/t pressure from the dialysate

High Risk for Ineffective Individual Coping r/t disability requiring change in lifestyle

High Risk for Infection: Peritoneal r/t invasive procedure, presence of catheter, dialysate

Impaired Home Maintenance Management r/t complex home treatment of client

Knowledge Deficit r/t home maintenance management

Pain r/t instillation of dialysate, temperature of dialysate

Refer to Renal Failure, Oliguric; Renal Failure Acute/Chronic, Child; Hospitalized Child; Child with Chronic Condition

Peritonitis

Altered Nutrition: Less than Body Requirements r/t nausea, vomiting

Constipation r/t inadequate intake, decrease of peristalsis

Fluid Volume Deficit r/t retention of fluid in bowel with loss of circulating blood volume

High Risk for Ineffective Breathing Pattern r/t pain, increased abdominal pressure

Pain r/t inflammation and stimulation of somatic nerves

Persistent Fetal Circulation

Refer to Congenital Heart Disease/Cardiac Anomalies

Personal Identity Problems

Personal Identity Disturbance r/t situational crisis, psychological impairment; chronic illness; pain

Personality Disorder

Chronic Low Self-Esteem r/t inability to set and achieve goals

Decisional Conflict r/t low self-esteem; feelings that choices will always be wrong

Impaired Adjustment r/t ambivalent behavior towards others and testing of others loyalty

Impaired Social Interaction r/t knowledge/skill deficit about ways to interact effectively with others; self-concept disturbances

Ineffective Family Coping: Compromised r/t lack of ability of client to provide positive feedback to family; chronicity exhausting family

Personal Identity Disturbance r/t lack of consistent positive self image

Spiritual Distress r/t lack of identifiable values, no meaning to life

Refer to Antisocial; Borderline Personality

Pertussis (Whooping Cough)

Refer to Respiratory Infections, Acute Childhood

Petechiae

Refer to Clotting Disorder

Phobia

Anxiety r/t inability to control emotions when dreaded object or situation is encountered

Ineffective Individual Coping r/t transfer of fears from self to dreaded object situation

Powerlessness r/t anxiety over encountering unknown or known entity

Refer to Anxiety

PID (Pelvic Inflammatory Disease)

Altered Sexuality Patterns r/t medically imposed abstinence from sexual activities until the acute infection subsides, change in reproductive potential

High Risk for Infection r/t insufficient knowledge to avoid exposure to pathogens; poor hygiene, nutrition, and other health habits

Knowledge Deficit r/t lack of exposure to information or unfamiliarity with information resources

Pain r/t biological injury; inflammation, edema, and congestion of pelvic tissues

Refer to Adolescence Maturational Issues

PIH (Pregnancy Induced Hypertension/Preeclampsia)

Altered Family Processes r/t situational crisis

Altered Parenting r/t bedrest

Altered Role Performance r/t change in physical capacity to assume role of pregnant woman or resume other roles

Anxiety r/t fear of the unknown; threat to self and infant; change in role functioning

Diversional Activity Deficit r/t bedrest

Fluid Volume Excess r/t decreased renal function

High Risk for Injury (Fetal) r/t decreased uteroplacental perfusion

High Risk for Injury (Maternal) r/t vasospasm and high blood pressure

Impaired Home Maintenance Management r/t bedrest

Impaired Physical Mobility r/t medically prescribed limitations

Impaired Social Interaction r/t imposed bedrest

Knowledge Deficit r/t lack of experience with situation

Powerlessness r/t complication threatening pregnancy and medically prescribed limitations

Situational Low Self-Esteem r/t loss of idealized pregnancy

Piloerection

Hypothermia r/t exposure to cool environment

Placenta Previa

Altered Family Processes r/t maternal bedrest or hospitalization

Altered Role Performance r/t maternal bedrest or hospitalization

Altered Tissue Perfusion: Placental r/t dilation of cervix and loss of placental implantation site

Body Image Disturbance r/t negative feelings about body and reproductive ability; feelings of helplessness

Diversional Activity Deficit r/t long-term hospitalization

Fear r/t threat to self and fetus, unknown future

High Risk for Altered Parenting r/t maternal bedrest or hospitalization

High Risk for Fluid Volume Deficit r/t maternal blood loss

Impaired Home Maintenance Management r/t maternal bedrest or hospitalization

Impaired Physical Mobility r/t medical protocol, maternal bedrest

Ineffective Individual Coping r/t threat to self and fetus

Situational Low Self-Esteem r/t situational crisis

Spiritual Distress r/t inability to participate in usual religious rituals, situational crisis

Pleural Effusion

Fluid Volume Excess r/t compromised regulatory mechanisms; heart, liver, or kidney failure

Hyperthermia r/t increased metabolic rate secondary to infection

Ineffective Breathing Pattern r/t pain

Pain r/t inflammation, fluid accumulation

Pleural Friction Rub

Ineffective Breathing Pattern r/t pain

Pain r/t inflammation, fluid accumulation

Refer to cause of Pleural Friction Rub

Pleurisy

High Risk for Ineffective Airway Clearance r/t increased secretions; ineffective cough because of pain

High Risk for Impaired Gas Exchange r/t ventilation perfusion imbalance

High Risk for Impaired Physical Mobility r/t activity intolerance; inability to "catch breath"

Ineffective Breathing Pattern r/t pain

Pain r/t pressure on pleural nerve endings associated with fluid accumulation or inflammation

PMS (Premenstrual Tension Syndrome)
Fatigue r/t hormonal changes
Fluid Volume Excess r/t alterations of hormonal levels inducing fluid retention
Knowledge Deficit r/t methods to deal with and prevent syndrome
Pain r/t hormonal stimulation of gastrointestinal structures

Pneumonia
Altered Oral Mucous Membranes r/t dry mouth from mouth breathing, decreased fluid intake
Activity Intolerance r/t imbalance between oxygen supply and demand
Altered Nutrition: Less than Body Requirements r/t loss of appetite
High Risk for Fluid Volume Deficit r/t inadequate intake of fluids
Hyperthermia r/t dehydration; increased metabolic rate; illness
Impaired Gas Exchange r/t decreased functional lung tissue
Ineffective Airway Clearance r/t inflammation and presence of secretions
Knowledge Deficit r/t risk factors predisposing person to pneumonia, treatment
Refer to Respiratory Infections, Acute Childhood for child with Pneumonia

Pneumothorax
Fear r/t threat to own well-being; difficulty breathing
High Risk for Injury r/t possible complications associated with closed chest drainage system
Impaired Gas Exchange r/t ventilation perfusion imbalance
Pain r/t recent injury; coughing, deep breathing

Poisoning: High Risk For
High Risk for Poisoning r/t Internal: reduced vision; verbalization of occupational settings without adequate safeguards; lack of safety or drug education; lack of proper precaution; cognitive or emotional difficulties; insufficient finances. External: large supplies of drugs in house; medicines stored in unlocked cabinets accessible to children or confused persons; dangerous products placed or stored within the reach of children or confused persons; availability of illicit drugs potentially contaminated by poisonous additives; flaking, peeling paint or plaster in presence of young children; chemical contamination of food and water; unprotected contact with heavy metals or chemicals; paint, lacquer, etc., in poorly ventilated areas or without effective protection; presence of poisonous vegetation; presence of atmospheric pollutants

Polydipsia
Refer to Diabetes Mellitus

Polyphagia
Refer to Diabetes Mellitus

Polyuria
Refer to Diabetes Mellitus

Postoperative Care
Refer to Surgery, Postoperative

Postpartum Blues
Altered Parenting r/t hormone-induced depression
Altered Role Performance r/t new responsibilities of parenting
Anxiety r/t new responsibilities of parenting
Body Image Disturbance r/t normal postpartum recovery
Fatigue r/t childbirth and postpartum
Impaired Adjustment r/t lack of support systems

Impaired Home Maintenance Management r/t fatigue and care of the newborn

Impaired Social Interaction r/t change in role functioning

Ineffective Individual Coping r/t hormonal changes and maturational crisis

Knowledge Deficit r/t lifestyle changes

Sexual Dysfunction r/t fears of another pregnancy

Postpartum Hemorrhage

Activity Intolerance r/t anemia from loss of blood

Body Image Disturbance r/t loss of ideal childbirth

Decreased Cardiac Output r/t hypovolemia

Fear r/t threat to self and unknown future

Fluid Volume Deficit r/t uterine atony and loss of blood

High Risk for Altered Parenting r/t weakened maternal condition

High Risk for Infection r/t loss of blood and depressed immunity

Impaired Home Maintenance Management r/t lack of stamina

Knowledge Deficit r/t lack of exposure to situation

Postpartum, Normal Care

Altered Role Performance r/t new responsibilities of parenting

Altered Urinary Elimination r/t effects of anesthesia or tissue trauma

Anxiety r/t change in role functioning and parenting

Constipation r/t hormonal effects on smooth muscles, fear of straining with defecation, effects of anesthesia

Effective Breastfeeding r/t basic breastfeeding knowledge, partner and health care provider support

Family Coping: Potential for Growth r/t adaptation to new family member

Fatigue r/t Childbirth, new responsibilities of parenting and body changes

Health Seeking Behaviors r/t postpartum recovery and adaptation

High Risk for Altered Parenting r/t lack of role models and knowledge deficit

High Risk for Infection r/t tissue trauma and blood loss

Impaired Skin Integrity r/t episiotomy or lacerations

Ineffective Breastfeeding r/t lack of knowledge, lack of support, or lack of motivation

Knowledge Deficit: Infant Care r/t lack of preparation for parenting

Sexual Dysfunction r/t fear of pain or pregnancy

Post-Trauma Response

Post-Trauma Response r/t disaster; wars epidemics; rape; assault; torture; catastrophic illness; accident

Potassium, Increase or Decrease
Refer to Hyperkalemia or Hypokalemia

Powerlessness

Powerlessness r/t prolonged activity restriction creating isolation; failing or deteriorating physiological condition; long-term stress; abandonment; lost belief in transcendent values/God

Pregnancy-Cardiac Disorders
Refer to Cardiac Disorders in Pregnancy

Pregnancy Induced Hypertension/Preeclampsia (see PIH)

Pregnancy Loss

Altered Role Performance r/t inability to take on parenting role

Altered Sexuality Patterns r/t self-esteem disturbance due to pregnancy loss and anxiety about future pregnancies

Anxiety r/t threat to role functioning, health status, and situational crisis

High Risk for Dysfunctional Grieving r/t loss of pregnancy

High Risk for Fluid Volume Deficit r/t blood loss

High Risk for Infection r/t retained products of conception

Ineffective Family Coping: Compromised r/t lack of support by significant other due to personal suffering

Ineffective Individual Coping r/t situational crisis

Pain r/t surgical intervention

Spiritual Distress r/t intense suffering

Pregnancy—Normal

Altered Family Process r/t developmental transition of pregnancy

Altered Nutrition: More than Body Requirements r/t frequent, closely spaced pregnancies

Body Image Disturbance r/t altered body function and appearance

Family Coping: Potential for Growth r/t satisfying partner relationship, attention to gratification of needs, effective adaptation to developmental tasks of pregnancy

Fear r/t labor and delivery

Health Seeking Behaviors r/t desire to promote optimal fetal/maternal health

Ineffective Individual Coping r/t personal vulnerability, situational crisis

Knowledge Deficit r/t primiparity

Sleep Pattern Disturbance r/t sleep deprivation secondary to discomfort of pregnant state

Sexual Dysfunction r/t altered body function, self-concept, and body image with pregnancy

Refer to Discomforts of Pregnancy

Premature Dilation of the Cervix (Incompetent Cervix)

Altered Role Performance r/t inability to continue usual patterns of responsibility

Anticipatory Grieving r/t potential loss of infant

Diversional Activity Deficit r/t bedrest

Fear r/t potential loss of infant

High Risk for Infection r/t invasive procedures to prevent preterm birth

High Risk for Injury (fetal) r/t preterm birth, use of anesthesia

High Risk for Injury (maternal) r/t surgical procedures to prevent preterm birth

Impaired Physical Mobility r/t imposed bedrest to prevent preterm birth

Impaired Social Interaction r/t bedrest

Ineffective Individual Coping r/t bedrest and threat to fetus

Knowledge Deficit r/t treatment regimen and prognosis for pregnancy

Powerlessness r/t inability to control outcome of pregnancy

Sexual Dysfunction r/t fear of harm to fetus

Situational Low Self-Esteem r/t inability to complete normal pregnancy

Premature Infant (Child)

Altered Growth and Development: Developmental Lag r/t prematurity, environmental and stimulation deficiencies, multiple caretakers

Altered Nutrition: Less than Body Requirements r/t delayed or under stimulated rooting reflex and easy fatigue during feeding, diminished endurance

High Risk for Infection r/t inadequate (or immature/undeveloped) acquired immune response

High Risk for Injury r/t prolonged mechanical ventilation, retrolental fibroplasia (RLF) secondary to 100% oxygen environment

Impaired Gas Exchange r/t effects of cardiopulmonary insufficiency

Impaired Swallowing r/t decreased or absent gag reflex, fatigue

Ineffective Thermoregulation r/t large body surface/weight ratio; immaturity of thermal regulation or state of prematurity

Sensory/Perceptual Alterations r/t noxious stimuli, noisy environment

Sleep Pattern Disturbance r/t noisy and noxious intensive care environment

Premature Infant (Parent)

Anticipatory Grieving r/t loss of "perfect child"; may lead to dysfunctional grieving (prolonged) r/t unresolved conflicts

Decisional Conflict r/t support system deficit or multiple sources of information

Ineffective Breastfeeding r/t disrupted establishment of effective pattern secondary to prematurity or insufficient opportunities

Ineffective Family Coping: Compromised r/t disrupted family roles and disorganization; prolonged condition exhausting supportive capacity of significant people

Parental Role Conflict r/t expressed concerns, expressed inability to care for child's physical/emotional developmental needs

Spiritual Distress r/t challenged belief/value systems regarding moral/ethical implications of treatment plans

Refer to Hospitalized Child; Child With Chronic Condition

Premature Rupture of Membranes

Anticipatory Grieving r/t potential loss of infant

Anxiety r/t threat to infants health status

Body Image Disturbance r/t inability to carry pregnancy to term

High Risk for Infection r/t rupture of membranes

High Risk for Injury (fetal) r/t risk of premature birth

Ineffective Individual Coping r/t situational crisis

Situational Low Self-Esteem r/t inability to carry pregnancy to term

Premenstrual Tension Syndrome
Refer to PMS

Prenatal Care/Normal

Altered Nutrition: Less than Body Requirements r/t nausea from normal hormonal changes

Altered Family Processes r/t developmental transition

Altered Urinary Elimination r/t frequency caused by increased pelvic pressure and hormonal stimulation

Constipation r/t decreased GI motility secondary to hormonal stimulation

Fatigue r/t increased energy demands

High Risk for Activity Intolerance r/t enlarged abdomen and increased cardiac workload

High Risk for Injury (Maternal) r/t knowledge deficit

High Risk for Sexual Dysfunction r/t enlarged abdomen and fear of harm to infant

Ineffective Breathing Pattern r/t increased intrathoracic pressure and decreased energy secondary to enlarged uterus

Knowledge Deficit r/t lack of experience with pregnancy and care

Sleep Pattern Disturbance r/t discomforts of pregnancy and fetal activity

Prenatal Testing

Anxiety r/t unknown outcome and delayed test results

High Risk for Infection r/t invasive procedures during amniocentesis or chorionic villi sampling

High Risk for Injury (fetal) r/t invasive procedures

Knowledge Deficit r/t need for diagnostic procedure, how procedure is done, and interpretation of results

Pre-operative Teaching

Knowledge Deficit r/t preoperative regimes, postoperative precautions, expectations of role of client during preoperative/postoperative time

Refer to Surgery, Preoperative

Pressure Ulcer

Altered Nutrition: Less than Body Requirements r/t limited access to food; inability to absorb nutrients due to biological factors; anorexia

High Risk for Infection r/t physical immobility; mechanical factors (shearing forces, pressure, restraint); altered circulation; skin irritants

Impaired Tissue Integrity r/t altered circulation, impaired physical mobility

Pain r/t tissue destruction and exposure of nerves

Total Incontinence r/t neurological dysfunction

Preterm Labor

Altered Role Performance r/t inability to carry out normal roles secondary to bedrest/hospitalization; change in expected course of pregnancy

Anticipatory Grieving r/t loss of idealized pregnancy and potential loss of fetus

Anxiety r/t threat to fetus; change in role functioning; change in environment and interaction patterns

Diversional Activity Deficit r/t long-term hospitalization

High Risk for Maternal Injury r/t use of tocolytic drugs

Impaired Home Maintenance Management r/t medical restrictions

Impaired Physical Mobility r/t medically imposed restrictions

Impaired Social Interaction r/t prolonged bedrest/hospitalization

Ineffective Individual Coping r/t situational crisis, preterm labor

Sexual Dysfunction r/t actual/perceived limitation imposed by preterm labor and/or prescribed treatment/separation from partner due to hospitalization

Situational Low Self-Esteem r/t threatened ability to carry pregnancy to term

Sleep Pattern Disturbance r/t change in usual pattern secondary to contractions, hospitalization, or treatment regimen

Projection

Anxiety r/t threat to self-concept

Chronic Low Self-Esteem r/t failure at life events

Impaired Social Interaction r/t self-concept disturbance; confrontive communication style

Defensive Coping r/t inability to acknowledge that own behavior may be a problem and blames others

Prolapsed Umbilical Cord

Altered Tissue Perfusion: (fetal) r/t interruption in umbilical blood flow

Fear r/t threat to fetus and impending surgery

High Risk for Injury: (fetal) r/t cord compression and altered tissue perfusion

Prolonged Gestation

Altered Nutrition: Less than Body Requirements (fetal) r/t aging of placenta

Anxiety r/t potential change in birthing plans; need for increased medical intervention; unknown outcome for fetus

Defensive Coping r/t underlying feeling of inadequacy about ability to give birth normally

Powerlessness r/t perceived lack of control over outcome of pregnancy

Prostatectomy

Refer to Transurethral Prostatectomy (TURP)

Prostatic Enlargement

Altered Pattern of Urinary Elimination r/t anatomical obstruction

High Risk for Infection r/t urinary residual after voiding, bacterial invasion of bladder

Knowledge Deficit r/t treatment and avoidance of possible causes

Sleep Pattern Disturbance r/t nocturia

Urinary Retention r/t obstruction

Protection, Altered

Altered Protection r/t extremes of age; inadequate nutrition; alcohol abuse; abnormal blood profiles (leukopenia, thrombocytopenia, anemia, coagulation); drug therapies (antineoplastic, corticosteroid, immune, anticoagulant, thrombolytic); treatments (surgery, radiation) and diseases such as cancer and immune disorders

Pruritis

Altered Comfort: Pruritis r/t inflammation in tissues

High Risk for Impaired Skin Integrity r/t scratching from pruritis

Knowledge Deficit r/t methods to treat and prevent itching

Psychosis

Alteration in Family Process r/t inability to express feelings, impaired communication

Alteration in Nutrition: Less than Body Requirements r/t unaware of hunger; disinterest toward food

Alteration in Thought Process r/t inaccurate interpretations of environment

Altered Health Maintenance r/t cognitive impairment; ineffective individual and family coping

Anxiety r/t unconscious conflict with reality

High Risk for Violence: Self-Directed or Directed at Others r/t lack of trust, panic, hallucinations, delusional thinking

Impaired Home Maintenance Management r/t impaired cognitive/emotional functioning; inadequate support systems

Impaired Social Interaction r/t impaired communication patterns; self-concept disturbance; altered thought process

Impaired Verbal Communication r/t psychosis; inaccurate perception; hallucinations; delusions

Ineffective Individual Coping r/t inadequate support systems; unrealistic perceptions; altered thought processes; impaired communication

Fear r/t altered contact with reality

Self-Care Deficit r/t loss of contact with reality; impairment in perception

Self-Esteem Disturbance r/t excessive use of defense mechanisms: projection, denial, rationalization

Sleep Pattern Disturbance r/t sensory alterations contributing to fear and anxiety

Social Isolation r/t lack of trust, regression, delusional thinking, represses fears

Refer to Schizophrenia

Pulmonary Embolism

Altered Tissue Perfusion: Pulmonary r/t interruption of pulmonary blood flow secondary to lodged embolus

Fear r/t severe pain and possible death

High Risk for Altered Cardiac Output r/t right ventricular failure secondary to obstructed pulmonary artery

Impaired Gas Exchange r/t altered blood flow to alveoli secondary to lodged embolus

Knowledge Deficit r/t activities to prevent embolism; self-care after diagnosis of embolism

Pain r/t biological injury; lack of oxygen to cells

Refer to Anticoagulant Therapy

Pulse Oximetry

Knowledge Deficit r/t use of oxygen monitoring equipment

Refer to Hypoxia

Pulse Pressure, Increased

Refer to Intracranial Pressure, Increased

Pulse Pressure, Narrowed

Refer to Shock

Pulses, Absent or Diminished-Peripheral

Altered Tissue Perfusion: Peripheral r/t interruption of arterial flow

High Risk for Peripheral Neurovascular Dysfunction r/t fractures; mechanical compression; orthopedic surgery trauma; immobilization; burns; vascular obstruction

Refer to cause of Absent or Diminished Peripheral Pulses

Pulmonary Stenosis

Refer to Congenital Heart Disease/Cardiac Anomalies

Purpura

Refer to Clotting Disorder

Pyelonephritis

Altered Comfort r/t chills and fever
Altered Health Maintenance r/t lack of knowledge regarding hygiene (toileting/bathing)
Altered Urinary Elimination r/t irritation of urinary tract
Pain r/t inflammation/irritation of urinary tract
Sleep Pattern Disturbance r/t urinary frequency

Pyloric Stenosis

Altered Health Maintenance r/t parental knowledge deficit regarding home care feeding regimen, wound care
Altered Nutrition: Less than Body Requirements r/t vomiting secondary to pyloric sphincter obstruction
Fluid Volume Deficit r/t vomiting and dehydration
Pain r/t surgical incision
Refer to Hospitalized Child

Quadraplegia

Anticipatory Grieving r/t loss of normal lifestyle, severity of disability
High Risk for Dysreflexia r/t bladder distention; bowel distention; skin irritation; lack of patient, and caregiver knowledge
Ineffective Breathing Pattern r/t inability to utilize intercostal muscles
Refer to Spinal Cord Injury

R

Radiation Therapy

Alteration in Nutrition: Less than Body Requirements r/t anorexia, nausea, vomiting; irradiation of areas of pharynx and esophagus

Alteration in Oral Mucous Membranes r/t irradiation effects

Diarrhea r/t irradiation effects

Altered Protection r/t suppression of bone marrow

High Risk for Activity Intolerance r/t fatigue from possible anemia

High Risk for Body Image Disturbance r/t change in appearance; hair loss

High Risk for Impaired Skin Integrity r/t irradiation effects

Knowledge Deficit r/t what to expect with radiation therapy

Social Isolation r/t possible limitations of time exposure of caregivers and significant others to client

Radical Neck

Refer to Laryngectomy

Rage

High Risk for Violence: Directed at Others r/t panic state; manic excitement; organic brain syndrome

High Risk for Self-Mutilation r/t command hallucinations

Rape-Trauma Syndrome

Rape-Trauma Syndrome r/t forced, violent sexual penetration against the victim's will and consent

Rape-Trauma Syndrome: Compound Reaction r/t forced,violent sexual penetration against the victim's will and consent; previous disruptions in health are activated (physical illness, psychiatric illness or substance abuse)

Rape-Trauma Syndrome: Silent Reaction r/t forced violent sexual penetration against the victim's will and consent; demonstrating repression of the incident

Rash

Altered Comfort: Pruritus r/t inflammation in skin

High Risk for Infection r/t traumatized tissue; broken skin

Impaired Skin Integrity r/t mechanical trauma

Rationalization

Defensive Coping r/t situational crisis; inability to accept blame for consequences of own behavior

Ineffective Denial r/t fear of consequences; actual or perceived loss

Rats, Rodents in the Home

Impaired Home Maintenance Management r/t lack of knowledge or insufficient finances

Raynaud's Disease

Altered Tissue Perfusion: Peripheral r/t transient reduction of blood flow

Knowledge Deficit r/t lack of information about disease process; possible complications; self-care needs regarding disease process, medication

Respiratory Distress Syndrome (RDS)

Refer to Respiratory Conditions of the Neonate

Rectal Pain/Bleeding

Constipation r/t pain on defecation

High Risk for Fluid Volume Deficit: Bleeding r/t untreated rectal bleeding

Knowledge Deficit r/t possible causes of rectal bleeding; pain; treatment modalities

Pain r/t pressure of defecation

Regression
Altered Role Performance r/t powerlessness over health status
Anxiety r/t threat to or change in health status
Defensive Coping r/t denial of obvious problems/ weaknesses
Powerlessness r/t health care environment
Refer to Hospitalized Child; Separation Anxiety

Rehabilitation
Altered Comfort r/t difficulty in performing reha- bilitation tasks
Impaired Physical Mobility r/t injury, surgery, psychosocial condition warranting rehabilitation
Ineffective Individual Coping r/t loss of normal function
Self-Care Deficit r/t impaired physical mobility

Relaxation Techniques
Health-Seeking Behaviors r/t requesting knowl- edge on ways to relieve stress

Religious Concern
Spiritual Distress r/t separation from religious/ cultural ties

Relocation Stress Syndrome
Relocation Stress Syndrome r/t past, concurrent, and recent losses, losses involved with decision to move; feeling of powerlessness; lack of ade- quate support system; little or no preparation for the impending move; moderate to high de- gree of environmental change; history and types of previous transfers; impaired psychosocial health status; decreased physical health status; advanced age

Renal Failure
Activity Intolerance r/t effects of anemia and con- gestive heart failure
Altered Comfort: Pruritus r/t effects of uremia

Altered Nutrition: Less than Body Requirements r/t anorexia, nausea, vomiting, altered taste sensa- tion, dietary restrictions
Altered Urinary Elimination r/t effects of disease and need for dialysis
Decreased Cardiac Output r/t effects of congestive heart failure
Fatigue r/t effects of chronic uremia and anemia
Fluid Volume Excess r/t decreased urine output, sodium retention or inappropriate fluid intake
High Risk for Altered Oral Mucous Membranes r/t dehydration, effects of uremia
High Risk for Infection r/t altered immune func- tioning
High Risk for Injury r/t bone changes, neuropathy, and muscle weakness
High Risk for Noncomplinace r/t complex medical therapy
Ineffective Individual Coping r/t depression sec- ondary to chronic disease

Renal Failure , Acute/Chronic, Child
Body Image Disturbance r/t growth retardation, bone changes, and visibility of dialysis access devices (graft, fistula), edema
Diversional Activity Deficit r/t immobility during dialysis
Refer to Renal Failure: Hospitalized Child; Child With Chronic Illness

Renal Failure, Non-oliguric
Anxiety r/t change in health status
High Risk for Fluid Volume Deficit r/t loss of large volumes of urine
Refer to Renal Failure

Renal Transplantation, Donor
Decisional Conflict r/t harvesting of kidney from traumatized donor
Spiritual Distress r/t anticipatory grieving from loss of significant person
Refer to nephrectomy for living donor

93

Renal Transplantation Recipient

Altered Protection r/t immunosupression therapy

Alteration in Urinary Elimination r/t possible impaired renal function

Anxiety r/t possible rejection; procedure

High Risk for Infection r/t use of immunosuppressive therapy to control rejection

Knowledge Deficit r/t specific nutritional needs; possible paralytic ileus, fluid, sodium restrictions

Impaired Health Maintenance r/t long-term home treatment after transplantation; diet, signs of rejection, use of medications

Spiritual Distress r/t obtaining transplanted kidney from someone's traumatic loss

Respiratory Conditions of the Neonate (RDS, Meconium Aspiration, Diaphragmatic Hernia)

Fatigue r/t increased energy requirements and metabolic demands

High Risk for Infection r/t tissue destruction/ irritation secondary to aspiration of meconium fluid

Impaired Gas Exchange r/t decreased surfactant and immature lung tissue

Ineffective Airway Clearance r/t sequelae of attempts to breathe in utero (resulting in meconium aspiration)

Ineffective Breathing Patterns r/t prolonged ventilator dependence

Refer to Hospitalized Child; Premature Infant; Bronchopulmonary Dysplasia

Respiratory Distress Syndrome (RDS)

Refer to Respiratory Conditions of the Neonate

Respiratory Infections, Acute Childhood (Croup, Epiglottitis, Pertussis, Pneumonia, RSV)

Activity Intolerance r/t generalized weakness, dyspnea, fatigue, poor oxygenation

Altered Nutrition: Less than Body Requirements r/t anorexia, fatigue, generalized weakness, poor sucking/breathing coordination, dyspnea

Anxiety/Fear r/t oxygen deprivation, difficulty breathing

Fluid Volume Deficit r/t insensible losses (fever, diaphoresis); inadequate oral fluid intake

High Risk for Aspiration r/t inability to coordinate breathing, coughing, and sucking

High Risk for Infection: Transmission to Others r/t virulent infectious organisms

High Risk for Injury (To Pregnant Others) r/t exposure to aerosolized medications, e.g. Ribavirin, Pentamadine, and resultant potential fetal toxicity

High Risk for Suffocation r/t inflammation of larynx, epiglottis

Hyperthermia r/t infectious process

Impaired Gas Exchange r/t insufficient oxygenation secondary to inflammation, edema of epiglottis, larynx, bronchial passages

Ineffective Airway Clearance r/t excess tracheobronchial secretions

Ineffective Breathing Patterns r/t inflamed bronchial passages, coughing

Refer to Hospitalized Child

Respiratory Distress

Refer to Dyspnea

Respiratory Syncytial Virus (RSV)

Refer to Respiratory Infections, Acute Childhood

Retina Detachment

Anxiety r/t change in vision; threat of loss of vision

Knowledge Deficit r/t symptoms of and need for early intervention to prevent permanent damage

High Risk for Impaired Home Maintenance Management r/t postoperative care; activity limitations, care of affected eye

Sensory Perceptual Alteration: Visual r/t changes in vision; sudden flashes of light, floating spots, blurring of vision

Reye's Syndrome
Altered Health Maintenance r/t knowledge deficit regarding use of salicylates during viral illness of child
Altered Nutrition: Less than Body Requirements r/t effects of liver dysfunction, vomiting
Altered Thought Processes r/t degenerative changes in fatty brain tissue
Anticipatory Grieving r/t uncertain prognosis and sequelae
Fluid Volume Deficit r/t vomiting, hyperventilation
Fluid Volume Excess (cerebral) r/t cerebral edema
High Risk for Injury r/t combative behavior, seizure activity
Impaired Gas Exchange r/t hyperventilation and sequelae of increased intracranial pressure
Impaired Skin Integrity r/t effects of decorticate/decerebrate posturing, seizure activity
Ineffective Breathing Patterns r/t neuromuscular impairment
Ineffective Family Coping: Compromised r/t acute situational crisis
Sensory-Perceptual Alterations r/t cerebral edema
Situational Low Self-Esteem (Family) r/t negative perceptions of self and perceived inability to manage family situation; expressions of guilt
Refer to Hospitalized Child

Rh Incompatibility
Anxiety r/t unknown outcome of pregnancy
Health Seeking Behaviors r/t prenatal care and compliance with diagnostic and treatment regimen
High Risk for Fetal Injury r/t intrauterine transfusions
Knowledge Deficit r/t treatment regimen from lack of experience with situation
Powerlessness r/t perceived lack of control over outcome of pregnancy

Rheumatic Fever
Refer to Endocarditis

Rheumatoid Arthritis, Juvenile (JRA)
Altered Growth and Development r/t effects of physical disability, chronic illness
Fatigue r/t chronic inflammatory disease
High Risk for Impaired Skin Integrity r/t splints, adaptive devices
High Risk for Injury r/t impaired physical mobility; splints, adaptive devices; increased bleeding potential secondary to antiinflammatory medications
Impaired Physical Mobility r/t pain and restricted joint movement
Pain r/t swollen, inflamed joints, restricted movement, physical therapy
Self-Care Deficits: Feeding, Bathing/Hygiene, Dressing/Grooming, Toileting r/t restricted joint movement, pain
Refer to Child With Chronic Condition; Hospitalized Child

Role Performance, Altered
Altered Role Performance r/t inability to perform role as anticipated

Respiratory Synctical Virus (RSV)
Refer to Respiratory Infection, Acute Childhood

Rubella
Refer to Communicable Diseases, Childhood

Rubor of Extremities
Altered Tissue Perfusion: Peripheral r/t interruption of arterial flow
Refer to Peripheral Vascular Disease

95

S

Sadness
Dysfunctional Grieving r/t actual or perceived loss

Safety, Childhood
Health Seeking Behavior: Enhanced Parenting r/t adequate support systems; requests help appropriately; desire and request for safety information; seeks information/assistance regarding parenting skills

High Risk for Altered Health Maintenance r/t parental knowledge deficit regarding appropriate safety needs per developmental stage, childproofing house, infant/child car restraints, water safety, teaching child how to avoid molestation

High Risk for Altered Parenting r/t lack of available, effective role model; lack of knowledge; misinformation from other family members ("old wives' tales")

High Risk for Aspiration and/or Suffocation r/t pillow or propped bottle placed in infant's crib; sides of playpen/crib wide enough that child can get head through; child left in car with engine running, enclosed areas; plastic bags or small objects used as toys; toys with small, break-away parts; refrigerators/freezers with doors not removed left accessible as play areas for children; children left unattended in or near bathtubs/pools/spas; low-slung clotheslines or electric garage doors without automatic stop/reopen; pacifier hung around infant's neck; food not cut into small, bite-size pieces appropriate for age of child; balloons, hot dogs, nuts, popcorn given to infants/young children (especially under 1 year of age); use of baby powder

High Risk for Injury/Trauma r/t developmental age; altered home maintenance management (house not "childproofed"); altered parenting; hot liquids within child's reach; nonuse of infant/child car restraints; no gates at top of stairs; lack of immunizations for age; no fences/pool/spa covers; leaving child in car unattended with windows up in hot weather; firearms loaded, in reach of child

High Risk for Poisoning r/t use of lead-based paint; presence of asbestos or radon gas; licit and illicit drugs not locked in cabinet; household products left in accessible area (bleach, detergent, drain cleaners, household cleaners); alcohol and perfume within reach of child; presence of poisonous plants; atmospheric pollutants

Knowledge Deficit: Potential for Enhanced Health Maintenance r/t parental knowledge/skill acquisition regarding appropriate safety measures

Salmonella
Refer to Gastroenteritis

Scabies
Refer to Communicable Diseases, Childhood

Schizophrenia
Alteration in Family Process r/t inability to express feelings, impaired communication

Alteration in Nutrition: Less than Body Requirements r/t fear of eating; unaware of hunger; disinterest toward food

Alteration in Thought Process r/t inaccurate interpretations of environment

Altered Health Maintenance r/t cognitive impairment; ineffective individual and family coping; lack of material resources

Anxiety r/t unconscious conflict with reality

Diversional Activity Deficit r/t social isolation; possible regression

Fear r/t altered contact with reality

High Risk for Caregiver Role Strain r/t bizarre behavior of client; chronicity of condition

High Risk for Violence: Self-Directed or Directed at Others r/t lack of trust, panic, hallucinations, delusional thinking

Impaired Home Maintenance Management r/t
impaired cognitive/emotional functioning; insufficient finances; inadequate support systems

Impaired Social Interaction r/t impaired communication patterns; self-concept disturbance; altered
thought process

Impaired Verbal Communication r/t psychosis;
disorientation; inaccurate perception; hallucinations; delusions

Ineffective Individual Coping r/t inadequate support systems; unrealistic perceptions; inadequate
coping skills; altered thought processes; impaired communication

Self-Care Deficit r/t loss of contact with reality;
impairment in perception

Self-Esteem Disturbance r/t excessive use of defense mechanisms: projection, denial, rationalization

Sleep Pattern Disturbance r/t sensory alterations
contributing to fear and anxiety

Social Isolation r/t lack of trust, regression, delusional thinking, represses fears

Scoliosis

Altered Health Maintenance r/t knowledge deficits
regarding treatment modalities, restrictions;
home care; postoperative activities

Body Image Disturbance r/t use of therapeutic
braces/scars after surgery; restricted physical
activity

High Risk for Infection r/t surgical incision

Impaired Adjustment r/t lack of developmental
maturity to comprehend long-term consequences of noncompliance with treatment procedures

Impaired Gas Exchange r/t restricted lung expansion secondary to severe curvature of spine
before surgery; immobilization

Impaired Physical Mobility r/t restricted movement; dyspnea secondary to severe curvature of
spine

Impaired Skin Integrity r/t braces/casts, surgical
correction

Ineffective Breathing Patterns r/t restricted lung
expansion secondary to severe curvature of
spine

Pain r/t musculoskeletal restrictions, surgery, re-
ambulation with cast/spinal rod

Refer to Hospitalized Child; Maturational Issues—
Adolescent

Seizure Disorders, Adult

Altered Health Maintenance r/t lack of knowledge
regarding anticonvulsive therapy

High Risk for Altered Thought Processes r/t
effects of anticonvulsant medications

High Risk for Ineffective Airway Clearance r/t
accumulation of secretions during seizure

High Risk for Injury r/t uncontrolled movements
during seizure or falls; drowsiness secondary to
anticonvulsants

Social Isolation r/t unpredictability of seizures and
imposed by community (social stigma)

Refer to Epilepsy

Seizure Disorders, Childhood (Epilepsy, Febrile Seizure, Infantile Spasms)

Altered Health Maintenance r/t lack of knowledge
regarding anti-convulsive therapy, fever reduction (febrile seizures)

High Risk for Altered Growth and Development r/t
effects of seizure disorder, parental overprotection

High Risk for Altered Thought Processes r/t
effects of anticonvulsant medications

High Risk for Ineffective Airway Clearance r/t
accumulation of secretions during seizure

High Risk for Injury r/t uncontrolled movements
during seizure or falls; drowsiness secondary to
anticonvulsants

Social Isolation r/t unpredictability of seizures and
imposed by community (social stigma)

Refer to Epilepsy

97

Self-Care Deficit, Bathing/Hygiene

Self-Care Deficit: *Bathing/Hygiene* r/t intolerance to activity, decreased strength and endurance; pain, discomfort; perceptual or cognitive impairment; neuromuscular impairment; musculoskeletal impairment; depression, severe anxiety

Self-Care Deficit, Dressing/Grooming

Self-Care Deficit: *Dressing/Grooming* r/t intolerance to activity, decreased strength and endurance; pain, discomfort; perceptual or cognitive impairment; neuromuscular impairment; musculoskeletal impairment; depression, severe anxiety

Self-Care Deficit, Feeding

Self-Care Deficit: *Feeding* r/t intolerance to activity, decreased strength and endurance; pain, discomfort; perceptual or cognitive impairment; neuromuscular impairment; musculoskeletal impairment; depression, severe anxiety

Self-Care Deficit, Toileting

Self-Care Deficit: *Toileting* r/t impaired transfer ability; impaired mobility status; intolerance to activity; decreased strength and endurance; pain, discomfort; perceptual or cognitive impairment; neuromuscular impairment; musculoskeletal impairment; depression, severe anxiety

Self-Destructive Behavior

High Risk for Self-Mutilation r/t feelings of depression, rejection, self-hatred, depersonalization; command hallucinations

High Risk for Violence: Self-Directed r/t panic state, history of child abuse, toxic reaction to medication

Post Trauma Response r/t unresolved feelings related to traumatic event

Self-Esteem: Chronic Low

Chronic Low Self-Esteem r/t long-standing negative self-evaluation

Self-Esteem Disturbance

Self-Esteem Disturbance r/t inappropriate learned negative feelings about self

Self-Esteem, Situational Low

Situational Low Self-Esteem r/t situational crisis

Self-Mutilation, High Risk For

High Risk for Self-Mutilation r/t inability to cope with increased psychological/physiological tension in a healthy manner; feelings of depression, rejection, self-hatred, separation anxiety, guilt, and depersonalization; fluctuating emotions, command hallucinations, need for sensory stimuli; parental emotional deprivation, dysfunctional family

Senile Dementia

Refer to Dementia

Sensory/Perceptual Alterations

Sensory/Perceptual Alterations (Visual, Auditory, Kinesthetic, Gustatory, Tactile, Olfactory) r/t altered environmental stimuli, excessive or insufficient; altered sensory reception, transmission and/or integration; chemical alterations, endogenous (electrolyte), exogenous (drugs, etc.); psychological stress

Separation Anxiety

Ineffective Individual Coping r/t maturational and situational crises; vulnerability secondary to developmental age; hospitalization; separation from family and familiar surroundings; multiple caregivers

Refer to Hospitalized Child

Sepsis—Child

Altered Comfort: increased sensitivity to environmental stimuli r/t sensory-perceptual alterations: visual, auditory, kinesthetic

Altered Tissue Perfusion: Cardiopulmonary, Peripheral r/t arterial/venous blood flow exchange problems; septic shock

Altered Nutrition: Less than Body Requirements r/t anorexia, generalized weakness; poor sucking reflex

High Risk for Impaired Skin Integrity r/t desquamation secondary to disseminated intravascular coagulation

Ineffective Thermal Regulation r/t infectious process; septic shock

Refer to Hospitalized Child; Premature Infant

Septicemia

Altered Nutrition: Less than Body Requirements r/t anorexia, generalized weakness

Altered Tissue Perfusion r/t increased systemic vascular resistance

Fluid Volume Deficit r/t vasodilatation of peripheral vessels, leaking of capillaries

Refer to Sepsis—Child; Shock; Septic Shock

Sexuality, Adolescent

Body Image Disturbance r/t anxiety secondary to unachieved developmental milestone (puberty) or knowledge deficit regarding reproductive maturation, as manifested by amenorrhea, expressed concerns regarding lack of growth of secondary sex characteristics

Decisional Conflict: Sexual Activity r/t undefined personal values or beliefs; multiple or divergent sources of information; lack of relevant information

High Risk for Rape Trauma Syndrome secondary to date rape, campus rape, insufficient knowledge regarding self-protection mechanisms

Knowledge Deficit: Potential for Enhanced Health Maintenance r/t multiple or divergent sources of information; lack of relevant information regarding sexual transmission of disease, contraception, prevention of toxic shock syndrome

Refer to Maturational Issues—Adolescent

Sexual Dysfunction

Sexual Dysfunction r/t biopsychosocial alteration of sexuality; ineffectual or absent role models; physical abuse, e.g., harmful relationships; vulnerability; values conflict; lack of privacy; lack of significant other; altered body structure or function (pregnancy, recent childbirth, drugs, surgery, anomalies, disease process, trauma, radiation); misinformation or lack of knowledge

Sexuality Patterns, Alteration in

Altered Sexuality Patterns r/t knowledge/skill deficit about alternative responses to health-related transitions, altered body function or structure, illness or medical; lack or privacy; lack of significant other; ineffective or absent role models; pregnancy or of acquiring a sexually transmitted disease; impaired relationship with a significant other

Sexually Transmitted Disease
Refer to STD

Shame

Self-Esteem Disturbance r/t inability to deal with past traumatic events; blames self for events not responsible for

Shivering

Hypothermia r/t exposure to cool environment

Shock

Altered Tissue Perfusion: Cardiopulmonary, Peripheral r/t arterial/venous blood flow exchange problems

Altered Urinary Elimination r/t decreased blood flow to the kidneys

Fear r/t serious threat to health status

High Risk for Injury r/t prolonged shock causing multiple organ failure, death

Refer to Shock, Cardiogenic; Shock, Hypovolemic; Shock, Septic

Shock, Cardiogenic

Decreased Cardiac Output r/t decreased myocardial contractility, dysrhythmias
Refer to Shock

Shock, Hypovolemic

Fluid Volume Deficit r/t abnormal loss of fluid
Refer to Shock

Shock, Septic

Altered Protection r/t inadequately functioning immune system
Fluid Volume Deficit r/t abnormal loss of fluid through capillaries, pooling of blood in peripheral circulation
Refer to Shock; Sepsis, Child; Septicemia

Sickle Cell Anemia/Crisis

Activity Intolerance r/t fatigue and effects of chronic anemia
Fluid Volume Deficit r/t decreased intake and increased fluid requirements during sickle cell crisis, decreased ability of kidneys to concentrate urine
High Risk for Altered Tissue Perfusion (renal, cerebral, cardiac, GI, peripheral) r/t effects of red cell sickling and infarction of tissues
High Risk for Infection r/t alterations in splenic function
Impaired Physical Mobility r/t pain and fatigue
Pain r/t viscous blood and tissue hypoxia
Refer to Hospitalized Child; Child With Chronic Condition

SIDS

Altered Family Processes r/t stress secondary to special care needs of infant with apnea
Anticipatory Grieving r/t potential loss of infant
Anxiety/Fear (parental) r/t life-threatening event
Knowledge Deficit: Potential for Enhanced Health Maintenance r/t knowledge/skill acquisition of CPR and home apnea monitoring

Sleep Pattern Disturbance (Parental, Infant) r/t home apnea monitoring
Refer to Terminally Ill Child/Death of Child

Skin Disorders

Impaired Skin Integrity r/t External; hyperthermia or hypothermia; chemical substance; mechanical factors (shearing forces, pressure, restraint); radiation; physical immobilization; humidity. *Internal*: medication; altered nutritional state (obesity, emaciation); altered metabolic state; altered circulation; altered sensation; altered pigmentation; skeletal prominence; developmental factors; immunological deficit; alterations in turgor (change in elasticity)

Skin Integrity, High Risk for Impaired

High Risk for Impaired Skin Integrity r/t (see Skin Disorders)

Skin Turgor, Change in Elasticity

Fluid Volume Deficit r/t active fluid loss
Note: decreased skin turgor can be normal finding in the elderly

Sleep Pattern Disorders

Sleep Pattern Disturbance r/t sensory alterations; internal (illness, psychological stress); external (environmental changes, social cues)

Sleep Pattern Disturbance (Parent/Child)

Sleep Pattern Disturbance (Child) r/t anxiety/apprehension secondary to parental deprivation (Refer to SCAN); fear/night terrors; enuresis; inconsistent parental responses to child's requests to alter bedtime rules; frequent nighttime awakening; inability to wean from parent's bed, hypervigilance
Sleep Pattern Disturbance (Parental) r/t time intensive home treatments; increased caretaker demands

Smell, Loss of

Sensory-Perceptual Alteration: Olfactory r/t altered sensory reception, transmission, or integration

Smoking Behavior

Altered Health Maintenance r/t denial of effects of smoking, lack of effective support for smoking withdrawal

Social Interaction, Impaired

Social Interaction, Impaired r/t knowledge/skill deficit about ways to enhance mutuality; communication barriers, self-concept disturbance; absence of available significant others or peers; limited physical mobility; therapeutic isolation; sociocultural dissonance; environmental barriers; altered thought processes

Social Isolation

Social Isolation r/t factors contributing to the absence or satisfying personal relationships, such as delay in accomplishing developmental tasks; immature interests; alterations in physical appearance; alterations in mental status; unaccepted social behavior; unaccepted social values; altered state of wellness; inadequate personal resources; inability to engage in satisfying personal relationships; fear

Sodium, Decrease, Increase

Refer to Hyponatremia, Hypernatremia

Somatoform Disorder

Anxiety r/t unresolved conflicts being channeled into physical complaints, conditions
Chronic Pain r/t unexpressed anger; multiple physical disorders and depression
Ineffective Individual Coping r/t lack of insight into underlying conflicts

Sore Nipples: Breastfeeding

Ineffective Breastfeeding r/t knowledge deficit about correct feeding procedure

Sore Throat

Impaired Swallowing r/t irritation of oropharyngeal cavity
Knowledge Deficit r/t treatment to relieve cause of discomfort
Pain r/t inflammation; irritation; dryness

Sorrow

Anticipatory Grieving r/t impending loss of significant person, object
Grieving r/t loss of significant person; object; role

Speech Disorders

Anxiety r/t difficulty with communication
Impaired Verbal Communication r/t anatomical defect, cleft palate; psychological barriers; decrease in circulation to brain

Spina Bifida

Refer to Neurotube Defects

Spinal Cord Injury

Altered Urinary Elimination r/t sensory/motor impairment
Body Image Disturbance r/t change in body function
Constipation r/t immobility; loss of sensation
Diversional Activity Deficit r/t long-term hospitalization; frequent lengthy treatments
Dysfunctional Grieving r/t loss of usual body function
Fear r/t powerlessness over loss of body function
High Risk for Altered Tissue Perfusion r/t dysreflexia
High Risk for Disuse Syndrome r/t paralysis
High Risk for Dysreflexia r/t bladder, bowel distension; skin irritation; knowledge deficit, patient and caregiver

High Risk for Ineffective Breathing Pattern r/t neuromuscular impairment

High Risk for Infection r/t chronic disease; stasis of body fluids

High Risk for Impaired Skin Integrity r/t immobility; paralysis

Impaired Health Maintenance r/t change in health status from injury; insufficient family planning, finances; knowledge deficit; inadequate support systems

Impaired Physical Mobility r/t neuromuscular impairment

Knowledge Deficit r/t self-care; complications; home maintenance

Reflex Incontinence r/t spinal cord lesion interfering with conduction of cerebral messages

Urinary Retention r/t inhibition of reflex arc

Self-Care Deficit r/t neuromuscular impairment

Sexual Dysfunction r/t altered body function

Refer to Hospitalized Child; Child with Chronic Condition; Neurotube Defects

Spiritual Distress

Spiritual Distress r/t separation from religious/cultural ties; challenged belief and value system, e.g., due to moral/ethical implications of therapy; due to intense suffering

STD Sexually Transmitted Disease)

Altered Sexuality Patterns r/t illness; altered body function

Fear r/t altered body function; high risk for social isolation; fear of incurable illness

High Risk for Infection r/t lack of knowledge concerning transmission of disease

Knowledge Deficit r/t transmission, symptoms and treatment of sexually transmitted disease

Pain r/t biological, psychological injury

Social Isolation r/t fear of contracting the disease or spreading the disease

Refer to Maturational Issues—Adolescence

Stertorous Respirations

Ineffective Airway Clearance r/t pharyngeal obstruction

Stoma

Refer to Ostomy

Stomatitis

Altered Oral Mucous Membranes r/t pathological conditions of oral cavity

Stone, Kidney

Refer to Kidney Stone

Straining with Defecation

Colonic Constipation r/t less than adequate fluid intake or less than adequate dietary intake

High Risk for Decreased Cardiac Output r/t vagal stimulation secondary to valsalva maneuver

Stress

Anxiety r/t feelings of helplessness; feelings of being threatened

Fear r/t powerlessness over feelings

Ineffective Individual Coping r/t ineffective use of problem-solving process; feelings of apprehension or helplessness

Self-Esteem Disturbance r/t inability to deal with life events

Stress Incontinence

Stress Incontinence r/t degenerative change in pelvic muscles

Refer to Incontinence of Urine

Stridor

Ineffective Airway Clearance r/t obstruction; tracheobronchial infection; trauma

Stuttering

Impaired Verbal Communication r/t anxiety; psychological problems

Subarachnoid Hemorrhage
Pain: *Headache* r/t irritation of meninges from blood, increased intracranial pressure
Refer to Intracranial Pressure, Increased

Substance Abuse
Altered Nutrition: Less than Body Requirements r/t anorexia
Altered Protection r/t malnutrition, sleep deprivation
Anxiety r/t loss of control
Compromised/Dysfunctional Family Coping r/t codependency issues
High Risk for Injury r/t alteration in sensory-perception
High Risk for Violence r/t reactions to substances used; impulsive behavior, disorientation, impaired judgment
Ineffective Individual Coping r/t use of substances to cope with life events
Powerlessness r/t substance addiction
Self-Esteem Disturbance r/t failure at life events
Sleep Pattern Disturbance r/t irritability, nightmares, tremors
Social Isolation r/t unacceptable social behavior; values
Refer to Maturational Issues—Adolescence

Substance Abuse, Adolescent
Refer to Alcohol Withdrawal; Substance Abuse; Maturational Issues—Adolescence

Substance Abuse in Pregnancy
High Risk for Altered Parenting r/t lack of ability to meet infant's needs
High Risk for Infection r/t intravenous drug use, lifestyle
High Risk for Fetal Injury r/t effects of drugs on fetal growth and development
High Risk for Maternal Injury r/t drug use
Knowledge Deficit r/t lack of exposure to information about effects of substance abuse in pregnancy

Noncompliance r/t differing value system, cultural influences, addiction
Refer to Substance Abuse

Sudden Infant Death Syndrome (SIDS) Near Miss, (Infant Apnea)
Refer to SIDS

Suffocation: High Risk for
High Risk for Suffocation r/t Internal: reduced olfactory sensation; reduced motor abilities; lack of safety education; lack of safety precautions; cognitive or emotional difficulties; disease or injury process. External: pillow placed in an infant's crib; propped bottle place in an infant's crib; vehicle warming in closed garage; children playing with plastics bags or inserting small objects into their mouths or noses; discarded or unused refrigerators or freezers without removed doors; children left unattended in bathtubs or pools; household outside; low-strung clothesline; pacifier hung around infant head; person who eats large mouthfuls of food

Suicide Attempt
High Risk for Violence: *Self-Directed* r/t suicidal ideation; feelings of hopelessness, worthlessness, lack of impulse control; feelings of anger or hostility (self-directed)
Hopelessness r/t perceived or actual loss; substance abuse; low self-concept; inadequate support systems
Ineffective Individual Coping r/t anger; dysfunctional grieving
Post Trauma Response r/t history of traumatic event: abuse, rape, incest, war, torture
Self-Esteem Disturbance r/t guilt; inability to trust; feelings of worthlessness/rejection
Social Isolation r/t inability to engage in satisfying personal relationships
Spiritual Distress r/t hopelessness; despair

Surgery, Pre-Operative Care

Anxiety r/t threat to or change in health status; situational crisis; fear of unknown

Knowledge Deficit r/t preoperative procedures; postoperative expectations

Sleep Pattern Disturbance r/t anxiety about upcoming surgery

Surgery, Postoperative Care

Activity Intolerance r/t pain, surgical procedure

Altered Nutrition: Less than Body Requirements r/t anorexia; nausea, vomiting; decreased peristalsis

Anxiety r/t change in health status; hospital environment

High Risk for Altered Pattern of Urinary Elimination r/t anesthesia; pain; fear; unfamiliar surroundings; or the client's position

High Risk for Altered Tissue Perfusion: Peripheral r/t hypovolemia; circulatory stasis; obesity and prolonged immobility; decreased coughing and deep breathing

High Risk for Colonic Constipation r/t decreased activity; decreased food and or fluid intake; anesthesia; pain medication

High Risk for Fluid Volume Deficit r/t hypermetabolic state; fluid loss during surgery; presence of indwelling tubes

High Risk for Infection r/t invasive procedure, pain, anesthesia, location of incision, weakened cough due to aging

High Risk for Ineffective Breathing Pattern r/t pain; location of incision; effects of anesthesia/narcotics

Knowledge Deficit r/t postoperative expectations; lifestyle changes

Pain r/t inflammation/injury in surgical area

Suspected Child Abuse and Neglect (SCAN)—Child

Altered Growth and Development: Regression vs Delayed r/t diminished/absent environmental stimuli, inadequate caretaking, inconsistent responsiveness by caretaker

Altered Nutrition: Less than Body Requirements r/t inadequate caretaking

Anxiety/Fear (child) r/t threat of punishment for perceived wrongdoing

Chronic Low Self-Esteem r/t lack of positive feedback or excessive negative feedback

Diversional Activity Deficit r/t diminished/absent environmental/personal stimuli

High Risk for Poisoning r/t inadequate safeguards, lack of proper safety precautions, accessibility of illicit substances secondary to impaired home maintenance management

High Risk for Suffocation secondary to aspiration r/t propped bottle, unattended child

High Risk for Trauma r/t inadequate precautions; cognitive or emotional difficulties

Impaired Skin Integrity r/t altered nutritional state; physical abuse

Pain r/t physical injuries

Post Trauma Response r/t physical abuse, incest/rape/molestation

Rape-Trauma Syndrome (Compound/Silent Reaction) r/t altered lifestyle secondary to abuse and changes in residence

Sleep Pattern Disturbance r/t hypervigilance, anxiety

Social Isolation, Family Imposed r/t fear of disclosure of family dysfunction and abuse

Refer to Hospitalized Child; Maturational Issues, Adolescent

Suspected Child Abuse and Neglect (SCAN)—Parent

Altered Health Maintenance r/t knowledge deficit of parenting skills secondary to unachieved developmental tasks

Altered Parenting r/t unrealistic expectations of child; lack of effective role model; unmet social/emotional maturation needs of parents; interruption in bonding process

Chronic Low Self-Esteem r/t lack of successful parenting experiences

High Risk for Violence Towards Child r/t inadequate coping mechanisms; unresolved stressors; unachieved maturational level by parent

Impaired Home Maintenance Management r/t disorganization, parental dysfunction; neglect of safe and nurturing environment

Ineffective Family Coping: Disabling r/t dysfunctional family; underdeveloped, nurturing parental role; lack of parent support systems/role models

Powerlessness r/t inability to perform parental role responsibilities

Suspicion

High Risk for Violence: Directed at Self or Others r/t inability to trust

Impaired Social Interaction r/t altered thought process; paranoid delusions, hallucinations

Powerlessness r/t repetitive paranoid thinking

Swallowing Difficulties

Impaired Swallowing r/t neuromuscular impairment (e.g., decreased or absent gag reflex, decreased strength or excursion of muscles involved in mastication, perceptual impairment facial paralysis); mechanical obstruction (e.g., edema, tracheostomy tube, tumor); fatigue; limited awareness; reddened, irritated oropharyngeal cavity; improper feeding, positioning

Syncope

Altered Tissue Perfusion: Cerebral r/t interruption of blood flow

Anxiety r/t fear of falling

Decreased Cardiac Output r/t dysrhythmias

High Risk for Injury r/t altered sensory-perception; transient loss of consciousness; risk for falls

Impaired Physical Mobility r/t fear of falling

Social Isolation r/t fear of falling

105

T

T & A

Altered Comfort r/t effects of anesthesia (nausea and vomiting)

High Risk for Altered Nutrition: Less than Body Requirements r/t hesitation/reluctance to swallow

High Risk for Aspiration/Suffocation r/t postoperative drainage and impaired swallowing

High Risk for Fluid Volume Deficit r/t decreased intake secondary to painful swallowing, effects of anesthesia (nausea and vomiting); hemorrhage

Ineffective Airway Clearance r/t hesitation/reluctance to cough secondary to pain

Knowledge Deficit: Potential for Enhanced Health Maintenance r/t sufficient knowledge regarding postoperative nutrition and rest requirements, signs and symptoms of complications, positioning

Pain r/t surgical incision

Tachycardia

Refer to Dysrhythmias

Tachypnea

Ineffective Breathing Pattern r/t pain; anxiety

Refer to cause of Tachypnea

Taste Abnormality

Sensory/Perceptual Alteration: Gustatory r/t medication side effects; altered sensory reception, transmission and/or integration; aging changes

Traumatic Brain Injury (TBI)

Refer to Intracranial Pressure, Increased

Temperature, Decreased

Hypothermia r/t exposure to cool environment

Temperature, Increased

Hyperthermia r/t dehydration; illness; trauma

Tension

Anxiety r/t threat to or change in health status; situational crisis

Terminally Ill Child/Death of Child—Parental

Altered Family Processes r/t situational crisis

Altered Parenting r/t high risk for overprotection of surviving siblings

Anticipatory Grieving r/t possible/expected/imminent death of child

Decisional Conflict r/t continuation/discontinuation of treatment, DNR status, ethical issues regarding organ donation

Family Coping: Potential for Growth r/t impact of crisis on family values, priorities, goals, or relationships; expressed interest or desire to attach meaning to child's life and death

Grieving r/t death of child

High Risk for Dysfunctional Grieving r/t prolonged, unresolved, or obstructed progression through stages of grief and mourning

Hopelessness r/t overwhelming stresses secondary to terminal illness

Impaired Social Interaction r/t dysfunctional grieving

Ineffective Denial r/t dysfunctional grieving

Ineffective Family Coping: Compromised r/t inability or unwillingness to discuss impending death and feelings with child, or support child through terminal stages of illness

Powerlessness r/t inability to alter course of events

Sleep Pattern Disturbance r/t grieving process

Social Isolation, Imposed by Others r/t feelings of inadequacy in providing support to grieving parents

Social Isolation, Self-Imposed r/t unresolved grief; perceived inadequate parenting skills

Spiritual Distress r/t sudden, unexpected death; prolonged suffering prior to death; questioning the death of youth; questioning meaning of own existence

Terminally Ill Child—Infant/Toddler
Ineffective Individual Coping r/t separation from parents and familiar environment secondary to inability to grasp external meaning of death

Terminally Ill Child—Pre-School Child
Fear r/t perceived punishment, bodily harm, feelings of guilt secondary to magical thinking (thoughts cause events)

Terminally Ill Child—School-Age Child/ Preadolescent
Fear r/t perceived punishment, body mutilation, feelings of guilt

Terminally Ill Child—Adolescent
Altered Body Image r/t effects of terminal disease; already critical feelings of group identity and self-image
Impaired Social Interaction/Social Isolation r/t forced separation from peers
Ineffective Individual Coping r/t inability to establish personal and peer identity secondary to threat of being different or "not being"; inability to achieve maturational tasks
Refer to Hospitalized Child; Child With Chronic Condition

Tetralogy of Fallot
Refer to Congenital Heart Disease/Cardiac Anomalies

Therapeutic Regimen, Ineffective Management of
Ineffective Management of Therapeutic Regimen r/t complexity of health care system; complexity of therapeutic regimen; decisional conflicts; economic difficulties; excessive demands made on individual or family; family conflict; family patterns of health care; inadequate number and types of cues to action; knowledge deficits; mistrust of regimen and/or health care personnel; perceived seriousness; perceived susceptibility; perceived barriers; perceived benefits, powerlessness; social support deficits

Thermoregulation, Ineffective
Ineffective Thermoregulation r/t trauma or illness; immaturity; aging; fluctuating environmental temperature

Thoracotomy
Activity Intolerance r/t pain; imbalance between oxygen supply and demand; presence of chest tubes
High Risk for Infection r/t invasive procedure
High Risk for Injury r/t disruption of closed-chest drainage system
Ineffective Airway Clearance r/t drowsiness, pain with breathing and coughing
Ineffective Breathing Pattern r/t decreased energy,fatigue; pain
Pain r/t surgical procedure; coughing and deep breathing
Knowledge Deficit r/t self-care; effective breathing exercises; pain relief

Thought Disorders
Altered Thought Processes r/t disruption in cognitive thinking, processing

Thrombophlebitis
Altered Tissue Perfusion: Peripheral r/t interruption of venous blood flow
Colonic Constipation r/t inactivity; bedrest
Diversional Activity Deficit r/t bedrest
High Risk for Injury r/t possible embolus
Impaired Physical Mobility r/t pain in extremity; forced bedrest
Knowledge Deficit r/t pathophysiology of condition; self-care needs; treatment regimen, outcome
Pain r/t vascular inflammation; edema
Refer to Anticoagulant Therapy

Thyroidectomy
High Risk for Altered Verbal Communication r/t edema; pain; vocal cord/laryngeal nerve damage
High Risk for Ineffective Airway Clearance r/t edema/hematoma formation, airway obstruction
High Risk for Injury r/t possible parathyroid damage, or removal
Refer to Surgery

TIA (Transient Ischemic Attack)
Altered Tissue Perfusion: Cerebral r/t lack of adequate oxygen supply to the brain
Health Seeking Behavior r/t obtaining knowledge regarding treatment and prevention of inadequate oxygenation
High Risk for Decreased Cardiac Output r/t dysrhythmias contributing to inadequate oxygen supply to brain
High Risk for Injury r/t possible syncope
Refer to syncope

Tinnitus
Altered Comfort: Tinnitus r/t edema; pressure on nerve endings
Knowledge Deficit r/t treatment of condition
Sensory/Perceptual Alteration: Auditory r/t altered sensory reception, transmission, or integration

Tissue Damage; Corneal, Integumentary, or Subcutaneous
Impaired Tissue Integrity r/t altered circulation; nutritional deficit/excess; fluid deficit/excess; knowledge deficit; impaired physical mobility; irritants, chemical (including body excretions, secretions, medications); thermal (temperature extremes); mechanical (pressure, shear, friction); radiation (including therapeutic radiation)

Tissue Perfusion, Decreased
Altered Tissue Perfusion r/t interruption of flow, arterial; interruption of flow, venous; exchange problems; hypovolemia; hypervolemia

Toileting Problems
Toileting Self-Care Deficit r/t impaired transfer ability; impaired mobility status; intolerance to activity; neuromuscular impairment; cognitive impairment

Toilet Training
Health Seeking Behavior: Bladder/Bowel Training r/t achievement of developmental milestone secondary to enhanced parenting skills

Tonsillectomy and Adenoidectomy (T & A)
Refer to T & A

Total Anomalous Pulmonary Venous Return (TAPVR)
Refer to Congenital Heart Disease/Cardiac Anomalies

Total Joint Replacement
High Risk for Infection r/t invasive procedure, anesthesia, immobility
High Risk for Injury: Neurovascular r/t altered peripheral tissue perfusion, altered mobility, prosthesis
Impaired Physical Mobility r/t musculoskeletal impairment; surgery; prosthesis
Knowledge Deficit r/t self-care; treatment regimen, outcomes
Pain r/t possible edema; physical injury, surgery

Total Parenteral Nutrition (TPN)
Refer to TPN

Toxemia
Refer to PIH

TPN (Total Parenteral Nutrition)
Altered Nutrition: Less than Body Requirements r/t inability to ingest or digest food or absorb nutrients due to biological/psychological factors
High Risk for Fluid Volume Excess r/t rapid administration of TPN

108

High Risk for Infection r/t concentrated glucose solution, invasive administration of fluids

High Risk for Injury r/t possible hyperglycemia/ hypoglycemia

Tracheoesophageal Fistula (TEF)

Altered Nutrition: Less than Body Requirements r/t difficulties in swallowing

High Risk for Aspiration r/t common passage of air/food

Ineffective Airway Clearance r/t aspiration of feeding secondary to inability to swallow

Refer to Respiratory Conditions of the Neonate; Hospitalized Child

Tracheostomy

Anxiety r/t impaired verbal communication; ineffective airway clearance

Body Image Disturbance r/t abnormal opening in neck

High Risk for Ineffective Airway Clearance r/t increased secretions; mucous plugs

High Risk for Infection r/t invasive procedure; pooling of secretions

Impaired Verbal Communication r/t presence of mechanical airway

Knowledge Deficit r/t self-care; home maintenance management

Pain r/t edema; surgical procedure

Traction and Casts

Constipation r/t immobility

Diversional Activity Deficit r/t immobility

High Risk for Disuse Syndrome r/t mechanical immobilization

High Risk for Impaired Skin Integrity r/t contact of traction/cast with skin

High Risk for Peripheral Neurovascular Dysfunction r/t mechanical compression

Impaired Physical Mobility r/t imposed restrictions on activity secondary to bone/joint disease injury

Pain r/t immobility, injury/disease

Self-Care Deficit: Feeding, Dressing/Grooming, Bathing/Hygiene, Toileting r/t degree of impaired physical mobility and body area affected by traction/cast

Transient Ischemic Attack (TIA)

Refer to TIA

Transposition of the Great Vessels

Refer to Congenital Heart Disease/Cardiac Anomalies

Transurethral Resection of the Prostrate (TURP)

Refer to TURP

Trauma; High Risk for

High Risk for Trauma r/t <u>Internal</u>: weakness; poor vision; balancing difficulties; reduced temperature and/or tactile sensation reduced large or small muscle coordination; reduced hand-eye coordination; lack of safety education; lack of safety precautions; insufficient finances to purchase safety equipment or effect repairs; cognitive or emotional difficulties; history of previous trauma. <u>External</u>: slippery floors, walkways; unanchored rugs; bathtub without hand grip or antislip equipment; use of unsteady ladders or chairs; entering unlighted rooms; unsturdy or absent stair rails; unanchored electric wires; litter or liquid spills on floors or stairways; high beds; children playing without gates at the top of the stairs; obstructed passageways; unsafe window protection in home with young children; inappropriate call-for-aid mechanisms for bedresting client; pot handles facing toward front of stove; bathing in very hot water, unsupervised bathing of young children; potential igniting gas leaks; delayed lighting of gas burner or oven; experimenting with chemical or gasoline; unscreened fires or heaters; wearing plastic apron or flowing clothes around open flame; children playing with matches, candles, cigarettes; inadequately stored combustible or corrosives; highly flammable children's toys or clothing overloaded fuse box; contact with rapidly moving machinery, industrial belts, or pulleys; sliding on coarse bed linen or struggling within bed restraints; faulty electrical plugs, frayed wires, or defective appliances; contact with acids or alkali; playing with fireworks or gunpowder; contact with intense cold; overexposure to sun, sun lamps, radiotherapy; use of cracked dishware or glasses; knives stored uncovered; guns or ammunition stored unlocked; large icicles hanging from the roof; exposure to dangerous machinery; children playing with sharp-edged toys; high crime neighborhood and vulnerable clients; driving a mechanically unsafe vehicle; driving after partaking of alcoholic beverages or drugs; driving at excessive speeds; driving without necessary visual aids; children riding in the front seat in car; smoking in bed or near oxygen; overloaded electrical outlets; grease waste collected on stoves; use of thin or worn potholders; misuse of necessary headgear for motorized cyclists or young children carried on adult bicycles; unsafe road or road-crossing conditions; play or work near vehicle pathways; nonuse or misuse of seat restraints

Trauma in Pregnancy
Anxiety r/t threat to self/fetus and unknown outcome
High Risk for Fluid Volume Deficit r/t blood loss
High Risk for Infection r/t traumatized tissue
High Risk for Fetal Injury r/t premature separation of the placenta
Impaired Skin Integrity r/t trauma
Knowledge Deficit r/t lack of exposure to situation
Pain r/t trauma

Traumatic Brain Injury
Refer to Intracranial Pressure, Increased

Traumatic Event
Post Trauma Response r/t previously experienced trauma

Tricuspid Atresia
Refer to Congenital Heart Disease/Cardiac Anomalies

Truncus Arteriosus
Refer to Congenital Heart Disease/Cardiac Anomalies

Tube Feeding
High Risk for Altered Nutrition: Less than Body Requirements r/t intolerance to tube feeding; inadequate calorie replacement to meet metabolic needs
High Risk for Aspiration r/t improperly administered feeding; improper placement of tube; improper positioning of client during and after feeding; excessive residual feeding (or lack of digestion)
High Risk for Fluid Volume Deficit r/t inadequate water administration with concentrated feeding

TURP (Transurethral Resection of the Prostate)
High Risk for Fluid Volume Deficit r/t fluid loss and possible bleeding
High Risk for Infection r/t invasive procedure; route for bacteria
High Risk for Urinary Retention r/t obstruction of urethra or catheter with clots
Knowledge Deficit r/t self-care postoperative; home maintenance management
Pain r/t incision; irritation from catheter; bladder spasms; kidney infection

U

Ulcer, Peptic or Duodenal
Altered Health Maintenance r/t lack of knowledge
  of health practices to prevent ulcer formation
Pain r/t irritated mucosa from acid secretion
Fatigue r/t loss of blood, chronic illness
Refer to GI Bleed

Ulcerative Colitis
Refer to IBS

Unilateral Neglect of One Side of Body
Unilateral Neglect r/t effects of disturbed perceptual abilities, e.g., hemianopsia; one-sided
  blindness; neurologic illness or trauma

Unsanitary Living Conditions
Impaired Home Maintenance r/t impaired cognitive or emotional functioning; lack of knowledge; insufficient finances

Urgency to Urinate
Urge Incontinence r/t decreased bladder capacity;
  irritation of bladder stretch receptors causing
  spasm; alcohol; caffeine; increased fluids; increased urine concentration; overdistention of
  bladder

Urinary Diversion
Refer to Ileal Conduit

Urinary Elimination, Altered
Altered Urinary Elimination r/t anatomical obstruction; sensory motor impairment; urinary tract
  infection

Urinary Retention
Urinary Retention r/t high urethral pressure caused
  by weak detrusor; inhibition of reflex arc;
  strong sphincter; blockage

Urinary Tract Infection (UTI)
Refer to UTI

Uterine Bleeding
Refer to Hemorrhage, Shock

UTI (Urinary Tract Infection)
Altered Pattern of Urinary Elimination: Frequency
  r/t urinary tract infection
Knowledge Deficit r/t methods to treat and prevent
  UTIs
Pain: Dysuria r/t inflammatory process in bladder

V

Vaginal Hysterectomy

High Risk for Altered Urinary Elimination r/t edema in area

High Risk for Infection r/t surgical site

Urinary Retention r/t edema at surgical site

Refer to Hysterectomy

Vaginitis

Altered Pattern of Sexuality r/t abstinence during acute stage; pain

High Risk for Infection r/t spread of infection, risk of reinfection

Knowledge Deficit r/t proper hygiene; preventive measures

Pain: Pruritus r/t inflamed tissues; edema

Varicose Veins

Altered Tissue Perfusion: Peripheral r/t venous stasis

Chronic Pain r/t impaired circulation

High Risk for Impaired Skin Integrity r/t altered peripheral tissue perfusion

Knowledge Deficit r/t health care practices; prevention/treatment regimen

Venereal Disease

Refer to STD

Ventilation, Inability to Sustain Spontaneous

Inability to Sustain Spontaneous Ventilation r/t metabolic factors; respiratory muscle fatigue

Ventilator Client

Dysfunctional Ventilatory Weaning Response (DVWR) r/t inability to sustain respirations without mechanical support

Fear r/t inability to breathe on own; difficulty communicating

High Risk for Infection r/t presence of endotracheal tube; pooled secretions

Impaired Gas Exchange r/t ventilation perfusion imbalance

Impaired Verbal Communication r/t presence of endotracheal tube; decreased mentation

Inability to Sustain Spontaneous Ventilation r/t metabolic factors, respiratory muscle fatigue

Ineffective Airway Clearance r/t increased secretions; decreased cough/gag reflex

Ineffective Breathing Pattern r/t decreased energy/fatigue secondary to possible alteration in nutrition: less than body requirements

Powerlessness r/t health treatment regimen

Social Isolation r/t impaired mobility r/t ventilator dependence

Refer to Child with Chronic Condition; Hospitalized Child; Respiratory Conditions of the Neonate

Ventilatory, Dysfunctional Weaning Response (DVWR)

Dysfunctional Ventilatory Weaning Response (DVWR) r/t inability to sustain respirations without mechanical support

Vertigo

Decreased Cardiac Output r/t possible dysrhythmias

High Risk for Injury r/t altered sensory-perception

Sensory/Perceptual Alteration: Kinesthetic r/t altered sensory reception, transmission or integration; medications

Violent Behavior

High Risk for Violence: Self-Directed or Directed at Others r/t antisocial character; battered women; catatonic excitement; child abuse; manic excitement; organic brain syndrome; panic states; rage reactions; suicidal behavior; temporal lobe epilepsy; toxic reactions to medication

Vision Impairment

Fear r/t loss of sight

High Risk for Injury r/t sensory-perceptual alteration

Self-Care Deficit: Specify r/t perceptual impairment

Sensory/Perceptual Alteration: Visual r/t altered sensory reception related to impaired vision

Social Isolation r/t altered state of wellness/inability to see

Vomiting

Altered Comfort: *Nausea, Retching* r/t tension on abdominal muscles

High Risk for Altered Nutrition: Less than Body Requirements r/t inability to ingest food

High Risk for Fluid Volume Deficit r/t decreased intake; loss of fluids with vomiting

W

Weakness
Fatigue r/t decreased/increased metabolic energy production

Weight Gain
Altered Nutrition: More than Body Requirements r/t excessive intake in relation to metabolic need

Weight Loss
Altered Nutrition: Less than Body Requirements r/t inability to ingest food due to biological, psychological, or economic factors

Wellness Seeking Behavior
Health Seeking Behavior r/t expressed desire for increased control of health practice

Wheezing
Ineffective Airway Clearance r/t tracheobronchial obstruction, secretions

Withdrawal from Alcohol
Refer to Alcohol Withdrawal

Withdrawal from Drugs
Refer to Drug Withdrawal

Wound Debridement
High Risk for Infection r/t open wound, presence of bacteria
Impaired Skin Integrity r/t presence of bacteria on skin
Pain r/t debridement of wound

Wound Dehisence, Evisceration
Altered Nutrition: Less than Body Requirements r/t inability to digest nutrients, need for increased protein for healing
Fear r/t client fear of body parts falling out, surgical procedure not going as planned

High Risk for Fluid Volume Deficit r/t inability to ingest nutrients; obstruction; fluid loss
High Risk for Injury r/t exposed abdominal contents

Wound Infection
Altered Nutrition: Less than Body Requirements r/t biological factors; infection; hyperthermia
Body Image Disturbance r/t unsightly open wound
High Risk for Infection (Spread of) r/t altered nutrition; less than body requirements
High Risk for Impaired Skin Integrity r/t presence of bacteria on skin
High Risk for Fluid Volume Deficit r/t increased metabolic rate
Hyperthermia r/t increased metabolic rate; illness/infection

SECTION III

Guide to Planning Care

ACTIVITY INTOLERANCE

Definition
A state in which an individual has insufficient physiological or psychological energy to endure or complete required or desired daily activities.

Defining Characteristics
*Verbal report of fatigue or weakness
Abnormal heart rate or blood pressure response to activity
Exertional discomfort or dyspnea
Electrocardiographic changes reflecting dysrhythmias or ischemia
(*Critical)

Related Factors (r/t)
Bedrest/immobility
Generalized weakness
Sedentary lifestyle
Imbalance between oxygen supply/demand

Client Outcomes/Goals
✓ Participates in prescribed physical activity with no or minimal change in heart rate, blood pressure, monitor pattern, breathing rate.
✓ Walks specified distance of _____ feet ___ times per day.
✓ Verbalizes increased comfort during activity.

Nursing Interventions
- Observe the cause of activity intolerance (see Related Factors above), determine if physical or psychological basis.
- Monitor and record client's ability to tolerate activity, noting pulse rate, blood pressure, monitor pattern, dyspnea, use of accessory muscles, skin color before and after activity.
- Observe for pain before activity and treat pain before activity if possible.
- Obtain any assistive devices or equipment needed before ambulation, such as walking belt, walker, cane, crutches, portable oxygen.
- Refer to physical therapy for help in increasing amount of activity.
- Work with client to set goals that increase level of activity.
- Space activities and allow for rest between activities.
- Provide passive range of motion if client is unable to tolerate activity.
Geriatric
- Slow the pace of care, allow the client extra time to carry out activities, provide rest periods as needed.
- Schedule treatments and diagnostic procedures allowing for periods of rest.

Client/Family Teaching

- Instruct client in use of relaxation techniques to utilize during activity.
- Teach client how to utilize assistive devices or medications before or during activity.
- Help client set up activity log to record exercise and ability to tolerate exercise.

HIGH RISK FOR ACTIVITY INTOLERANCE

Definition
A state in which an individual is at risk of experiencing insufficient physiological or psychological energy to endure or complete required or desired daily activities.

Defining Characteristics
Presence of risk factors such as:
History of previous intolerance to activity
Deconditioned status
Presence of circulatory/respiratory problems
Inexperience with activity

Related Factors (r/t)
See risk factors.

Client Outcomes/Goals, Nursing Interventions, and Client/Family Teaching
Refer to care plan for *Activity Intolerance.*

IMPAIRED ADJUSTMENT

Definition
The state in which the individual is unable to modify his/her lifestyle/behavior in a manner consistent with a change in health status.

Defining Characteristics
Major: Verbalization of nonacceptance of health status change
Nonexistent or unsuccessful ability to be involved in problem solving or goal setting
Minor: Lack of movement toward independence
Extended period of shock, disbelief, or anger regarding health status change
Lack of future-oriented thinking

Related Factors (r/t)
Disability requiring change in lifestyle
Inadequate support systems
Impaired cognition

Sensory overload
Assault to self-esteem
Altered locus of control
Incomplete grieving

Client Outcomes/Goals
✓ States acceptance of health status change.
✓ States personal goals to achieve in dealing with change in health status.
✓ Lists behaviors needed to adjust to health status change and moves towards independence.
✓ Experiences a period of grief over loss that is in proportion to the actual or perceived effect of the loss.

Nursing Interventions
- Monitor the degree of the health status change; physical/psychological.
- Allow the client time to express feelings about the health status change.
- Assist in working through the stages of grief with denial the usual initial response; acknowledge that grief takes time and give permission to grieve; accept crying.
- Discuss resources that have worked for the client in the past in dealing with changes in lifestyle or health.
- Use open-ended questions to allow freer expression, e.g., "Tell me about your last hospitazliation" "How does this time compare?"
- Discuss what the client's goals are at this time; if appropriate, have him list them so they can be referred to and steps taken to accomplish them.
- List things client may need assistance with and things that can be done independently.
- Allow client choices in daily care, e.g., "What time you would like your shower?"
- Allow client time to adjust to new situation, introduce new material gradually to prevent overload; ask for frequent feedback.

- Give positive feedback for accomplishments no matter how small.
- Manipulate environment to decrease stress.
- Maintain consistency and continuity in daily schedule to provide some constancy in client's life.

Geriatrics
- Maximize the client's remaining functional abilities.

Client/Family Teaching
- Assist client to list strengths (focus on the here and now).
- Allow client to proceed at their own pace in learning; provide time for return demonstrations, e.g., self-injection of insulin.
- Initiate community referrals as needed; grief counseling, self-help groups, peer counseling programs.
- Involve significant others in planning and teaching.

INEFFECTIVE AIRWAY CLEARANCE

Definition
A state in which an individual is unable to clear secretions or obstructions from the respiratory tract to maintain airway patency.

Defining Characteristics
Abnormal breath sounds (rales [crackles], rhonchi [wheezes])
Changes in rate or depth of respiration
Tachypnea
Cough, effective/ineffective, with or without sputum
Cyanosis
Dyspnea

Related Factors (r/t)
Decreased energy/fatigue
Tracheobronchial infection, obstruction, secretions
Perceptual/cognitive impairment
Trauma

Client Outcomes/Goals
✓ Demonstrate effective coughing and clear breath sounds, free of cyanosis and dyspnea.
✓ Maintains a patent airway at all times.
✓ Relates methods to enhance secretion removal.
✓ Relates the significance of changes in sputum to include color, character, amount, and odor.

Nursing Interventions
- Auscultate breath sounds every _____ hours.
- Monitor respiratory pattern to include rate, depth, and effort.
- Monitor arterial blood gas values.
- Position patient to optimize respiration, e.g., elevating head of bed 30 to 45 degrees, reposition at least every 2 hours.
- Assist client to deep breathe and cough; reposition and suction when indicated.
- Document results of coughing/suctioning particularly client tolerance and secretion characteristics.
- Encourage activity and ambulation as tolerated.
- Encourage fluids if not contraindicated to liquefy secretions; monitor client's fluid/hydration status.
- Administer oxygen per appropriate devices as ordered.
- Administer medications, such as bronchodilators, as indicated.
- Provide comfort measures to decrease anxiety, which promotes more effective breathing, e.g., reassurance, backrubs.

Client/Family Teaching

- Instruct client how to deep breath and cough effectively.
- Teach client to utilize a small pillow or bath blanket for support while coughing if painful abdomen.
- Teach client the significance of rest periods between short periods of exertion.
- Educate client and family about the significance of changes in sputum production to include color, character, amount, and odor.

ANXIETY

Definition
A vague uneasy feeling whose source is often nonspecific or unknown to the individual.

Defining Characteristics

Subjective: Increased tension
Apprehension
Painful and persistent feelings
Increased helplessness
Uncertainty
Fearful
Scared
Regretful
Overexcited
Rattled
Distressed
Jittery
Feelings of inadequacy
Shakiness
Fear of unspecific consequences
Expressed concerns re change in life events

Worried
Anxious
Objective: Sympathetic
stimulation—cardiovascular excitation, superficial vasoconstriction, pupil dilation
Restlessness
Insomnia
Glancing about
Poor eye contact
Trembling/hand tremors
Extraneous movement (foot shuffling, hand/arm movements)
Facial tension
Voice quivering
Focus "self"
Increased wariness
Increased perspiration

Related Factors (r/t)

Unconscious conflict about essential values/goals of life
Threat to self-concept
Threat of death
Threat to or change in health status

Threat to or change in environment
Threat to or change in interaction patterns
Situational/maturation crises
Interpersonal transmission/contagion
Unmet needs

Client Outcomes/Goals

✓ States relief of tension, control over feelings of helplessness, not fearful or scared, not worried or anxious.
✓ Looks realistically at consequences; accepts change in life events.
✓ Heart rate and rhythm normal for client; pupils appropriate to environment; no signs of superficial vasoconstriction.
✓ Posture relaxed, makes eye contact, able to focus on speaker or object.
✓ Facial expression relaxed, voice normal for client, no extraneous movements of hands or feet.
✓ Focuses on events "outside of self."

✓ Expresses trust; return of problem-solving ability.

Nursing Interventions

- Observe level of anxiety and physical reaction to anxiety: tachycardia, tachypnea, nonverbal expressions of anxiety.
- Stay with the client, reassure him that he is safe and he can ask for help if he feels threatened; speak slowly and calmly with client, use active listening skills, focus on the here and now, encourage expression of feelings, validate your observations, "Are you feeling tense now?"
- Use self, presence, touch (with permission).
- Accept defenses, rationalizations, do not confront or argue, allow talking, crying, physical activity, nonverbal expressions if incapable of verbal.
- Encourage client to express needs, ask questions, and seek clarification of unknowns/concerns.
- Help the client identify the reality of own health care situation; allow expression of pain or discomfort; reinforce individuals personal reaction to pain or threat to well-being.
- Explain all procedures and surgical routines; use short, simple sentences and explanations, validate understanding.
- Explore coping skills used previously to relieve anxiety; reinforce them.
- Encourage ambulation or physical movement within client's capabilities; explore other outlets.
- Allow uninterrupted sleep; help client reestablish normal sleep pattern.
- Encourage client to participate in own care; include client in development of nursing care plan.
- If pharmacological therapy is indicated, consult a physician and offer medications PRN as ordered.
- Limit amount of caffeine intake.

Geriatric
- Monitor for depression; anxiety often accompanies depression in elderly adults because of worry about illness, finances, and accumulated losses.
- Provide protective, safe environment; use consistent caregivers; maintain accustomed environmental structure.
- Observe for behavioral changes if antianxiety drugs are taken; elderly are more sensitive to both clinical and toxic effects.

Client/Family Teaching

- Teach progressive muscle relaxation technique.
- Teach breathing technique: breathe in through nose, think "re," breathe out through mouth, think "lax."
- Teach to visualize restful scenes (beach, forest, favorite place) sight, sounds, smells.
- Teach to suppress negative thoughts: say "Stop," substitute a positive thought for the negative one.
- Teach relationship between healthy physical lifestyle and positive mental attitude; diet, exercise.
- Teach use of appropriate community resources in emergency situations: Hotline, emergency rooms, help of law enforcement agency if abusive situation.
- Encourage use of community self-help groups in nonemergency situations.

HIGH RISK FOR ASPIRATION

Definition
The state in which an individual is at risk for entry of gastrointestinal secretions, oropharyngeal secretions, or solids, fluids, or small objects into the tracheobronchial passages.

Defining Characteristics
Presence of risk factors such as:
Reduced level of consciousness
Depressed cough and gag reflexes
Presence of tracheostomy or endotracheal tube
Incomplete lower esophageal sphincter
Gastrointestinal tubes
Tube feeding

Medication administration
Situations hindering elevation of upper body
Increased gastrointestinal motility
Delayed gastric emptying
Impaired swallowing
Facial/oral/neck surgery or trauma
Wired jaws

Related Factors (r/t)
See risk factors.

Client Outcomes/Goals
✓ Swallows/digests oral, nasogastric or gastric feeding without aspiration.
✓ Maintains patent airway.

Nursing Interventions
- Monitor respiratory rate, depth and effort; note any signs of aspiration: dyspnea, cough, cyanosis, wheezing, fever.
- Auscultate lung sounds q____ hours, noting any new onset of crackles, wheezing.
- Take vital signs q_____ hours.
- Explore any history of aspiration; check gag reflex before initiating oral feeding.
- Have suction machine available for high risk clients.
- Consult dietitian for best diet for client, e.g., may need thickening agent to make food easier to swallow.
- Note presence of any nausea, vomiting, or diarrhea.
- Listen to bowel sounds q ____hours, note new onset of abdominal distention, increased rigidity of abdomen.
- Check to make sure initial feeding tube placement was confirmed by x-ray, keep feeding tube securely taped.
- Determine placement of feeding tube before each feeding, every 4 hours if continuous feeding.
- If client has a tracheostomy, check for inflation of the tracheostomy cuff before iniating feeding.
- Check for gastric residual at least every 8 hours and before feedings, if greater than 100 cc, follow hospital protocol on holding feeding.

- Position client with head of bed elevated at least 30 degrees during feeding; turn on right side if can not elevate head of bed.
- Stop continual feeding temporarily when turning or moving client.
- Feed or hydrate client only during formal rest periods from restraints.
- If client shows symptoms of nausea and vomiting position on side.
- If the client needs to be fed, feed slowly and allow adequate time for chewing and swallowing; make sure food is cut into small pieces for ease in chewing and swallowing.

Geriatric
- Use CNS depressants cautiously; elderly clients have altered metabolism, distribution and excretion of drugs.

Client/Family Teaching
- Teach client/family how to administer tube feeding safely.
- Teach client/family precautions should take to prevent aspiration, signs of aspiration.

BODY IMAGE DISTURBANCE

Definition
Disruption in the way one perceives one's body image.

Defining Characteristics
Objective: Missing body part
Actual change in structure or function
Not looking at or touching body part
Hiding or overexposing body part (intentional or unintentional)
Trauma to nonfunctioning part
Change in social involvement
Change in ability to estimate spatial relationship of body to environment
Subjective verbalization of: Change in lifestyle
Fear of rejection or of reaction by others
Focus on past strength, function, or appearance
Negative feelings about body and feelings of helplessness, hopelessness, or powerlessness
Preoccupation with change or loss
Emphasis on remaining strengths, heightened achievement
Extension of body boundary to incorporate environmental objects
Personalization of part or loss by name
Depersonalization of part or loss by impersonal pronouns
Refusal to verify actual change

Related Factors (r/t)
Biophysical change
Cognitive/perceptual change
Psychosocial change
Cultural or spiritual change

Client Outcomes/Goals
✓ States/demonstrates an ability to adjust to lifestyle change by accepting change or loss.
✓ Calls body part or loss by appropriate name.
✓ Looks at and touches changed or missing body part.
✓ Cares for changed or nonfunctioning part without inflicting trauma.
✓ Returns to previous social involvement.

Nursing Interventions
- Observe client's usual coping mechanisms under extreme times of stress and reinforce their use in this crisis.
- Acknowledge feelings of denial, anger, or depression as normal feelings in adjusting to changes in body/lifestyle.

- Encourage client/family to discuss and share feelings regarding health problem, treatment, progress, or prognosis.
- Explore strengths and resources with client; discuss possible changes in weight and hair loss (select a wig before hair loss occurs).
- Encourage client to discuss interpersonal, social, spiritual, and cultural conflicts that may arise.
- Encourage client to make own decisions and participate in plan of care; accept self, both inadequacies/strengths.
- Encourage the acceptance of help from others and provide list of appropriate community resources (i.e., Reach to Recovery, Ostomy Association)
- Help client describe self-ideal and identify self-criticisms, be accepting of self.
- Allow client sufficient time to accept change, while reinforcing strengths.
- Avoid look of distaste when caring for client with disfiguring surgery or injury; provide privacy.
- Encourage client to maintain usual grooming routine and own clothing if possible.
- Assist with the resolution of a alteration in body image by encouraging looking at change, and touching change if appropriate.

Client/Family Teaching
- Teach appropriate care of altered body part (mastectomy, amputation, ostomy).
- Teach client what community support groups are available; offer to make initial phone call.

EFFECTIVE BREASTFEEDING

Definition
A state in which a mother-infant dyad exhibits adequate proficiency and satisfaction with breastfeeding process.

Defining Characteristics
Major: Mother able to position infant at breast to promote a successful latch-on response
Infant is content after feeding
Regular and sustained suckling/swallowing at the breast
Appropriate infant weight patterns for age
Effective mother-infant communication patterns (infant cues, maternal interpretation and response)
Minor: Signs or symptoms of oxytocin release (let-down or milk ejection reflex)
Adequate infant elimination patterns for age
Eagerness of infant to nurse
Maternal verbalization of satisfaction with the breastfeeding process

Related Factors (r/t)
Basic breastfeeding knowledge
Normal maternal breast structure
Normal infant oral structure
Infant gestational age greater than 34 weeks
Support sources
Maternal confidence

Outcomes/Goals
✓ Maintains effective breastfeeding.
✓ Infant will maintain normal growth patterns.
✓ Verbalizes satisfaction with the breastfeeding process.

Nursing Interventions
- Assess knowledge base regarding basic breastfeeding.
- Observe breast and nipple structure.
- Assist with the first attachment at the breast within the first hour after birth.
- Determine knowledge of prevention/treatment of common breastfeeding problem.
- Monitor breastfeeding process.
- Avoid nipple shields, supplemental bottle feeding.
- Encourage rooming-in with breastfeeding on demand around the clock.
- Evaluate adequacy of infant intake.
- Observe support person network.
- Give praise for positive mother-infant interactions.
- Do not provide samples of formula at discharge.

Client/Family Teaching

- Reinforce and add to knowledge base regarding breastfeeding.
- Provide education to support persons as needed.
- Teach to observe for infant's subtle hunger cues (quiet alert state, rooting, sucking, and hand-to-mouth activity) and to nurse whenever signs are apparent.
- Review guidelines for frequency of feeding (every 2 to 3 hours or at least 8 feeding per 24 hours).
- Review guidelines for duration of feeding until suckling and swallowing slow down.
- Teach how to use a breast pump to provide breast milk for infant when alternate infant care is required.
- Provide anticipatory guidance about common infant behaviors (infant growth spurts, temperament, sleep/wake cycles, and introduction of other foods).
- Provide information about additional breastfeeding resources.

INEFFECTIVE BREASTFEEDING

Definition
The state in which a mother, infant, or child experiences dissatisfaction or difficulty with the breast-feeding process.

Defining Characteristics
Major: Unsatisfactory breastfeeding process.
Minor: Actual or perceived inadequate milk supply
Infant inability to attach on to maternal breast correctly
No observable signs of oxytocin release
Observable signs of inadequate infant intake
Nonsustained suckling at the breast
Insufficient emptying of each breast per feeding
Persistence of sore nipples beyond the first week of breastfeeding
Insufficient opportunity for suckling at the breast
Infant exhibiting fussiness and crying within the first hour after breastfeeding
Unresponsive to other comfort measures
Infant arching and crying at the breast
Resisting latching on

Related Factors (r/t)
Prematurity
Infant anomaly
Maternal breast anomaly
Previous breast surgery
Previous history of breastfeeding failure
Infant receiving supplemental feedings with
    artificial nipple

Poor infant sucking reflex
Nonsupportive partner/family
Knowledge deficit
Interruption in breastfeeding
Maternal anxiety or ambivalence

Client Outcomes/Goals
✓ Achieves effective breastfeeding.
✓ Verbalizes/demonstrates techniques to manage breastfeeding problems.
✓ Infant manifests signs of adequate intake at the breast.
✓ Manifests positive self-esteem in relation to the infant feeding process.
✓ Explains a safe alternative method of infant feeding if unable to continue exclusive breastfeeding.

Nursing Intervention
- Observe for presence/absence of related factors or conditions that would preclude breastfeeding.
- Evaluate and record the mother's ability to position, give cues and help the infant latch-on.

- Evaluate and record the infant's ability to properly grasp and compress the areola with lips, tongue, and jaw.
- Evaluate and record the infant's suckling and swallowing pattern at the breast.
- Evaluate and record signs of oxytocin release.
- Evaluate and record infant's state at the time of feeding.
- Observe knowledge base regarding psychophysiology of lactation and specific treatment measures for underlying problems.
- Monitor psychosocial factors that may contribute to ineffective breastfeeding (e.g., anxiety, goals, values, or lifestyle that contribute to ambivalence about breastfeeding).
- Promote comfort and relaxation to reduce pain and anxiety.
- Use alerting techniques (provide variety in auditory, visual, and kinesthetic stimuli, such as unwrapping, placing upright, or talking to the infant) or consoling techniques as needed to bring the infant to a quiet alert state.
- Enhance the flow of milk: when infant's swallowing slows down teach mother to massage breast or burp infant and switch to other breast.
- Discourage supplemental bottle feeding and encourage exclusive, effective breastfeeding.
- Strengthen new mother's self-esteem by acknowledging her frustration and disappointment and supporting her decision to continue or choose an alternate plan.
- Make appropriate referrals.
- If unsuccessful in achieving effective breastfeeding, help client accept and learn an alternate method of infant feeding.

Client/Family Teaching
- Provide instruction in correct positioning.
- Reinforce and add to knowledge base regarding psychophysiology of lactation and specific treatment measures for underlying problem.
- Teach how to use the breast pump for times the mother must be parted from the infant.
- Provide education to support persons as needed.

INTERRUPTED BREASTFEEDING

Definition
A break in the continuity of the breastfeeding process as a result of inability or inadvisability to put baby to breast for feeding.

Defining Characteristics
Major: Infant does not receive nourishment at the breast for some or all of feedings
Minor: Maternal desire to maintain lactation and provide (or eventually provide) her breast milk for her Infant's nutritional needs
Separation of mother and infant
Lack of knowledge regarding expression and storage of breast milk

Related Factors (r/t)
Maternal or infant illness
Prematurity
Maternal employment
Contraindications to breastfeeding (e.g., drugs, true breast milk jaundice)
Need to abruptly wean infant

Client Outcomes/Goals
Infant: Client will receive mother's breastmilk (if not contraindicated by maternal or infant condition).
Maternal: Client will initiate or maintain lactation.
✓ Client will achieve effective breastfeeding or satisfaction with the breastfeeding experience.
✓ Client will demonstrate effective methods of breastmilk collection and storage.

Nursing Interventions
- Determine and record mother's desire to begin or continue breastfeeding.
- Determine advisability of initiating or reinstituting breastfeeding.
- Evaluate infant's ability and interest in breastfeeding.
- Evaluate mother's social support for continuing to breastfeed.
- Assess mother's emotional response to events that caused interruption.
- Develop with mother a satisfactory feeding plan to allow for continued breastfeeding.
- Determine and record mother's knowledge of how to handle (store, transport) breastmilk safely.
- Determine equipment needs.
- Provide resource information (support groups, equipment, and supply rental or sales).
- Promote emotional resolution through encouragement to verbalize frustrations and disappointment.

Client/Family Teaching
- Teach mother effective methods of express breastmilk.
- Teach mother safe breastmilk handling techniques.
- Provide anticipatory guidance for common problems associated with interrupted breastfeeding (i.e., diminishing milk supply, infant difficulty with resuming breastfeeding).
- Provide education to support persons as needed.

INEFFECTIVE BREATHING PATTERN

Definition
The state in which an individual's inhalation or exhalation pattern does not enable adequate pulmonary inflation or emptying.

Defining Characteristics
Dyspnea, shortness of breath, tachypnea, fremitus
Abnormal arterial blood/gas
Cyanosis
Cough
Nasal flaring
Respiratory depth changes

Assumption of 3-point position
Pursed-lip breathing/prolonged expiratory phase
Increased anteroposterior diameter
Use of accessory muscles
Altered chest excursion

Related Factors (r/t)
Neuromuscular impairment
Musculoskeletal impairment
Perception/cognitive impairment

Pain
Anxiety
Decreased energy/fatigue

Client Outcomes/Goals
✓ Demonstrates a breathing pattern that supports blood gas results within the client's normal parameters.
✓ Free of signs of hypoxia, hypercapnea.
✓ Free of cyanosis, uses normal muscles of respiration.

Nursing Interventions
- Monitor breath sounds, respiratory rate, depth, and effort.
- Note and report any tachypnea, nasal flaring, retractions, irritability.
- Observe skin and mucous membrane color.
- Monitor for dyspnea.
- Observe sputum noting color, odor and characteristics.
- Evaluate laboratory values to include hemoglobin and hematocrit, ABGs, electrolytes, total protein and albumin.
- Observe for pain; provide pain medication as ordered to facilitate adequate deep breathing and coughing
- Promote client sleep.
- Increase client's activity as tolerated.
- Plan for adequate rest periods before and after activity.
- Suction to remove pulmonary secretions as indicated.
- Position client in upright position as tolerated to facilitate chest expansion.
- Consider small frequent feeding to avoid compromising ventilatory effort and conserve energy.

Client/Family Teaching

- Educate client and family about physiological effects of an altered breathing pattern.
- Inform client and family about necessity of laboratory tests and assessment techniques.
- Teach pursed-lip breathing techniques, relaxation techniques, guided imagery, breathing exercises.
- Teach use of incentive spirometer if ordered.

DECREASED CARDIAC OUTPUT

Definition
A state in which the blood pumped by an individual's heart is sufficiently reduced that it is inadequate to meet the needs of the body's tissues.

Defining Characteristics
Variations in blood pressure readings
Dysrhythmias
Fatigue
Jugular vein distention
Color changes of skin and mucous membranes
Oliguria ↓ in urine output
Decreased peripheral pulses
Cold clammy skin
Crackles
Dyspnea, orthopnea pain c̄ breathing

Change in mental status
Shortness of breath
Syncope
Vertigo dizziness
Edema
Cough
Frothy sputum
Gallop rhythm
Weakness

Related Factors (r/t)
Myocardial infarction or ischemia
Valvular disease: cardiomyopathy
Serious dysrhythmias
Ventricular damage
Altered preload and/or afterload
Pericarditis
Sepsis

Congenital heart defects
Vagal stimulation
Stress
Anaphylaxis
Cardiac tamponade (Adapted from Doenges and
    Moorhouse)

Client Outcomes/Goals
✓ Demonstrates adequate cardiac output as evidenced by blood pressure, pulse rate, and rhythm within normal parameters; strong peripheral pulses; able to tolerate activity without symptoms of dyspnea, syncope, chest pain.
✓ Free of side effects from the medications used to accomplish adequate cardiac output.
✓ Explains actions and precautions should take to live with cardiac disease.

Nursing Interventions
■ Observe for chest pain; note location, radiation, severity, quality, duration, precipitating, and relieving factors.
■ If chest pain present, monitor, run EKG strip, medicate for pain as ordered, notify the physician.
■ Listen to heart sounds; rate, rhythm, S3,S4, rub, new onset systolic murmur.
■ Monitor for dysrhythmias.

- Monitor hemodynamic parameters for: increase in pulmonary wedge pressure, increased systemic vascular resistance, decrease in cardiac index.
- Observe for: neck vein distension, quality of peripheral pulses, crackles in lungs, edema (sacral edema if on bedrest), skin color and temperature, capillary refill, mental status, presence of nausea.
- Monitor intake and output, observe for decreased output.
- Note test results to correlate with severity of disease, need for restrictions: CPK-MB,LDH, WBC, ABG, ECG, Echocardiogram.
- Administer oxygen as needed per physicians order.
- Schedule periods of rest between activities.

Geriatrics

- Observe for atypical pain; elderly often have jaw pain instead of chest pain because of diminished responses of neurotransmitters.
- Observe for syncope, dizziness, palpitations, or feelings of weakness with cardiac disease; dysrhythmias are common in elderly.
- Observe for toxicities from medications; elderly may have difficulty with metabolism and excretion of medications.

Client/Family Teaching

- Teach symptoms of cardiovascular disease and appropriate action to take if client is symptomatic.
- Teach stress reduction: imagery, controlled breathing, and other relaxation techniques.
- Explain restrictions necessary, including diet, fluids, avoiding valsalva maneuver, exercise designed for client, and changes in lifestyle.
- Teach client the action and side-effects of cardiovascular medications.
- Teach family how to perform CPR.

CAREGIVER ROLE STRAIN

Definition
A caregiver's felt difficulty in performing the family caregiver role.

Defining Characteristics*
Caregivers report they:

Do not have enough resources (time, emotional strength, physical energy, or help from others) to provide the
care needed

Find it hard to do specific caregiving activities, such as bathing, cleaning up after incontinence, having to
manage behavior problems, and having to manage pain

Worry about the care receiver's health and emotional state, having to put the care receiver in
an institution, and who will care for the care receiver if something should happen to the caregiver

Feel that caregiving interferes with other important roles in their lives, such as being a worker, parent, spouse,
or friend

Feel loss because the care receiver is like a different person compared with before caregiving began or, in
the case of a child, that the care receiver was never the child the caregiver expected

Feel family conflict around issues of providing care, feeling that other family members do not do their share
in providing care to the receiver or that not enough appreciation is shown for what the caregiver does

Feel stress or nervousness in their relationship with the care receiver

Feel depressed

*80 % of caregivers report one or more of defining characteristics

Related Factors (r/t)
Pathophysiological: Illness severity of the care receiver

Addiction or codependency; premature birth/congenital defect

Discharge of family member with significant home care needs

Caregiver health impairment

Unpredictable illness course or instability in the care receiver's health

Caregiver is female

Psychological or cognitive problems in care receiver

Developmental: Caregiver is not developmentally ready for caregiver role, e.g., young adult needing to
provide care for a middle-aged parent

Developmental delay or retardation of the care receiver or caregiver

Psychosocial: Marginal family adaptation or dysfunction before the caregiving situation

Marginal caregiver's coping patterns

Past history of poor relationship between caregiver and care receiver

Caregiver is spouse

139

Care receiver exhibits deviant, bizarre behavior

Situational: Presence of abuse or violence

Presence of situational stressors that normally affect families, such as significant loss, disaster, or crisis

Poverty or economic vulnerability, major life events, e.g., birth, hospitalization, leaving home, returning home, marriage, divorce, employment, retirement, or death

Duration of caregiving required

Inadequate physical environment for providing care, e.g., housing, transportation, community services, equipment

Family/caregiver isolation

Lack of respite and recreation for caregiver

Inexperience with caregiving

Caregiver's competing role commitments

Complexity/amount of caregiving tasks

Client Outcomes/Goals
✓ Caregiver is physically and psychologically healthy.
✓ Caregiver is able to identify resources available to help in giving care.
✓ Carereceiver is receiving appropriate care.

Nursing Interventions
- Monitor quality of care being given for adequacy, need for improvement.
- Determine physical and psychological health of caregiver and refer to resources as needed.
- Observe for signs of addiction or codependency in caregiver or care receiver.
- Provide for home health services as needed to help with significant home care needs.
- Arrange for respite care for caregiver at intervals.
- Help caregiver to identify supports and decide on how to best utilize them.
- Clarify things caregiver has no control over, such as other persons, life, and health; allow time for grief over situations that can not be changed.
- Identify with caregiver those things they have control over.
- Assist caregiver to find time for personal time to meet own needs.
- Encourage caregiver to talk about feelings, concerns, and fears.
- Acknowledge frustration associated with caregiver responsibilities.
- Give caregiver permission to share angry feelings in a safe environment.
- Give caregiver permission to arrange custodial care in an institution if necessary and support both through this transition.

Geriatric
- Recognize that it is hard for elderly to accept any change in caregivers or environment.
- Assist caregiver in identifying ways to equitably distribute workload among family/significant others.

140

Client/Family Teaching
- Teach caregiver methods to provide care more efficiently as needed.
- Teach caregiver that she/he must ask for help from other people at intervals.
- Refer to counseling support groups to assist in adjustment to caregiver role.
- Refer to support groups that deal with issues of addiction/codependency: Alcoholics Anonymous, or Adult Children of Alcoholics.

HIGH RISK FOR CAREGIVER ROLE STRAIN

Definition
A caregiver is vulnerable for felt difficulty in performing the family caregiver role.

Related Factors (r/t)
Refer to related factors for *Caregiver Role Strain*

Client Outcomes/Goals, Nursing Interventions, and Client/Family Teaching
Refer to care plan for *Caregiver Role Strain*

ALTERED COMFORT

Definition
The state in which an individual experiences an uncomfortable sensation in response to a noxious stimulus (Carpenito).

Defining Characteristics
Major: The person reports or demonstrates discomfort
Minor: Guarded position
Cutaneous irritation
Abdominal heaviness
Itching
Retching

Related Factors (r/t)
Visceral disorders
Inflammation
Musculoskeletal disorders
Treatment related

Personal situation (pregnancy, overactivity)
Chemical irritants
(Adapted from Carpenito)

Client Outcomes/Goals
✓ States is comfortable.
✓ Explains methods to decrease itching.
✓ Explains methods to decrease nausea/vomiting.
✓ States relief or discomfort of nausea.

Nursing Interventions
Pruritus
- Determine cause of pruritus: dry skin, contact with irritating substance, medication effect, insect bite.
- Apply cool washcloths or ice as helpful.
- Provide tepid bath or soak affected part.
- Keep fingernails trimmed short.
- Leave pruritus area open to the air if possible.
- Avoid use of soaps, drying agents.
- Keep skin well-lubricated.
- Provide distraction to keep mind off itching.
- Consult with physician for medication to relieve itching.

Geriatric
- Limit number of complete baths, alternating with daily perineal care; dry well after bathing.
- Use bath oil in water instead of soap.
- Increase fluid intake within cardiac/renal limits, minimum of 1500 cc/day.

143

Nausea/Vomiting
- Determine cause of nausea/vomiting: medication effect; viral illness; food poisoning; extreme anxiety.
- Keep clean emesis basin and tissues within reach.
- Provide oral care after client vomits.
- Stay with client to give support and assistance when vomiting.
- Provide distraction from sensation of nausea.
- Maintain quiet environment.
- Keep head of bed elevated if not contraindicated and avoid sudden changes in position; if lower level of consciousness, position on side.
- Medicate for nausea/vomiting as needed and ordered.
- Have suction available for immobilized/wired jaw client.
- After vomiting is controlled, begin with small amounts of clear fluids (carbonated beverages with carbonation gone), then dry toast or crackers as tolerated.
- When client is nauseated, remove meal tray from room (smells stimulate nausea).
- Provide pain relief measures (pain can trigger nausea).

Client/Family Teaching
- Teach distraction techniques can use when uncomfortable.
- Teach not to scratch the skin.
- Teach progressive muscle relaxation technique.
- If nausea, vomiting occurs at home, teach client to stop all food and fluids until the acute phase passes.

IMPAIRED VERBAL COMMUNICATION

Definition
The state in which an individual experiences a decreased or absent ability to use or understand language in human interaction.

Defining Characteristics
*Unable to speak dominant language
*Speaks or verbalizes with difficulty
*Does not or cannot speak
Stuttering
Slurring
Difficulty forming words or sentences

Difficulty expressing thoughts verbally
Inappropriate verbalization
Dyspnea
Disorientation
(* Critical)

Related Factors (r/t)
Decrease in circulation to brain
Brain tumor
Physical barrier (tracheostomy, intubation)
Anatomical defect
Impaired hearing

Cleft palate
Psychological barriers (psychosis, lack of
   stimuli)
Cultural difference
Developmental or age related

Client Outcomes/Goals
✓ Uses effective communication techniques.
✓ Uses alternate methods of communication effectively.
✓ Client's verbal and nonverbal behavior are congruent.

Nursing Interventions
- Determine language spoken, obtain interpreter if possible or language dictionary.
- Listen carefully; validate verbal and nonverbal expressions and repeat and rephrase thoughts as needed
- Anticipate needs until effective communication is possible.
- Use simple communication; short sentences, nonverbal gestures; do not shout at client.
- Maintain eye contact at client's level; read client's lips as able; use touch as appropriate.
- Spend time with client; allow time for responses; keep call light readily available.
- Obtain communication devices, such as electronic device, letterboard, picture board, magic slate, or pencil and paper.
- Establish an alternative communication method, such as writing, pointing to letter, word phrase, or picture cards.
- Obtain order for speech therapy; supplement work of speech therapist with appropriate exercises.
- Give praise for progress noted, ignore mistakes, and watch for frustration, or fatigue.
- Encourage family to bring in familiar pictures, calendar.
- Establish understanding of client's use of symbolic speech (especially with schizophrenic clients).

Geriatric
- Encourage client to wear prescribed eyeglasses and hearing aid.
- Provide sufficient light, decrease background noise, and remove any distractions to increase communication.
- Allow time for thought comprehension when communicating with client.

Client/Family Teaching
- Teach client/family techniques to increase communication.
- Teach client how to utilize communication devices.

CONSTIPATION

Definition
A state in which an individual experiences a change in normal bowel habits characterized by a decrease in frequency or passage of hard dry stools.

Defining Characteristics
Decreased frequency of defecation, less than usual pattern
Hard, formed stool
Straining at stool
Feeling of rectal fullness and pressure
Abdominal pain
Palpable mass
Appetite impairment
Back pain
Headache
Interference with daily living
Use of laxatives

Related Factors (r/t)
Decreased activity level
Decreased fluid intake
Inadequate fiber in diet
Emotional disturbances
Lack of privacy
Embarrassment about defecating in hospital environment
Decreased peristalsis from hypokalemia, hypothyroidism
Side effects from antidepressant/antipsychotic therapy

Client Outcomes/Goals
✓ Soft, formed stool without straining every other day.
✓ States relief from discomfort of constipation.
✓ Identifies measures that prevent/treat constipation.

Nursing Interventions
- Observe usual pattern of defecation: time of day, usual stimulus, consistency, amount and frequency of stool.
- Monitor laxative use, diet, exercise pattern, and personal remedies for constipation.
- Palpate for abdominal distention, auscultate bowel sounds twice a day.
- Observe for medication cause of constipation: narcotics, antacids, iron, barium, antidepressants, or neuroleptics.
- Assess for anxiety, embarrassment regarding defecation.
- Force fluids to 3,000 cc/day within cardiac and renal reserve.
- Encourage ambulation; daily exercise program.
- Sprinkle bran over food at each meal as allowed by client and prescribed diet.
- Encourage intake of foods containing fiber: fresh fruits, vegetables, bran cereals.
- Check for impaction—digital removal per physician's order.
- Provide privacy for defecation, on commode or toilet, if possible.

147

- Provide laxative, suppository, or enema as needed per orders.
- Neurological client—consider putting on bowel routine of suppository every other day with physician's permission.

Geriatric

- Determine client's perception of normal bowel elimination; promote adherence to regular schedule.
- Explain valsalva maneuver and why it should be avoided.
- Respond quickly to client's call for help with toileting after laxative or suppository.
- If impaction, break up digitally and remove gently according to protocol, or physicians order.

Client/Family Teaching

- Encourage client to heed warning signs of need to defecate and develop a schedule of defecation at regular time, utilizing stimulus such as warm drink or prune juice.
- Recommend client avoid long-term use of laxatives, and enemas if they have been used consistently; withdraw their use gradually.
- Teach client how to do bent-leg situps, if not contraindicated, to increase abdominal tone; encourage to contract abdominal muscles frequently through the day.
- Teach need for foods with increased roughage and need for increased fluids.
- Develop with the client a daily exercise program to increase peristalsis.

COLONIC CONSTIPATION

Definition
The state in which an individual's pattern of elimination is characterized by hard, dry stools that result from a delay in passage of food residue.

Defining Characteristics

Major: Decreased frequency of defecation
Hard, dry stool
Straining at stool
Abdominal distention
Painful defecation
Palpable mass

Minor: Rectal pressure
Headache
Appetite impairment
Abdominal pain

Related Factors (r/t)

Inadequate fluid intake
Inadequate fiber in diet
Inadequate dietary intake
Decreased activity level
Immobility
Emotional disturbances
Stress
Lack of privacy
Change in daily routine

Decreased peristalsis from hypokalemia,
   hypocalcemia, or hypothyroidism
Decreased gastrointestinal motility from
   hormonal changes of pregnancy
Hesitancy or reluctance to pass stool secondary
   to previous experience with rectal fissures
   and/or bleeding
(Adapted from NANDA)

Client Outcomes/Goals, Nursing Interventions, and Client/Family Teaching
Refer to care plan for Constipation

PERCEIVED CONSTIPATION

Definition
The state in which an individual makes a self-diagnosis of constipation and ensures a daily bowel movement through abuse of laxatives, enemas, and suppositories.

Defining Characteristics
Expectation of a daily bowel movement with the resulting overuse of laxatives, enemas, and suppositories; expected passage of stool at same time every day.

Related Factors (r/t)
Cultural-family beliefs
Faulty appraisal
Impaired thought processes

Client Outcomes/Goals
✓ Defecates soft, formed stool without use of aids on usual schedule.
✓ Explains the need to decrease/eliminate use of laxatives, suppositories, enemas.
✓ Identifies measures that can ensure defecation other than laxatives, enemas, or suppositories.

Nursing Interventions
- Observe usual pattern of defecation: timing consistency, amount, and frequency of stool.
- Determine client's perception of appropriate defecation pattern.
- Monitor use of laxatives, suppositories, or enemas.
- Observe exercise pattern and diet, including intake of fluids.
- Observe motivation for abuse of laxatives, etc; allow to ventilate feelings about the subject.
- Force fluids to 3,000 cc/day within cardiac and renal reserve.
- Encourage increased activity; work with client to set daily activity goals.
- Sprinkle bran over food at each meal as allowed by client and prescribed diet.
- Obtain a dietary referral for analysis and input on diet.
- Provide privacy for defecation, avoiding use of bedpan if possible.
- Observe for potential body image disturbance; use of laxatives to control or decrease weight.

Geriatric
- Encourage prompt response to defecation reflex.
- Explain valsalva maneuver and why it should be avoided.
- Teach that it is not necessary to have daily bowel movements and that normal people range from 3 stools a day to 3 stools a week.

Client/Family Teaching
- Work with client/family to develop a diet that fits lifestyle and includes increased roughage-fiber.
- Explain to client the harmful effects of continued use of aids to defecation.

150

- Encourage client to gradually decrease use of usual laxatives or enemas; set date when client will be free of all aids to defecation.
- Determine how to increase fluid intake and fit practice into client's lifestyle.
- Work with client/family to design a bowel training routine based on previous pattern (before laxative, or enema abuse) with ingestion of warm fluid, privacy, predictable routine.

DEFENSIVE COPING

Definition
The state in which an individual repeatedly projects falsely positive self-evaluation based on a self-protective pattern that defends against underlying perceived threats to positive self-regard.

Defining Characteristics
Major: Denial of obvious problems/weakness
Projection of blame/responsibility
Rationalizes failures
Hypersensitive to slight/criticism
Grandiosity

Minor: Superior attitude toward others
Difficulty establishing and maintaining
  relationships
Hostile laughter or ridicule of others
Difficulty in reality testing perceptions
Lack of follow through or participation in
  treatment or therapy

Related Factors (r/t)
Situational crisis
Psychological impairment
Substance abuse

Client Outcomes/Goals
✓ Accepts responsibility for actions.
✓ Accepts constructive criticism of actions without personal rejection.
✓ Interacts with others in an appropriate fashion.
✓ Participates in treatment/therapy and establishes realistic goals.

Nursing Interventions
- Determine clients perception of the problem.
- Assist the client to identify the situations or people that trigger feelings of defensiveness.
- Monitor for symptoms of substance abuse: mood swings, changes in sleep patterns, personality changes, withdrawal, or gregarious behavior.
- Observe for anger, identify previous outlets for anger.
- Explore new outlets for anger: physical activity within client's capabilities, hitting a pillow, woodworking, sanding, or scrubbing floors.
- Encourage client to feel good about himself; use group therapy, individual therapy, role-playing, one-to-one interactions, and role modeling by the therapist.
- Provide feedback on others perception of client's behavior via group therapy, milieu therapy, or one-to-one interactions.
- Encourage client to use "I" statements and to accept responsibility for own actions and consequences of actions.

- Refer to community agency appropriate for dealing with substance abuse, such as Alcoholics Anonymous or Narcotics Anonymous.
- Refer client to appropriate therapist for grandiose symptoms that may be harmful, such as promiscuity, insomnia, euphoria, overspending, or alcohol/drug overuse.
- Work with client's support group to identify harmful behaviors and to seek help for client if they are unable to control behavior.

Geriatric
- Assess for signs of depression or dementia.

Client/Family Teaching
- If medications are indicated and ordered, teach action, side effects, and importance of taking medications daily as prescribed even when the client feels "good."
- Teach use of positive thinking; block negative thought with the word "stop" and insert positive thought, e.g., "I'm a good person, friend, student, and so on."

INEFFECTIVE INDIVIDUAL COPING

Definition

Impairment of adaptive behaviors and problem-solving abilities of a person in meeting life's demands and roles.

Defining Characteristics

*Verbalization of inability to cope or inability to ask for help

Inability to meet role expectations

Inability to meet basic needs

*Inability to problem solve

Alteration in societal participation

Destructive behavior toward self or others

Inappropriate use of defense mechanisms

Change in usual communication patterns

Verbal manipulation

High illness rate

High rate of accidents

(*Critical)

Related Factors (r/t)

Situational crises

Maturational crises

Personal vulnerability

Client Outcomes/Goals

✓ Verbalizes ability to cope and asks for help when needed.

✓ Demonstrates ability to solve problems and participates at usual level in society.

✓ Free of destructive behavior toward self or others.

✓ Able to communicate needs and negotiate with others to have them met.

✓ Able to discuss how recent life stress events have overwhelmed normal coping strategies.

✓ Illness and accident rate not excessive for age and developmental level.

Nursing Interventions

■ Observe causes, such as poor self-concept; grief; no problem-solving skills; lack of support; recent change in life situation.

■ Observe strengths, e.g., ability to relate facts; recognize source of stressors.

■ Monitor risk of self-harm or harming others and intervene appropriately. (Refer to nursing diagnosis *High Risk for Violence*.)

■ Assist client in setting realistic goals; identify personal skills and knowledge.

■ Encourage client to verbalize fears and express emotions.

■ Encourage client to participate in plan of care, schedule activities and make choices.

■ Provide mental and physical activities within client's ability, such as reading, exercise, TV, radio, or crafts.

■ Discuss changes with client before making them.

■ Discuss alternatives, power to change the situation, and the need to accept the situation.

- Help client to confront reality, e.g., equipment needed for care or viewing the dead body.
- Assist in expressing emotions, such as crying or anger (within appropriate limits).
- Avoid false reassurance, give honest answers, and provide only information requested.
- Encourage client to describe previous stress and coping mechanisms used.
- Be supportive of coping behaviors; allow time for relaxing.
- Refer for counseling as needed.

Geriatric
- Observe clients fear of illness and identify patterns elderly client has used in past response to stress; reinforce.
- Observe any physiological imbalance as a contributor to ineffective coping; take appropriate nursing actions to correct imbalance. (Notify physician of abnormal laboratory results; drug side effects or interactions.)
- Increase and mobilize support available to the older person.

Client/Family Teaching
- Teach problem solving: define the problem, the cause, and list the options, advantages, and disadvantages of choices made.
- Teach relaxation techniques.
- Teach about available community resources: therapist, minister, counselor, and self-help group.

DECISIONAL CONFLICT (SPECIFY)

Definition
The state of uncertainty about course of action to be taken when choice among competing actions involves risk loss or challenge to personal life values.

Defining Characteristics
Major: Verbalized uncertainty about choices
Verbalization of undesired consequences of alternative actions being considered
Vacillation between alternative choices
Delayed decision making
Minor: Verbalized feeling of distress while attempting a decision
Self-focusing
Physical signs of distress or tension (increased heart rate, increased muscle tension, restlessness)
Questioning personal values and beliefs while attempting a decision

Related Factors (r/t)
Unclear personal values/beliefs
Perceived threat to value system
Lack of experience or interference with decision making

Lack of relevant information
Support system deficit
Multiple or divergent sources of information

Client Outcomes/Goals
✓ Relates the advantages and disadvantages of choices.
✓ Shares fears and concerns regarding choices and responses of others.
✓ Makes an informed choice.

Nursing Interventions
- Observe causative/contributing factors to conflict, e.g., value conflict, fears of outcome, poor problem solving.
- Explore patient's perception of the future in relation to different decisions.
- Demonstrate unconditional respect and acceptance of client's values, spiritual beliefs, and cultural norms.
- Allow adequate time to make decisions.
- Encourage listing of advantages and disadvantages of alternatives.
- Initiate health teaching and referrals when indicated.
- Facilitate communication between family members regarding decision being made; offer support to person making final decision.
- Emphasize living/taking one day at a time.

Geriatric
- Explore with individual and family if have discussed and recorded client's end-of-life decisions.
- Describe the possible future dilemmas when these discussions are avoided.
- Discuss the purpose of a living will and durable power of attorney.
- Discuss choices to be made, e.g., moving into a nursing home, adult foster care home, or with adult children.
- Teach family members how to be supportive of final decision; if not able to be supportive, how to refrain from being destructive.

Client/Family Teaching
- Instruct the client and family members to provide directives in the following areas:
    Person to contact in an emergency
    Preference to die at home, hospital, or no preference
    Desire to sign a living will
    Decision on organ donation
    Funeral arrangements, burial, or cremation
- Help family identify long-term results and delayed decision making

INEFFECTIVE DENIAL

Definition
The state of a conscious or unconscious attempt to disavow the knowledge or meaning of an event to reduce anxiety/fear to the detriment of health.

Defining Characteristics
Major: Delays seeking or refuses health care attention to the detriment of health;
Does not perceive personal relevance of symptoms or danger
Minor: Uses home remedies (self-treatment) to relieve symptoms
Does not admit fear of death or invalidism
Minimizes symptoms
Displaces source of symptoms to other organs
Displaces fear of impact of the condition
Unable to admit impact of disease on life pattern
Makes dismissive gestures or comments when speaking of distressing events
Displays inappropriate affect

Related Factors (r/t)
Fear of consequences; chronic/terminal illness
Actual or perceived fear of possible loss of job, or significant other
Refusal to acknowledge substance abuse problem
Fear of the social stigma of disease

Client Outcomes/Goals
✓ Seeks out health care attention when needed.
✓ Uses home remedies only when appropriate.
✓ Displays appropriate affect, verbalizes fears.
✓ Recognizes relevance of symptoms and implications for well-being.
✓ Acknowledges substance abuse problem and seeks help.

Nursing Interventions
- Observe client's understanding of symptoms/illness.
- Spend one-on-one time with client to allow expression of use of denial; sit down at eye level and use touch if appropriate; touch client's hand or arm to convey empathy.
- Explain signs and symptoms of illness; reinforce use of prescribed treatment plan.
- Help client to recognize existing sources of support and additional sources of support; allow time for adjustment.
- Refer to skilled mental health counselor, if appropriate, for help in setting up planned "intervention" to confront client with continuing self destructive behavior: drinking, drugs, or eating disorder.
- Allow client to express feelings; acknowledge fear, e.g., "I sense that you may be feeling afraid."

- Give positive feedback when client follows appropriate treatment plan.
- Observe whether denial has been/is being used as coping mechanism in other areas of life.

Geriatric
- Identify recent losses of client; grieving may prolong denial.
- Encourage verbalization of feelings.

Client/Family Teaching
- Teach signs and symptoms of illness and appropriate response of client to illness of taking medication, going to the emergency room, calling the physician.
- If problem is substance abuse refer to appropriate community agency, e.g., Alcoholics Anonymous.

DIARRHEA

Definition
A state in which an individual experiences a change in normal bowel habits characterized by the frequent passage of loose, fluid, unformed stools.

Defining Characteristics
Abdominal pain and cramping

Increased frequency, urgency of defecation

Increased frequency of bowel sounds

Loose liquid stool with possible change in color

Related Factors (r/t)
Infection (viral, bacterial, protozoan)

Change in diet/food

Gastrointestinal disorders

Stress

Medication effect

Impaction

Client Outcomes/Goals
✓ Formed soft stool every other day.

✓ Rectal area free of irritation.

✓ States relief from cramping, decreased or no diarrhea.

✓ Explains cause of diarrhea and rationale for treatment.

✓ Good skin turgor, weight at usual level.

Nursing Interventions
- Observe cause of diarrhea: exposure to infected person, food, medication effect, tube feeding, antibiotics, abuse of laxatives. (Refer to Related Factors.)
- Observe and record number and consistency of stools per day.
- Inspect, palpate, percuss, and auscultate abdomen noting if frequent bowel sounds.
- Observe skin turgor over sternum and inspect oral cavity for longitudinal furrows of the tongue.
- Observe for symptoms of sodium and potassium loss: weakness, abdominal/leg cramping, dysrhythmias
- Monitor and record intake and output, note oliguria.
- Weigh daily and note decreased weight.
- Avoid use of medications that slow peristalsis if infectious diarrhea.
- Give clear fluids as tolerated: clear soda, Jell-O, Gatorade; serve fluids at lukewarm temperature.
- Add solid foods gradually, such as bananas, crackers, pretzels, rice, and applesauce. Avoid milk products and most fruits and vegetables.
- Provide readily available bed pan/commode/bathroom.
- Provide pericare and ointment to rectal area following each stool.
- If client is receiving tube feeding, note amount of sorbitol in liquid medications (causes diarrhea), dilute feeding per physicians order, note rate of infusion, prevent contamination of feeding by replacing container every 24 hours, rinsing container every 8 hours.

Geriatric
- Monitor closely to detect presence of impaction causing diarrhea; remove impaction as ordered.
- Seek medical attention if diarrhea is severe or persists more than 24 hours.
- Provide emotional support for client having trouble controlling unpredictable episodes of diarrhea.
- Observe for signs of dehydration and electrolyte imbalances.

Client/Family Teaching
- Encourage avoidance of coffee, spices, foods irritating or stimulating to GI tract.
- Teach appropriate method to take ordered antidiarrheal medications and explain side effects.
- Explain how to prevent spread of infectious diarrhea, e.g., careful handwashing and appropriate handling and storage of food.
- Assist client to determine causes of stress in life and set up appropriate stress reduction plan.
- Teach signs and symptoms of dehydration and electrolyte imbalance.

HIGH RISK FOR DISUSE SYNDROME

Definition
A state in which an individual is at risk for deterioration of body systems as the result of prescribed or unavoidable musculoskeletal inactivity.
Note: Complications from immobility can include pressure ulcer, constipation, stasis of pulmonary secretions, thrombosis, urinary tract infection/retention, decreased strength/endurance, orthostatic hypotension, decreased range of joint motion, disorientation, body image disturbance, and powerlessness.

Defining Characteristics
Presence of risk factors of:
Paralysis
Altered level of consciousness
Mechanical immobilization
Prescribed immobilization
Severe pain

Related Factors (r/t)
Refer to risk factors

Client Outcomes/Goals
✓ Maintains full range of motion in joints.
✓ Skin intact, good peripheral blood flow, normal pulmonary function.
✓ Maintains normal bowel and bladder function.
✓ Expresses feelings about imposed immobility.
✓ Explains methods that can be utilized to prevent complications of immobility.

Nursing Interventions
- Observe skin condition every two hours when turning client, assess thoroughly every 12 hours.
- Monitor peripheral circulation especially noting color, pulses, presence of any swelling in calf or thigh, check Homan's sign.
- Monitor respiratory function; note breath sounds, respiratory rate, percuss for new onset of dullness in lungs.
- Note bowel function daily.
- Apply antiembolism stockings if ordered, remove twice a day to provide skin care.
- Have client cough and deep breath or use incentive spirometry every 2 hours while awake.
- Provide pressure-relieving mattress; turn and position every 2 hours giving special attention to bony prominences.
- Do range of motion for all joints possible at least twice a day, preferably every 4 hours while awake (may vary with clients condition).

- Utilize high-top sneakers or specialized boots from Occupational Therapy to prevent footdrop; remove twice a day to provide foot care.
- Position so that joints are in normal anatomical alignment at all times.
- Get client up in chair as soon as appropriate, utilizing stretcher chair if necessary.
- Utilize tilt table to provide weight bearing on long bones if not contraindicated.
- Obtain assistive devices to help client reach and maintain as much mobility as possible.
- Force fluids to 2500 cc/day, within cardiac and renal reserve, to prevent kidney stones.
- Encourage intake of balanced diet with adequate amount of fiber and protein.

Note: Refer to *Constipation* for further nursing interventions to prevent constipation; *Alterations in Sensory Perception* for further interventions to prevent confusion; *Powerlessness* for further interventions for psychological impact of immobility.

Client/Family Teaching

- Teach complications of immobility.
- Teach to perform range of motion.
- Teach need to wiggle toes, do leg exercises, such as quadriceps, gluteal, and abdominal setting exercises every hour.
- Teach family how to turn and position client.

DIVERSIONAL ACTIVITY DEFICIT

Definition
The state in which an individual experiences a decreased stimulation from or interest or engagement in recreational or leisure activities.

Defining Characteristics
Client states is bored, wishes there was something to do
Usual hobbies cannot be undertaken in hospital

Related Factors (r/t)
Environmental lack of diversional activity, such as long-term hospitalization or frequent lengthy treatments.

Client Outcomes/Goals
Engages in personally satisfying diversional activities.

Nursing Interventions
- Observe ability to engage in activities requiring use of hands and good vision.
- Discuss activities that are interesting with client.
- Encourage client to share feelings about situation of inactivity away from usual hobbies.
- Encourage mix of physical and mental activities, e.g., crafts and watching videotapes.
- Encourage client to make a schedule of visitors so that not all present at once or at inconvenient times.
- Provide reading material, TV, radio, "Books on Tape."
- If able to write, have client keep a journal; if not able to write, have client tape record thoughts.
- Request occupational therapy referral to assist with providing diversional activities.
- Provide change in scenery and get client out of room as much as possible.
- If prolonged hospitalization, help client to "redecorate room," for example, with posters, banners, and balloons.
- Recommend participation in activities at home such as bird-watching or maintaining an aquarium; the client can watch and become involved with animals.
- Structure client's schedule around personal wishes for care and relaxing, fun activities.
- Schedule activities in gradually increasing time blocks; do not anticipate a total change in participation skills

Geriatric
- Encourage socialization with all age groups.
- Encourage involvement in senior citizen activities, such as AARP, YMCA, church groups, or Gray Panthers.
- Arrange transportation for elderly person to get to activities.
- Encourage client to use ability to help others with volunteer work.
- Provide environment that promotes activity, such as adequate lighting for crafts; allow periods of solitude with privacy.

- Utilize reminiscence therapy and provide time to listen.
- Encourage to learn a new skill or acquire new hobbies.

Client/Family Teaching
- Work with client/family to learn diversional activities that client desires, e.g., knitting, hooking rugs, or writing memoirs.

DYSREFLEXIA

Definition
The state in which an individual with a spinal cord injury at T7 or above experiences a life-threatening uninhibited sympathetic response of the nervous system to a noxious stimulus.

Defining Characteristics
Individual with spinal cord injury (T7 or above)

Major: Paroxysmal hypertension (sudden periodic elevated blood pressure >140/90 mm Hg), bradycardia or tachycardia (<60 or >100), diaphoresis (above the injury level), red splotches on skin above the injury, pallor on skin below the injury, or headache (diffuse pain in different portions of the head and not confined to any nerve distribution area)

Minor: Chilling

Conjunctival congestion

Horner's syndrome (contraction of pupil on one side, partial ptosis of the eyelid, recession of eyeball into the head, and sometimes loss of sweating over the affected side of the face)

Paresthesia

Pilomotor reflex (gooseflesh formation when skin is cooled)

Blurred vision

Chest pain

Metallic taste in mouth

Nasal congestion

Related Factors (r/t)
Bladder distention

Bowel distention

Skin irritation

Sexual stimulation

Lack of client's and caregiver's knowledge

Client Outcomes/Goals
✓ Vital signs normal or free of symptoms of dysreflexia.

✓ Explains symptoms, prevention, and treatment of dysreflexia.

Nursing Interventions
- Monitor for symptoms of dysreflexia. (Refer to defining characteristics of Dysreflexia.)
- Observe with physician cause of dysreflexia: distended bladder (most common cause), impaction, pressure sore, urinary calculi, bladder infection, acute abdomen, penile pressure, ingrown toenail, and so on.
- If present, place client in high-Fowlers position and remove all support hose or binders to promote venous pooling and decrease venous return, decreasing blood pressure.
- Initiate ordered antihypertensive therapy.

- Be careful not to increase stimuli; if ordered, use numbing agent on anus and 1 inch into rectum before an attempt is made to remove a fecal impaction; spray pressure sore with numbing agent, also use agent instilled into bladder.
- Monitor vital signs q _____ hours/minutes.
- Recognize that dysreflexia happens only when spinal shock has worn off and client is in spastic paralysis.

Client/Family Teaching
- Teach the pathophysiology of dysreflexia.
- Teach causes, prevention, symptoms, and treatment of dysreflexia.

INEFFECTIVE FAMILY COPING: COMPROMISED

Definition

A usually supportive primary person (family member or close friend) is providing insufficient, ineffective, or compromised support, comfort, assistance, or encouragement that may be needed by the client to manage or master adaptive tasks related to his or her health challenge.

Defining Characteristics

Subjective: Client expresses or confirms a concern or complaint about significant other's response to his or her health problem

Significant person describes preoccupation with personal reaction, (e.g., fear, anticipatory grief, guilt, anxiety, to client's illness, disability, or to other situational or developmental crises)

Significant person describes or confirms an inadequate understanding or knowledge base, which interfere with effective assistance or supportive behaviors

Objective: Significant person attempts assistive or supportive behaviors with less than satisfactory results

Significant person withdraws or enters into limited or temporary personal communication with the client at time of need

Significant person displays protective behavior disproportionate (too little or too much) to the client's abilities or need for autonomy

Related Factors (r/t)

Inadequate or incorrect information or understanding by a primary person

Temporary preoccupation by a significant person who is trying to manage emotional conflicts and personal suffering and is unable to perceive or act effectively in regard to clients needs

Temporary family disorganization and role changes

Other situational or developmental crises or situations the significant person my be facing

Little support provided by client, in turn, for primary person

Prolonged disease or disability progression that exhausts supportive capacity of significant people

Client Outcomes/Goals

✓ Family verbalizes resources within themselves to deal with situation.

✓ Family verbalizes knowledge and understanding of illness/disability/disease.

✓ Family provides support and assistance as needed.

✓ Family identifies need for and seeks outside support.

Nursing Interventions

- Observe for cause of family problems.
- Assess how family interacts.
- Help family to identify strengths; make a list that they can refer to for positive feedback.

- Encourage family members to verbalize feelings; spend time with them, sit down and make eye contact, offer coffee, and other nourishment (acceptance of nourishment indicates a beginning acceptance of situation).
- Talk with family about the importance of sharing feelings and ways to do this, such as role playing or writing a letter to significant other.
- Involve client and family in planning care as much as possible.
- Provide privacy during family visits; maintain flexible visiting hours, if possible, to accommodate more frequent family visits.
- Arrange staff assignments, if possible, so the same staff have contact with the family; familiarize other staff with the situation in the absence of usual staff spokesperson.
- Refer to appropriate resources for assistance as indicated, e.g., counseling, psychotherapy, financial, or spiritual.

Geriatric
- Assess needs of significant other, assist in meeting needs while visiting, e.g., diabetic—ensure meals are eaten.
- Assist in finding transportation to enable visiting family members.
- If unable to visit because homebound, encourage phone contact to provide ongoing scheduled progress reports.

Client/Family Teaching
- Provide information for family/significant others about specific illness/condition.

INEFFECTIVE FAMILY COPING: DISABLING

Definition

The behavior of a significant person (family member or other primary person) that disables his or her own capacities and the client's capacities to effectively address tasks essential to either person's adaptation to the health challenge.

Defining Characteristics

Neglectful care of the client in regard to basic human needs or illness treatment

Distortion of reality regarding the client's health problem, including extreme denial about its existence or severity

Intolerance

Rejection

Abandonment

Desertion

Carrying on usual routines, disregarding client's needs

Psychosomaticism

Taking on illness signs of client

Decisions and actions by family that are detrimental to economic or social well-being

Agitation, depression, aggression, or hostility

Impaired restructuring of a meaningful life for self

Impaired individualization, prolonged overconcern for client

Neglectful relationships with other family members

Client's development of helpless, inactive dependence

Related Factors (r/t)

Significant person with chronically unexpressed feelings of guilt, anxiety, hostility, or despair

Dissonant discrepancy of coping styles for dealing with adaptive tasks by the significant person and client or among significant people

Highly ambivalent family relationships

Arbitrary handling of family's resistance to treatment, which tends to solidify defensiveness as it fails to deal adequately with underlying anxiety

Client Outcomes/Goals

✓ Family and significant others express realistic understanding and expectations of the client.

✓ Family participates positively in the care of the client, within limits of their abilities.

✓ Significant other(s) are expressing feelings openly and honestly, as appropriate.

Nursing Interventions

■ Observe for causative, contributing factors.

■ Identify pre-illness behaviors/interactions of the family.

- Identify current behaviors of family members, e.g., withdrawal (not visiting, brief visits, or ignoring client when visiting), anger, and hostility toward client and others, as well as expressions of guilt.
- Note other stressors in family (inadequate finances, work stress).
- Encourage family to verbalize feelings.
- Provide a role model for those interpersonal skills that will assist the family to improve their verbal interaction.
- Provide structure for family interaction, such as length of visiting time, number of members at visiting, and content of interaction.
- Assist family to identify personal strengths and health care needs of client/family unit.
- Provide continuity of care by maintaining effective communication between staff members and initiate a multidisciplinary client care conference involving the client/family in problem solving.
- Explore available hospital and community resources with family.
- Observe for any symptoms of elder or child abuse or neglect.

Geriatric
- Refer family to appropriate community resources, e.g., senior centers, medicare assistance, and meal programs.
- If abuse or neglect is an issue, report to Social Services.
- Encourage family members to participate in appropriate support group, e.g., COPD, Arthritis, I Can Cope, or Alzheimer's Support Group.
- Teach family management techniques of common problems related to normal aging.

Client/Family Teaching
- Discuss with family appropriate ways to demonstrate feelings.
- Teach family those skills required for care of client.

FAMILY COPING: POTENTIAL FOR GROWTH

Definition

Effective managing of adaptive tasks by family member involved with the client's health challenge, who now is exhibiting desire and readiness for enhanced health and growth in regard to self and in relation to the client.

Defining Characteristics

Family member attempting to describe growth aspect of crisis on his or her own values, priorities, goals or relationships

Family member moving in direction of health promoting and enriching lifestyle that supports and monitors maturational processes, audits and negotiates treatment programs, and generally chooses experiences that optimize wellness

Individual expressing interest in making contact on a one-to-one basis or on a mutual aid group basis with another person who has experienced a similar situation

Related Factors (r/t)

Needs sufficiently gratified and adaptive tasks effectively addressed to enable goals of self-actualization to surface

Client Outcomes/Goals

✓ Family states a plan for family's growth.
✓ Family is able to perform tasks needed for change.
✓ Family states positive effects of changes made.

Nursing Interventions

- Observe skills family possesses to initiate change; positive attitude, and statement of hope that change is possible.
- Allow family time to verbalize their concerns; provide one-to-one interaction with the family.
- Have family share responsibilities for change and encourage all members to have input.
- Have family write down their goals.
- Explore with family ways to attain their goals, such as adult education classes, enrichment courses, and family activities, e.g, sports, cooking, reading, and sharing time together.
- Encourage "fun time," or time with no tasks, i.e., just time to enjoy each other's company. (Might need to set up a schedule to do this since most have busy lives).
- Help family to communicate with each other by using techniques they are comfortable with e.g., role-playing, letter writing, or tape recording messages.

Geriatric:

- Encourage family members of the elderly to reminisce with the older person.
- Start and maintain a log of anecdotal stories of older member of the family.
- Encourage children in family to spend time and share activities with older persons.

172

Client/Family Teaching
- Teach that it is normal for changes in families and family relationships to occur.
- Refer to parenting classes and classes for coping with older parents.
- Identify groups with similar problems and concerns, such as Al-Anon or I Can Cope.
- Teach family communication skills, e.g., use of "I" messages and actively listening to each other.
- Teach the importance of establishing and following rituals, such as special celebrations on birthdays, holidays, and trips together.

ALTERED FAMILY PROCESSES

Definition
The state in which a family that normally functions effectively experiences a dysfunction.

Defining Characteristics
Family system unable to meet physical, emotional, or spiritual needs of its members
Parents do not demonstrate respect for each other's views on child-rearing practices
Inability to express/accept wide range of feelings
Inability to express/accept feelings of members
Family unable to meet security needs of its members
Inability of the family members to relate to each other for mutual growth and maturation
Family uninvolved in community activities
Inability to accept/receive help appropriately
Rigidity in function and roles
A family not demonstrating respect for individuality and autonomy of its members
Family unable to adapt to change/deal with traumatic experience constructively
Family failing to accomplish current/past developmental tasks
Unhealthy family decision-making process
Failure to send and receive clear messages
Inappropriate boundary maintenance
Inappropriate/poorly communicated family rules, rituals, or symbols
Unexamined family myths
Inappropriate level and direction of energy

Related Factors (r/t)
Situation transition or crisis
Developmental transition or crisis

Client Outcomes/Goals
✓ Family members are able to express feelings.
✓ Family identifies ways to cope effectively; utilizes appropriate support systems.
✓ Family will treat impaired family member as normally as possible to avoid overdependence.
✓ Family states knowledge of illness/injury, treatment modalities, and prognosis.
✓ Impaired family member participates in the development of the plan of care to the best of his ability.
✓ Family able to define boundaries, rules, and appropriate rituals.

Nursing Interventions
▪ Observe cause of change in family's normal pattern of functioning.
▪ Spend time with family: sit down and allow them to verbalize feelings.

- Acknowledge the stages of grief when there is a change in health status of a family member and accept the stage family is in; tell them it is "normal" to be angry.
- Encourage family to list their personal strengths.
- Discuss with family how they handled crises in the past.
- Encourage the family to visit client, adjust visiting hours to accommodate family's schedule, e.g., work, school, or babysitting needs.
- Help to arrange sleeping areas if family is spending the night; provide a place to lie down, and pillows and blankets.
- Encourage the family to assist in the client's care.
- Have family participate in client conferences that involve all members of the health team.
- Refer to appropriate support if needed, e.g., counseling, social services, self-help groups, or pastoral care.

Geriatric
- Teach family members about impact of developmental events, e.g., retirement, death, change in health status, and household composition.
- Support group problem solving among family members, including the older or ill member.
- Refer for family counseling with a psychotherapist with knowledge of gerontology.

Client/Family Teaching
- Identify community agencies that might be helpful, such as Meals on Wheels, Respite care (agency to provide care for the caregiver), or I Can Cope (group for clients diagnosed with cancer).
- Teach family how to care for client, give medications, and administer treatments.

FATIGUE

Definition
An overwhelming sustained sense of exhaustion and decreased capacity for physical and mental work.

Defining Characteristics
Major: Verbalization of an unremitting and overwhelming lack of energy
Inability to maintain usual routines
Minor: Perceived need for additional energy to accomplish routine tasks
Increase in physical complaints
Emotionally labile or irritable
Impaired ability to concentrate
Decreased performance
Lethargic or listless
Disinterest in surroundings/introspection
Decreased libido
Accident prone

Related Factors (r/t)
Decreased/increased metabolic energy production
Overwhelming psychological or emotional demands
Increased energy requirements to perform activities of daily living
Excessive social or role demands
States of discomfort
Altered body chemistry (e.g., medications, drug withdrawal, or chemotherapy)

Client Outcomes/Goals
✓ Verbalizes the signs and symptoms of fatigue.
✓ Describes the effects of fatigue on activities of daily living, role responsibilities, and relationships.
✓ Has ability to maintain usual routines.
✓ Able to concentrate and has interest in surroundings.
✓ Identifies activities that reduce or decrease fatigue.

Nursing Interventions
- Observe client's fatigue patterns.
- Determine the effect of client's fatigue on daily activities.
- Schedule and coordinate procedures and activities to restrict energy outlay.
- Set realistic, attainable goals for increased activity.
- Schedule rest periods between activities.
- Provide assistance with ADL when necessary.

- Avoid procedures during scheduled rest periods; encourage family members to observe client's rest periods and to schedule visitations at other times.
- Enlist support of family members to assist client with activities that cause fatigue for the client.

Geriatric
- Identify recent losses; monitor for depression as a possible contributing factor to fatigue.

Client/Family Teaching
- Teach how to recognize the signs and symptoms of fatigue.
- Teach strategies for energy conservation (sitting instead of standing during activities, such as showering, planning activities ahead of time, having all materials assembled for a task to save steps, and storing items at waist level).
- Teach the importance of following a healthy lifestyle to decrease fatigue; need for adequate diet, rest, and exercise.
- Teach that it is OK to limit social and role demands and that sometimes it is better to just say no when there are multiple time demands.

FEAR

Definition
Feeling of dread related to an identifiable source that the person validates.

Defining Characteristics
Ability to identify object of fear
Wide-eyed, trembling, tachycardia, diaphoresis, hyperventilation (adapted from Carpenito)

Related Factors (r/t)
Stressor from the environment
Hospitalization
Treatments
Pain
Powerlessness

Separation from support system
Language barrier
Sensory impairment
Real or imagined threat to own well-being
Knowledge deficit
(Adapted from Carpenito)

Client Outcomes/Goals
✓ Verbalizes fears that are known.
✓ States accurate information about the situation.
✓ Demonstrates coping behaviors that may decrease fear.
✓ Demonstrates appropriate feelings and lessened fear.

Nursing Interventions
- Discuss situation with client and help him to distinguish between real and imagined threat to his well-being.
- Allow client to communicate the source of fear and convey acceptance of his perception; determine factors that stimulated fear originally.
- If possible, remove the source of the client's fear.
- Stay with the client when they express fear, provide verbal and nonverbal (touch and hug with permission) reassurances for their safety if it is within your control.
- Provide explanations for the client regarding hospital treatment and routines.
- Provide opportunity for questions and answer truthfully.
- Recognize the client's fear and convey acceptance for expression of feelings.
- Allow client to gain control by involving in planning of nursing care.

Geriatric
- Establish a trusting relationship so all fears are identified; an older persons response to a real fear may be immobilizing.
- Intervene to increase clients knowledge, competence, or awareness of the feared situation or object.
- Identify others who can be involved in resolving client's fear, e.g., social worker who can inform client of resources available.

Client/Family Teaching
- Teach reality and support for dealing with what's real.
- Assist client to learn and practice relaxation, visualization, and guided imagery if they are able.
- Instruct about social services available and crisis intervention if needed.
- If antianxiety medications are ordered, teach client appropriate use.

FLUID VOLUME DEFICIT

Definition
The state in which an individual experiences vascular, cellular, or intracellular dehydration.

Defining Characteristics
Change in urine output
Change in urine concentration
Sudden weight loss or gain
Decreased venous filling
Hemoconcentration
Change in serum sodium
Hypotension
Thirst

Increased pulse rate
Decreased skin turgor
Decreased pulse volume/pressure
Change in mental state
Increased body temperature
Dry skin
Dry mucous membranes
Weakness

Related Factors (r/t)
Active fluid volume loss
Failure of regulatory mechanisms

Client Outcomes/Goals
✓ Client's intake equals output.
✓ Blood pressure, pulse, CVP, PWP are within normal range.
✓ Good skin turgor, moist mucous membranes, +1200 cc urine output for 24 hours.
✓ Explains measures that can be taken to treat or prevent fluid volume loss.
✓ Laboratory values within normal limits.
✓ Free of dizziness with position change.

Nursing Interventions
- Observe cause of deficit, such as vomiting, nausea, diarrhea, difficulty swallowing or feeding self, active blood loss, high osmotic tube feeding, depression, fatigue, extreme heat, enemas or diuretics.
- Check vital signs frequently if unstable, especially pulse rate and blood pressure; take blood pressure lying and standing if client not too dizzy or weak.
- Check peripheral pulses; note quality and presence.
- Strict I & O, daily weight; note pattern of decreasing weight with I < O.
- Note amount, color, and specific gravity of urine; if fluid loss acute, do hourly urine measurement.
- Monitor mental status; note any confusion, restlessness, anxiety or syncope.
- Encourage fluid intake of 2000 to 3000 cc/day if not contraindicated; note taste preferences.
- Monitor laboratory values, such as sodium, potassium, hematocrit, serum and urine osmolarity, BUN, and creatinine.
- Check skin turgor, color, and warmth.

- Check for dryness in mouth especially longitudinal furrows on the tongue.
- Medicate for nausea, vomiting, or diarrhea promptly as ordered by physician.
- If receiving IVs at a rapid rate, assess carefully for onset of fluid overload with crackles in lungs, dyspnea, or bounding pulse.

Nursing Interventions for Client in Hypovolemic Shock
- If BP very low, position flat in bed with legs elevated.
- Monitor vital signs frequently, every 15 to 60 minutes as needed.
- Monitor hemodynamic parameters: CVP, RAP, PWP.
- Utilize pulse oximeter and note oxygen saturation continuously; administer oxygen as ordered.
- Do hourly urine; report if urine output is less than 30 cc/hour or greater than 200 cc/hour .
- Watch continuously for any further fluid loss from any source.
- Monitor continuously for worsening of shock, such as cold clammy skin, confusion, or absence of peripheral pulses.
- Administer fluids at rapid rate as ordered; recognize should replace fluid volume before giving vasoconstrictive medications such as dopamine.

Geriatric
- Offer fluid regularly with direct approach to clients with cognitive impairment; elderly have decreased thirst sensation.
- Incorporate regular hydration into daily routines, e.g., extra glass of fluid with medication, social activities.
- Recognize that elderly can easily go from fluid deficit to fluid overload because of decreased compensatory mechanisms.

Client/Family Teaching
- Teach importance of regular fluid intake.
- Teach symptoms of fluid volume deficit and steps to take if symptoms should occur.

HIGH RISK FOR FLUID VOLUME DEFICIT

Definition
The state in which an individual is at risk of experiencing vascular, cellular, or intracellular dehydration.

Defining Characteristics
Presence of risk factors such as:
Extremes of age
Extremes of weight
Excessive losses through normal routes, e.g., diarrhea
Loss of fluids through abnormal routes, e.g., indwelling tubes
Deviations affecting access to or intake or absorption of fluids, e.g., physical immobility
Factors influencing fluid needs, e.g., hypermetabolic state
Knowledge deficiency related to fluid volume
Medication effect, e.g., diuretics

Related Factors (r/t)
Refer to risk factors

Client Outcomes/Goals, Nursing Interventions, and Client/Family Teaching
Refer to Nursing Diagnosis *Fluid Volume Deficit*

FLUID VOLUME EXCESS

Definition
The state in which an individual experiences increased fluid retention and edema.

Defining Characteristics
Edema
Effusion
Anasarca
Weight gain
Dyspnea
Orthopnea
Crackles in lungs
S3 heart sound
Pulmonary congestion on chest x-ray
Intake greater than output

Jugular vein distention
Positive hepatojugular reflex
Decreased hemoglobin, hematocrit, or serum
   osmolarity
Specific gravity changes
Altered electrolytes
Oliguria
Azotemia
Restlessness and anxiety
(Adapted from NANDA)

Related Factors (r/t)
Compromised regulatory mechanism
Excess fluid intake
Excess sodium intake

Client Outcomes/Goals
✓ Clear breath sounds, vital signs within normal range.
✓ Free of edema and effusion; weight appropriate for client; intake equals output.
✓ Explains methods to use to prevent fluid volume excess.

Nursing Interventions
- Determine cause of fluid volume excess: excessive fluid or sodium intake, renal dysfunction, cardiac dysfunction, or hepatic cirrhosis.
- Daily weight, I & O; note any pattern of increased intake and decreased output, increasing weight.
- Take vital signs, noting especially increasing or decreasing blood pressure.
- Evaluate hemodynamic parameters; note especially increasing CVP, RAP, PWP, and change in cardiac output.
- Monitor for edema: feet, shins, puffy eyelids, and sacral area if on bedrest.
- Observe for heart failure, e.g., crackles in lungs, gallop rhythm, NVD, or dyspnea. If present, refer to Nursing Diagnosis *Decreased Cardiac output.*
- Monitor for ascites; note any abdominal distention, presence of shifting dulless on percussion, or fluid wave with palpation.
- Observe for confusion and restlessness from decreased sodium, use safety precautions if present.

- Note laboratory results of sodium, potassium, hemoglobin, hematocrit, BUN, creatinine, serum albumin, total protein, serum osmolarity, and urine osmolarity.
- Keep all IV fluids on IV control pump.
- Check to ensure receives low-sodium diet, encourage protein intake.
- Maintain ordered fluid restriction; have client help determine how restricted fluids can best be allotted during the 24 hours.

Geriatric
- Recognize that edema in the elderly can be caused by malnutrition, note serum albumin levels.

Client/Family Teaching
- Teach importance of fluid and sodium restriction, and how to live with restriction.
- Explain symptoms of fluid overload and actions to take if they occur.

IMPAIRED GAS EXCHANGE

Definition

The state in which an individual experiences decreased passage of oxygen or carbon dioxide between the alveoli of the lungs and the vascular system.

Defining Characteristics

Confusion
Somnolence
Restlessness
Irritability

Inability to move secretions
Hypercapnea
Hypoxia

Related Factors (r/t)

Ventilation perfusion imbalance

Client Outcomes/Goals

✓ Maintains a patent airway at all times.
✓ Blood gases within client's normal parameters.
✓ Lung fields clear and free of signs of respiratory distress.
✓ Verbalizes understanding of oxygen and other therapeutic interventions.

Nursing Interventions

- Maintain patent airway, position appropriately, provide oropharyngeal airway if tongue is obstructing airway.
- Monitor breath sounds and respiratory pattern.
- Monitor respiratory rate, depth, and effort to include use of accessory muscles and nasal flaring.
- Monitor mental status; changes in mentation are early signs of impaired gas exchange.
- Observe cough pattern.
- Monitor vital signs.
- Observe for cyanosis, especially of oral mucous membranes.
- Obtain and interpret blood gas results; utilize pulse oximeter to monitor oxygen saturation.
- Administer appropriate medications, e.g., bronchodilators, diuretics, steroids, antibiotics, and anticoagulants as ordered.
- Administer intravenous fluids as indicated.
- Encourage deep breathing and coughing, use of incentive spirometer every _____ hrs.
- Change positions at frequent intervals.
- Monitor the effects of sedation, narcotics, and analgesics on respiratory pattern.
- Schedule nursing care to provide rest and minimize fatigue.
- Administer humidified oxygen through appropriate device, e.g., nasal cannula or face mask per physicians order.
- Provide adequate fluids to liquefy secretions.

- Explain procedures to client to decrease anxiety.
- Keep environment free of pollutant and allergy causing substances; caregivers avoid use of perfume.

Geriatric

- Use CNS depressants carefully because elderly are more prone to respiratory depression.
- Monitor blood gases (elderly normally have somewhat lower saturation and PaO_2).
- Maintain low-flow oxygen therapy because elderly clients are more susceptible to oxygen-induced respiratory depression.

Client/Family Teaching

- Inform client and significant others of therapeutic plans and care approach.
- Teach client the importance of conserving energy and planning rest periods into activities.
- Teach client and family the importance of not smoking; refer to smoking cessation programs.
- Instruct client and family on home care regime and refer to social services if necessary for special home therapy.
- Instruct family about home oxygen therapy: maintenance of system, flow rate, and safety precautions. (Refer to care plan for *Ineffective Airway Clearance*.)

GRIEVING

Definition
A state in which an individual or group of individuals reacts to an actual or perceived loss. This loss may be of a person, object, function, status, relationship, or body part.

Defining Characteristics
Verbal expression of distress at loss
Anger
Sadness
Crying
Difficulty in expressing loss
Alterations in: eating habits, sleep patterns, dream patterns, activity level, libido
Reliving of past experiences
Interference with life functioning
Alterations in concentration and/or pursuits of tasks

Related Factors (r/t)
Actual or perceived object loss (object loss is used in the broadest sense)
Object may include: people, possessions, a job, status, home, ideals, parts, and processes of the body

Client Outcomes/Goals
✓ Expresses feelings of guilt, fear, anger, sadness.
✓ Identifies problems associated with grief: changes in appetite, insomnia, loss of libido, decreased energy, and alteration in activity level.
✓ Plans for future one day at a time; identifies personal strengths.
✓ Functions at normal developmental level and performs tasks of daily living.

Nursing Interventions, Teaching
• If grief is from dying loved one, encourage family members to stay with client during dying process.
• Allow family members to participate in care of the body as desired. Help survivors say good-bye in the most loving and caring way possible.
• Encourage and support sharing memories of loved one with others.
• Provide spiritual counseling if desired.
Refer to Nursing Interventions and Client/Family Teaching for *Anticipatory Grieving*.

Note: Grieving is not an official NANDA nursing diagnosis. The authors have used this nursing diagnosis because we feel that grieving is part of the normal human response to loss, and nurses can utilize interventions to help the client grieve.

ANTICIPATORY GRIEVING

Definition
The state in which an individual/group experiences feelings in response to an expected significant loss (Adapted from Carpenito).

Defining Characteristics
Potential loss of significant object
Expression of distress at potential loss
Denial of potential loss
Guilt
Anger
Sorrow

Choked feelings
Changes in eating habits
Alterations in sleep patterns
Alterations in activity level
Altered libido
Altered communication patterns

Related Factors (r/t)
Perceived or actual state of impending loss of object, people, possessions, a job, status, home, ideals, or parts and processes of the body (Adapted from Carpenito).

Client Outcomes/Goals
✓ Expresses feelings of guilt, anger, or sorrow.
✓ Identifies problems associated with anticipatory grief; changes in activity, eating, or libido.
✓ Seeks help in dealing with anticipated problems.
✓ Plans for the future one day at a time.

Nursing Interventions
- Observe cause/contributing factors of potential loss.
- Monitor the stage of grief, e.g., anger, denial, bargaining, depression, or acceptance.
- Use therapeutic communication; open-ended questions, such as "What are your thoughts and fears?" "How might this anticipated change affect your lifestyle?"
- Use silence, touch (with permission), or sit and make eye contact if possible.
- Review past experiences, role changes, coping skills, and strengths.
- Include family/significant others when providing support and helping to cope.
- Acknowledge that feelings are real; encourage expression.
- Permit expressions of anger, and fear, free of judgment.
- Be honest; do not give false reassurance.
- Expect client to meet responsibilities; give positive reinforcement.
- Discuss control issues, e.g., what is changeable or is outside of client's control.
- Identify problems of eating, activity level, sexual desire, sleep, and so on.
- Identify support systems: family, friends, groups, therapist, minister.

Geriatric
- Observe any changes in mood, physical condition, supportive contacts, or financial status.
- Use reminiscent therapy in conjunction with expression of emotions.

Client/Family Teaching
- Refer to community support, such as counseling, psychotherapy, or bereavement groups.
- Teach that use of sedatives/tranquilizers may delay the expression of loss.
- Instruct in the process of organ donation, if appropriate; refer to organ procurement group.

DYSFUNCTIONAL GRIEVING

Definition
A state in which an individual or group of individuals reacts to an actual or perceived loss. This loss may be a person, an object, a function, status, relationship, or body part. The reaction may be absent, delayed, exaggerated, or prolonged and the individual(s) may engage in detrimental activities (Adapted from Carpenito).

Defining Characteristics:
Verbal expression of distress at loss
Denial of loss
Expression of guilt, unresolved issues
Anger
Sadness
Crying
Difficulty in expressing loss
Alterations in: eating habits, sleep patterns, dream
    patterns, activity level, or libido

Idealization of lost object
Reliving of past experiences
Interference with life functioning
Developmental regression
Labile affect
Alterations in concentration or pursuit of tasks

Related Factors (r/t)
Actual or perceived object loss (object loss is used in the broadest sense)
Objects may include people, possessions, a job, status, home, ideals, or parts and processes of the body

Client Outcomes/Goals
✓ Expresses feelings of guilt, fear, anger, or sadness.
✓ Identifies problems associated with grief, such as changes in appetite, insomnia, nightmares, loss of libido, decreased energy, and alteration in activity level.
✓ Seeks help in dealing with problems associated with grief.
✓ Plans for future one day at a time; identifies personal strengths.
✓ Functions at normal developmental level and performs tasks of daily living.

Nursing Interventions
▪ Observe stage of grief, e.g., anger, denial, bargaining, depression, or acceptance.
▪ Review past experiences, role changes, and coping skills.
▪ Use therapeutic communication, e.g., active listening or silence.
▪ Include family/significant others in support or coping; help them express their feelings.
▪ Identify client's strengths, support systems; reinforce them.
▪ Encourage verbalization of feelings; be accepting and nonjudgmental.
▪ Assure that someone stays with client; be aware of own feelings.

- If grief from client death, allow family members to view the body and if they desire, encourage touching and holding.
- Expect client to meet responsibilities; give positive reinforcement.
- Identify problems of eating, activity level, or sexual desire.
- Do not give false reassurance; discuss issues honestly.
- Identify level of depression or suicide risk.

Geriatric
- Observe for following reactions:
  -Delayed: the bereaved exhibits little emotion and continues with a busy life
  -Inhibited: the bereaved exhibits various physical conditions and doesn't feel grief
  -Chronic: the behaviors of the normal grief periods continue
- Identify previous losses and assess client for depression; losses and changes in older age often occur in rapid succession without adequate recovery time.
- Refer as needed to specialist for assistance in dealing with abnormal grief; studies of the elderly bereaved show that those who have poor outcomes do not live with family members. Continued emotional support is needed; arrange for social support.
- Use reminiscent therapy in conjunction with expression of emotions.

Client/Family Teaching
- Refer to community support, such as Reach to Recovery, bereavement groups, or psychotherapy.
- Caution that use of sedatives may delay expressions of loss.
- Assist client to identify ways of modifying lifestyle to adapt to loss.
- Teach about stages of grief and that feelings associated with grief are normal.
- Assist with future planning or funeral arrangements.

ALTERED GROWTH AND DEVELOPMENT

Definition
The state in which an individual demonstrates deviations in norms from his/her age group.

Defining Characteristics
Major: Delay or difficulty in performing skills (motor, social, or expressive) typical of age group; altered physical growth; inability to perform self-care or self-control activities appropriate for age.
Minor: Flat affect; listlessness; decreased responses.

Related factors (r/t)
Inadequate caretaking
Indifference, inconsistent responsiveness, multiple caretakers
Separation from significant others
Environmental and stimulation deficiencies
Effects of physical disability
Prescribed dependence

Client Outcomes/Goals
✓ Caregivers will identify normal patterns of growth and development.
✓ Caregivers will provide child with activities which support age related developmental tasks.
✓ Child will demonstrate an increase in behaviors (social, interpersonal, cognitive) and motor activities appropriate to age.

Nursing Interventions
- Assist caregivers to identify possible causative, contributing factors (refer to related factors).
- Identify learning opportunities in child's environment and work with caregivers to utilize all resources.
- Involve child in decision making according to maturity.
- Encourage independence with positive feedback.
- Incorporate age-appropriate activities into plan of care: *Infants:* cuddling, rocking,mobiles, rattles, talk, sing, smile. Place on floor, protect child and allow to roll, sit, creep. *Toddler/Preschool:* sing alongs, stuffed toys, dolls, books, push-pull toys, coloring puzzles. Encourage self-feeding and dressing. *School-age:* bedside school work or school room, books, puzzles, crafts, board games, video games, same sex and age roommates. Encourage self-care. *Adolescent:* provide privacy. Encourage expression of feelings, ideas about condition and care. Identify and allow for hobbies, appropriate activities, such as music, movies, interaction with others of same age range. Encourage street clothes, personal self-care.

Client/Family Teaching
- Teach caregivers appropriate patterns of growth of growth and development; provide reading material or video on subject.

- Teach activities that are age-appropriate and support growth and development, including safety considerations.
- Assist family to identify regressive behaviors and how best to assist child to move on and through regression.
- Teach positive behavior modification techniques.
- Give information about community resources: support groups, parenting classes, child care professionals.

ALTERED HEALTH MAINTENANCE

Definition
Inability to identify, manage, or seek out help to maintain health.

Defining Characteristics
Demonstrated lack of knowledge regarding basic health practices
Demonstrated lack of adaptive behaviors to internal/external environmental changes
Reported or observed inability to take responsibility for meeting basic health practices in any or all functional pattern areas
History of lack of health seeking behavior
Expressed interest in improving health behaviors
Reported or observed lack of equipment, financial or other resources
Reported or observed impairment of personal support systems

Related Factors (r/t)
Lack of, or significant alteration in, communication skills (written, verbal, or gestural)
Lack of ability to make deliberate and thoughtful judgments
Perceptual-cognitive impairment (complete-partial lack of gross and/or fine motor skills)
Ineffective individual coping
Dysfunctional grieving
Unachieved developmental tasks
Ineffective family coping
Disabling spiritual distress
Lack of material resources
Substance abuse

Client Outcomes/Goals
✓ Follows mutually agreed on health care maintenance plan.
✓ Meets goals for health care maintenance.

Nursing Interventions
- Observe client's feelings, values, reasons for not following prescribed plan of care (refer to related factors).
- Encourage client to share feelings about change in health status and effects on life.
- Determine what the client feels is the most important aspect of the health care plan, and start teaching and reinforcement in that area if possible.
- Have client identify at least two significant support people and have them attend any teaching sessions if possible.
- Help client determine how he can fit change in health care plan into daily schedule, e.g., take pills before breakfast and dinner every day.

- Refer client to community agencies for appropriate follow-up care; day treatment or adult day health program.
- Observe client's knowledge of illness, treatment, and cognitive ability to follow through with treatment recommended.
- Obtain or design educational material that is appropriate for the client, utilizing pictures if possible.
- Make sure follow-up appointments are scheduled before client is discharged; discuss with client how to ensure he keeps the appointment(s).
- Refer to social services for financial assistance.

Geriatric

- Provide aids to assist with compliance, e.g., prepare medication schedules, and prepare week's medications in daily containers.
- Assess barriers to compliance, e.g., no transportation for follow-up visits.
- Recognize resistance to change in life-long patterns of personal health care.
- Set realistic goals with client's input for changes in health maintenance.

Client/Family Teaching

- Teach client/family prescribed health care treatment, e.g., medications, treatments, diet, ADL, methods of coping, and when to seek help.
- Teach nonthreatening material before more anxiety producing information is given.
- Have client/family give a return demonstration, at least twice, of any procedures to be done at home.
- Establish a written contract with client to follow agreed on health care plan.

HEALTH SEEKING BEHAVIORS (SPECIFY)

Definition
A state in which an individual in stable health is actively seeking ways to alter personal health habits, and/or the environment to move toward a higher level of health. *Note*: Stable health status is defined as age-appropriate illness prevention measures achieved, client reports good or excellent health, and signs and symptoms of disease, if present, are controlled.

Defining Characteristics
Major: Expressed or observed desire to seek a higher level of wellness for self or family
Minor: Expressed or observed desire for increased control of health practice
Expression of concern about current environmental conditions of health status
Stated or observed unfamiliarity with wellness community resources
Demonstrated or observed lack of knowledge in health promotion behaviors

Related Factors (r/t)
Role changes
Change in developmental level (marriage, parenthood, "empty-nest" syndrome, or retirement)
Lack of knowledge of need for preventive health behaviors, appropriate health screening, optimum nutrition and weight control, regular exercise program, stress management, supportive social network, and responsible role participation
(Adapted from Carpenito).

Client Outcomes/Goals
✓ Maintains ideal weight and is knowledgeable of nutritious diet.
✓ Explains how to fit newly prescribed change in health habits into lifestyle.
✓ Lists community resources available for assistance in achieving wellness.

Nursing Interventions
- Determine client/families health habits including diet, pattern of exercise, sleep pattern, amount of stress, smoking, drinking, preventative care for health.
- Determine with client the most important change in health behavior to be worked on at this time.

Nutrition
- Determine height, weight; compare with recommended weight for age, or size.
- Encourage to eat diet that is low in salt, fat, sugar, and preservatives; encourage intake of complex carbohydrates, fruits, vegetables, and appropriate amount of protein and fat.
- Refer to dietician or weight loss program for further assessment of diet; help with weight loss or gain if appropriate.

Exercise
- Determine amount of exercise client obtains per week and ability to tolerate exercise; refer to physician for testing to determine ability to tolerate exercise.

- Encourage aerobic exercise that increases heart rate within prescribed limit; exercise at least 3 times per week for 30 or more minutes, utilizing exercise that is preferable to client, e.g., walking, jogging, aerobics, swimming, and bicycling.
- Set up weight training program for client to increase muscle strength, and stamina.
- Help client determine how to include aerobic exercise into lifestyle pattern, set up support and reward system.

Stress Management

- Ask client to rate the amount of stress in life on a scale of 1 to 10.
- Determine usual ways the client relieves stress and discuss appropriateness.
- Determine amount of personal time client has and, if needed, decide how this could be increased.
- Determine the quality of client's social supportive network.
- Teach techniques to relieve stress, such as relaxation breathing, progress muscle relaxation, need for exercise, meditation, power strategies, problem-solving, imagery, gaining perspective, and spirituality.

Smoking, Drinking

- Determine frequency of destructive health habits.
- Smoking: refer to supportive withdrawal organization; discuss how client can deal with loss of significant habit and addiction in life; suggest client discuss use of nicotine patches with physician.
- Drinking: refer to Alcoholics Anonymous, preferably to a designated support person to help bring client into the organization.
- Determine if another person's drinking causes harm and refer to Al-Anon family groups.
- Refer to *Altered Health Maintenance*.

Health Screening, Appropriate Health Care

- Determine usual practice of health care, including frequency of physician visits and screening examinations.
- Female: encourage yearly Pap smears if sexually active, also mammogram as prescribed by physician, if over 40 yrs of age, especially if history of cancer in family, also stool for occult blood, glaucoma examination.
- Male: yearly health examination, if over 40, include prostate examination, stool for occult blood, glaucoma examination.
- Refer to *Altered Health Maintenance*.

Geriatric

- Give client information about community resources for the elderly.

Client/Family Teaching

- Provide and review pamphlets about health-seeking opportunities and wellness resources.

IMPAIRED HOME MAINTENANCE MANAGEMENT

Definition
Inability to independently maintain a safe growth-promoting immediate environment.

Defining Characteristics
Subjective: *Household members express difficulty in maintaining their home in a comfortable fashion
*Household members request assistance with home maintenance
*Household members describe outstanding debts or financial crises
Objective: Disorderly environment
*Unwashed or unavailable cooking equipment, clothes, or linen
*Accumulation of dirt, food wastes, or hygienic wastes
Offensive odors
Inappropriate household temperature
*Overtaxed family members, e.g., exhausted, or anxious
Lack of necessary equipment or aids
Presence of vermin or rodents
*Repeated hygienic disorders, infestations, or infections
(*Critical)

Related Factors (r/t)
Individual-family member disease or injury
Insufficient family organization or planning
Insufficient finances
Unfamiliarity with neighborhood resources
Impaired cognitive or emotional functioning
Lack of knowledge
Lack of role modeling
Inadequate support systems

Client Outcomes/Goals
✓ Family members have available clean clothing, nutritious meals, and sanitary/safe home.
✓ Have identified supports to help maintain home.
✓ Family members express satisfaction with home situation.

Nursing Interventions
- Assess cause of impaired home maintenance management (refer to Related Factors above).
- Assess family members concerns about maintenance of the home.
- Ask family to identify at least two support people to help in maintenance of the home.
- Obtain adaptive equipment to help family member continue to maintain home as appropriate.

- Initiate a referral to community agencies for help as needed including housekeeping aids, Meals on Wheels, or transportation.
- Work with family to determine plan to share household duties.
- Set up a system of relief for main caretaker in home so client has ability to get out of the house.
- Refer client to social services to help with debt consolidation, or financial concerns.

Geriatric
- Explore resources for seniors to assist with home care, e.g., Senior Centers, Department of Aging, and school volunteer programs.
- Ensure home is safe environment; remove any throw rugs, have safety bars installed in bathroom, and paint stair borders and stove know with bright paint.

Client/Family Teaching
- Teach how to perform activities to maintain the home as needed, e.g., cooking, cleaning, and rodent control.
- Teach caretaker the need to have some personal time every day to meet own needs.
- Encourage family to maintain contact with family and friends even if only by phone.
- Teach family first aid and CPR measures.

HOPELESSNESS

Definition
A subjective state in which an individual sees limited or no alternatives or personal choices available and is unable to mobilize energy on own behalf.

Defining Characteristics
Major: Passivity and decreased verbalization
Decreased affect
Verbal cues (despondent content, "I can't" or sighing)
Minor: Lack of initiative
Decreased response to stimuli
Decreased affect
Turning away from speaker
Closing eyes
Shrugging in response to speaker
Decreased appetite
Increased/decreased sleep
Lack of involvement in care or passively allowing care

Related Factors (r/t)
Prolonged activity restriction creating isolation
Failing or deteriorating physiological condition
Long-term stress
Abandonment
Lost belief in transcendent values/God

Client Outcomes/Goals
✓ Able to verbalize feelings; participates in care.
✓ Makes positive statements, "I can" or "I'll try."
✓ Makes eye contact and focuses on speaker.
✓ Appetite appropriate for age and physical health.
✓ Sleep time appropriate for age and physical health.

Nursing Interventions
- Monitor and document potential for suicide (refer to *High Risk for Violence: Self-Directed* for specific interventions).
- Spend one-to-one time with client.
- Acknowledge acceptance of expression of feelings (everyone is entitled to their own feelings).
- Give client time to initiate interactions; after time is allowed, approach client in accepting, nonjudgmental manner.

- Encourage client to participate in group activities to provide social support and alternate ways to problem solve.
- Review with the client their strengths; have client list them on a 3 by 5 card and carry it with him to refer to.
- Involve family/significant others in plan of care.
- Encourage family/significant others to express care and love for client.
- Use touch to demonstrate caring and encourage family to use touch.

Geriatric
- Assess for clinical signs and symptoms of depression, and differentiate from functional or organic dementia.
- Identify significant losses with client that might be leading to feelings of hopelessness.
- Discuss stages and emotional responses to multiple losses.
- Use reminiscence and life review to identify past coping behaviors.
- Express hope to client and give positive feedback whenever appropriate.
- Identify client's past sources of spirituality and help client explore his life and identify those experiences that are noteworthy.

Client/Family Teaching
- Teach stress reduction; relaxation; imagery.
- Refer to self-help groups, such as "I Can Cope", "Make Today Count."
- Supply crisis-line number and secure contract with client to use number if thoughts of harming self occur.

201

HYPERTHERMIA

Definition
A state in which an individual's body temperature is elevated above his/her normal range.

Defining Characteristics
Major: Increase in body temperature above normal range
Minor: Flushed, hot skin; increased respiratory rate, and tachycardia; seizures/convulsions

Related Factors (r/t)
Exposure to hot environment
Vigorous activity
Medications-anesthesia
Inappropriate clothing
Increased metabolic rate
Illness-trauma
Dehydration
Inability or decreased ability to perspire

Client Outcomes/Goals
✓ Temperature, pulse, and respirations within normal range.
✓ Skin normal temperature and color.
✓ Free of seizure activity, and neurological damage.

Nursing Interventions
- Observe cause/contributing factors, such as dehydration, infection, drug effect, hyperthyroidism (refer to related factors).
- Take vital signs q _____ hours, especially note temperature (take rectally if possible) and blood pressure.
- Observe for signs of hyperthermia, such as flushed, hot skin and diaphoresis.
- Monitor neurological function, noting mental status, reaction to stimuli, pupil reaction, presence of posturing, or seizures.
- Keep careful record of all fluid losses.
- Remove bedding over the client except for light sheet.
- Administer antipyretic medications as ordered when temperature is elevated.
- Support hypermetabolic state with adequate fluids and sufficient amounts of simple carbohydrates.
- Provide cool water sponging and an electric fan blowing over client.
- Administer medications to control shivering and seizures as ordered by physician.
- Place client on cooling blanket if high temperature with physician's order and regulate to bring temperature down slowly.
- Cooling blanket: take temperature hourly; turn cooling blanket off when temperature 1° C (2° F) above desired body temperature.

- If client on cooling blanket, keep skin well lubricated.

Geriatric
- If receiving IVs, carefully observe for symptoms of fluid overload or pulmonary edema.
- Give cool water sponge baths with massage to avoid peripheral vasoconstriction from the external cooling.
- Direct to seek air conditioned environment in extreme heat spells.

Client/Family Teaching
- Teach client to avoid physical activity during hotter parts of day and to wear a hat when exposed to direct sunlight.
- Recommend client drink liberal amounts of nonalcoholic fluids throughout the day if high environmental temperature.
- Explain symptoms of hyperthermia, indicating need for prompt intervention.

HYPOTHERMIA

Definition
The state in which an individual's body temperature is reduced below normal range.

Defining Characteristics
Major: Reduction in body temperature below normal range
Shivering (mild)
Cool skin
Pallor (moderate)
Minor: Slow capillary refill
Piloerection
Cyanotic nail beds
Bradycardia
Bradypnea
Decreased mentation
Drowsiness-confusion
(Adapted from NANDA, Carpenito)

Related Factors (r/t)
Exposure to cool or cold environment;
Illness-trauma
Damage to hypothalmus
Inability or decreased ability to shiver
Malnutrition
Inadequate clothing
Consumption of alcohol
Medications causing vasodilatation
Evaporation from skin in cool environment
Decreased metabolic rate
Inactivity; aging

Client Outcomes/Goals
✓ Body temperature within normal range.
✓ Warm pink skin with rapid capillary refill.
✓ States measures should take to prevent hypothermia.
✓ Identifies symptoms of hypothermia, action needed if hypothermia present.

Nursing Interventions
▪ Observe for cause of hypothermia (refer to related factors).
▪ Take temperature every _____ hour(s).

204

- Take vital signs every _____ hour(s) noting changes associated with hypothermia of decreased pulse, irregular pulse rhythm, decreased respiratory rate, or initially increased then decreased blood pressure.
- Monitor for signs of hypothermia, such as shivering, cool skin, piloerection, pallor, slow capillary refill, cyanotic nail beds, decreased mentation, or comatose.
- Rewarm passively: cover with blanket and supply warm fluid orally or parenterally with physician's order. Allow rewarming to occur at person's own pace.
- Rewarm actively with physicians order, place client on heating pads and monitor temperature-vital signs every _____ hour carefully.
- Apply extra blankets, additional clothing, such as socks, long underwear, and cap for head.
- Encourage good nutrition: have dietician see client or ask for order for parental/enteral feeding if necessary.
- Keep client covered with warm blankets; do not allow to get chilled from bath or other procedures.
- Request social service referral to help client obtain needed heat/shelter/food to maintain body temperature.

Geriatric
- Since older persons are more likely to become comatose as body temperature decreases, assess neurological signs frequently.
- Gradually warm body at a rate of about 0.5° C per hour.

Client/Family Teaching
- Teach client/family how to take a temperature and signs of hypothermia.
- Teach how to prevent hypothermia by wearing adequate clothing, warming when chilled and avoiding environmental extremes.
- Instruct family on how to wear layers of clothing to stay warm.
- Instruct family not to use heating pads or electric blankets with young infants/children or elderly with decreased sensation.

BOWEL INCONTINENCE

Definition
A state in which an individual experiences a change in normal bowel habits characterized by involuntary passage of stool.

Defining Characteristics
Involuntary passage of stool

Related Factors (r/t)
Loss of control of rectal sphincter
Neurological dysfunction
Severe regression
Gastrointestinal disorders (inflammatory bowel syndrome) colorectal surgery, anorectal trauma, or diarrhea
(Adapted from Carpenito)

Client Outcomes/Goals
✓ Formed continent stool at least every other day.
✓ Intact skin in rectal-sacral area.
✓ Decreased incidence of incontinence.
✓ Able to utilize commode/toilet at regular intervals without intervening episodes of incontinence.

Nursing Interventions
- Determine with client/family usual previous time and pattern of defecation.
- Document frequency and timing of incontinence.
- Provide ready access to bedpan-commode-bathroom.
- Respond immediately to client's call for bedpan or commode.
- Provide privacy; give nonjudgmental and accepting care.
- Assist on commode-bedpan at usual time of defecation daily.
- Cleanse skin thoroughly after each incontinent stool, utilize spray cleansers designed for this purpose.
- Apply petroleum-based ointment to skin around rectum after cleaning.
- If frequent incontinence, apply adult diaper or pad on bed.
- If obtunded or comatose and liquid stool, ask for physician's order to apply fecal incontinence pouch.
- Neurologically altered client—establish bowel routine with suppository every other day or digital stimulation with physician's order.

Geriatric
- Observe etiology and treat appropriately, e.g., modify environment for ease of toileting, toilet regularly after meals, and provide medications as prescribed.
- Check for impaction as ordered.
- Teach exercises to strengthen muscles, use behavior modification to help control bowel function.

Client/Family Teaching
- Establish bowel training program of using warm fluids in morning; private place for defecation.
- Teach how to deal with incontinence to decrease embarrassment of client or family.

FUNCTIONAL INCONTINENCE

Definition

The state in which an individual experiences a difficulty or inability to reach the toilet in time due to environmental barriers, disorientation, and physical limitations (Adapted from Carpenito).

Defining Characteristics

Major: Urge to void or bladder contractions sufficiently strong to result in loss of urine before reaching an appropriate receptacle

Related Factors (r/t)

Altered environment
Sensory, cognitive, or mobility deficits

Client Outcomes/Goals

✓ Free from urinary incontinence or reduced incidents of incontinence.
✓ Environmental barriers to utilization of bathroom are removed or minimized.

Nursing Interventions

- Determine if there is another cause leading to incontinence, such as urinary tract infection, urge, reflex, or stress incontinence, urinary retention.
- Observe obstacles to reaching appropriate receptacle, such as poor lighting, siderails, lack of privacy, or frequently occupied bathroom.
- Monitor frequency of incontinence and appropriate voiding to determine the pattern and environmental circumstances surrounding incontinence; have client keep record if possible.
- Provide rapid access to a urinary receptacle, especially when diuretics given.
- Ensure that client has ready access to call light at all times, answer light immediately.
- If decreased cognition, encourage client to void every 2 hours, after meals, and at bedtime.
- Encourage client to wear normal clothes if possible.

Geriatric

- Provide reality orientation when needed to increase awareness of time, place, and environment.
- If clothing a barrier to rapid urination, modify clothing with velcro fasteners.

Client/Family Teaching

- Work with client/family to set up schedule of voiding using environmental and behavioral cues, such as after meals, before bedtime, and before of after television shows.
- Have client/family keep record of voiding-incontinence to show progress.
- Discuss with client/family how to provide rapid access to urine receptacles.
- If incontinent on way to bathroom, teach to stop when feels urge, take several deep breaths, think of a dry environment such as the desert, and then proceed when urge is under control.
- Teach client how to perform Kegel exercises.

REFLEX INCONTINENCE

Definition
The state in which an individual experiences an involuntary loss of urine, occurring at somewhat predictable intervals when a specific bladder volume is reached.

Defining Characteristics
Major: No awareness of bladder filling
No urge to void or feelings of bladder fullness
Uninhabited bladder contraction/spasm at regular intervals

Related Factors (r/t)
Neurological impairment (e.g., spinal cord lesion that interferes with conduction of cerebral messages above the level of the reflex arc)

Client Outcomes/Goals
✓ Follows prescribed voiding schedule, urine clear.
✓ Able to perform intermittent self catheterization.
✓ Demonstrates successful use of triggering techniques to stimulate voiding.
✓ Perineal area free from irritation or breakdown.
Note: When client acutely ill in flaccid paralysis (lower motor neuron involvement) will generally need foley catheter or intermittent catheterization. When in spastic paralysis and stable, then voiding techniques can be used. It is very important that the bladder be regularly and adequately emptied to prevent UTIs and hydronephrosis.

Nursing Interventions
- Monitor pattern of urination, fluid intake, ability to urinate voluntarily, clarity of urine, incidences of incontinence of urine, and bladder distention.
- Regulate fluid intake; may be on limited fluids if intermittent catheterization; force fluids to 3000 cc/day once bladder training is started.
- Set up bladder training program when client ready.

Example bladder training program:
- Catheter removed at 7 AM.
- Glass of fluid—240 ml every hour.
- After 2 to 3 hours, attempt to void by using triggering mechanisms (upper motor neuron bladder) or using pressure mechanisms (lower motor neuron bladder).
- If client voids, catheterize for residual (physicians order).
- If residual less than 50 cc proceed with training program; if more than 50 cc, reinsert catheter and reschedule bladder training for a later date.

- Provide support and encouragement to accomplish bladder training.

- If self-catheterization not feasible, bladder training ineffective, and urine not retained, use external drainage device for male.
- Refer to rehabilitation nurse for further help in establishing appropriate urination schedule.

Client/Family Teaching
- Teach signs of a full bladder: sweating, restlessness, abdominal discomfort.
- Have client keep a written record of fluid intake, voiding pattern.
- Teach techniques to trigger voiding-upper motor neuron bladder: suprapubic tapping, stroking of penis, inner thigh, or abdomen, pulling pubic hair, stretching the anal sphincter with gloved finger or doing push-ups on the commode.
- Teach techniques to exert pressure on bladder causing voiding-lower motor neuron bladder: Crede's bladder; valsalva maneuver (if not contraindicated); or contracting abdominal muscles to exert pressure on the bladder.
- Teach client/family intermittent straight catheterization techniques, if ordered.

STRESS INCONTINENCE

Definition
The state in which an individual experiences a loss of urine of less than 50 ml occurring with increased abdominal pressure.

Defining Characteristics
Major: Reported or observed dribbling with increased abdominal pressure
Minor: Urinary urgency and frequency—more often than every two hours

Related Factors (r/t)
Degenerative changes in pelvic muscles and structural supports associated with increased age
High intraabdominal pressure (e.g., obesity, gravid uterus)
Incompetent bladder outlet
Overdistention between voidings
Weak pelvic muscles and structural supports

Client Outcomes/Goals
✓ Reports a decreased incidence or cessation of stress incontinence events.
✓ Verbalizes the cause and treatment of stress incontinence.
✓ Maintains dignity; free of odor and embarrassment associated with stress incontinence.

Nursing Interventions
- Monitor cause of stress incontinence: childbirth, prostate surgery, obesity, aging, or retention of urine.
- Monitor pattern of incontinence including frequency, timing, or precipitating events.
- Note color and clarity of urine; send urine for analysis if any signs of UTI.
- Encourage client to verbalize feelings about stress incontinence.
- Ensure rapid access to toilet or commode.
- Discuss and provide client small adhesive peri-pad to wear in underclothing.

Geriatric
- Develop an individualized toileting schedule with clients input.
- Assess feasibility of biofeedback treatments for incontinence.
- Refer client to a geriatric center that specializes in treatment of incontinence.

Client/Family Teaching
- Develop schedule of frequent voluntary voiding to avoid incontinence.
- Teach client how to perform Kegel exercises to increase perineal tone; work with client to develop schedule to do exercises.
- Encourage to increase fluid intake to 1500 to 2000 ml per day, since concentrated urine can irritate the urinary tract and cause dribbling.

- Encourage to avoid fluids containing caffeine, such as coffee, tea, caffeinated sodas (caffeine causes irritation of urinary tract); also alcohol because it serves as a diuretic.

TOTAL INCONTINENCE

Definition
The state in which an individual experiences a continuous and unpredictable loss of urine.

Defining Characteristics
Major: Constant flow of urine occurs at unpredictable times without distention or uninhibited bladder contractions-spasm

Urinary incontinence refractory to other treatments

Nocturia more than two times during sleep time

Minor: Lack of perineal or bladder filling awareness/unawareness of incontinence

Related Factors (r/t)
Neuropathy preventing transmission of reflex indicating bladder fullness

Neurological dysfunction causing triggering of micturation at unpredictable times

Independent contraction of detrusor reflex due to surgery, trauma or disease affecting spinal cord
    nerves

Anatomical incontinence (fistula)

Client Outcomes/Goals
✓ Perineal area free from irritation or breakdown.

✓ States feels dignity has been maintained.

✓ Explains measures can take to deal with incontinence of urine .

Nursing Interventions
- Observe voiding pattern and incidence of incontinence.
- Check for incontinence at frequent intervals.
- Clean perineal area after each incident of incontinence to prevent skin irritation.
- If male, consider use of external condom catheter connected to foley bag, change every 24 hours, observe for skin breakdown.
- Utilize incontinence briefs as needed.
- Pad the bed well with absorbent pads; place bath blanket over several incontinent pads to collect urine.
- Keep perineal-sacral area well lubricated with protective ointment.
- Avoid use of foley catheter unless client critically ill or severe skin breakdown.
- Place client on defined schedule of fluid intake with predictable voiding after; decrease fluid intake in the evening.
- Offer bedpan or urinal at intervals based on fluid intake.

Geriatric
- If possible, assess and modify drug regime that may be interfering with continence.
- Use meticulous infection control procedures if indwelling catheter is used.

Client/Family Teaching

- Teach how to deal with urine incontinence: padding, protecting clothing, and pattern of fluid intake and toileting.
- Teach how to perform intermittent self-catheterization, if appropriate.
- Teach measures to prevent UTIs.
- Refer to rehabilitation or gerontolog center for help dealing with incontinence.

URGE INCONTINENCE

Definition
The state in which an individual experiences involuntary passage of urine occurring soon after a strong sense of urgency to void.

Defining Characteristics
Major: Urinary urgency, frequency (voiding more often than every two hours)
Bladder contracture-spasm
Minor: Nocturia (more than two times per night);
Voiding in small amounts (less than 100 cc) or large amounts (more than 550 cc)
Inability to reach the toilet in time

Related Factors (r/t)
Decreased bladder capacity (e.g., history of PID, abdominal surgeries, or indwelling urinary catheter)
Irritation of bladder stretch receptors causing spasm (e.g., bladder infection); alcohol
Caffeine
Increased fluid
Increased urine concentration
Overdistention of the bladder

Client Outcomes/Goals
✓ Voids clear straw-colored urine in appropriate receptacle every 3 or more hours without distress.
✓ Follows mutually agreed on voiding plan.

Nursing Interventions
- Observe voiding pattern, urine characteristics, keep careful I & O.
- Monitor fluid intake and usual amount and kind of fluids ingested.
- Observe cause especially if new onset (refer to related factors).
- Provide convenient access to toilet or bathroom.
- Help client to bathroom in evening to help prevent nocturia.
- Encourage client that he can become continent again and not to isolate self.
- Refer to physician-nurse specialist in incontinence for further evaluation, use of biofeedback, medications, or further modalities.

Geriatric
- Check for impaction and remove following institution protocol.
- Develop regular toileting schedule.

Client/Family Teaching
- Teach need for fluids avoiding caffeine and alcohol.

215

- Work with client to establish voiding pattern-habit training to avoid incontinence.
- Teach how to do Kegel exercises to increase urinary control.
- If diminished bladder capacity, urine sterile, and too frequent voiding, use bladder training, and have client void at predetermined times increasing length of time between voiding using sphincter contraction, relaxation breathing, visualization of dry environment (e.g., driving through the desert), and positive reinforcement.
- Teach measures needed to prevent UTI.

INEFFECTIVE INFANT FEEDING PATTERN

Definition
A state in which an infant demonstrates an impaired ability to such or coordinate the suck-swallow response.

Defining Characteristics
Inability to initiate or sustain an effective suck
Inability to coordinate sucking, swallowing, and breathing

Related Factors (r/t)
Prematurity
Neurological impairment/delay

Oral hypersensitivity
Prolonged NPO

Client Outcomes/Goals
✓ Infant will receive adequate nourishment.
✓ Infant will progress to normal feeding pattern.
✓ Family will learn successful techniques for feeding the infant.

Nursing Interventions
- Assess infant's oral reflexes (i.e., root, gag, suck and swallow).
- Determine infant's ability to coordinate suck, swallow, and breathing reflexes.
- Collaborate with other health care providers (physician, neonatal nutritionist, and physical therapist) to develop feeding plan.
- Implement gavage feedings (or other alternative feeding methods) before infant's readiness for by mouth feedings.
- Evaluate feeding environment and minimize sensory stimuli.
- Position infant in a flexed feeding posture similar to a full-term infant.
- Attempt to nipple feed baby only when in a quiet/alert state.
- Allow appropriate time for nipple feeding to ensure safety without excess calorie expenditure.
- Monitor infant's physiological condition during feeding.
- Determine infant's active feeding behaviors without prodding.
- Assess infant's ability to take in enough calories to sustain temperature and growth.
- Encourage family to participate in feeding process.
- Refer to neonatal nutritionist, physical or occupational therapist, or lactation specialist as needed.

Client/Family Teaching
- Provide anticipatory guidance for infant's expected feeding course.
- Teach parents infant feeding methods.
- Teach parents how to recognize infant cues.
- Provide anticipatory guidance for infant's discharge.

HIGH RISK FOR INFECTION

Definition
The state in which an individual is at increased risk for being invaded by pathogenic organisms.

Defining Characteristics
Presence of Risk Factors of:

Inadequate primary defenses (broken skin, traumatized tissue, decrease in ciliary action, stasis of body fluids, change in pH secretions, and altered peristalsis)

Inadequate secondary defense (e.g., decreased hemoglobin, leukopenia, and suppressed inflammatory response) and immunosuppression

Inadequate acquired immunity

Tissue destruction and increased environmental exposure

Chronic disease

Malnutrition

Invasive procedures

Pharmaceutical agents

Trauma

Rupture of amniotic membranes

Insufficient knowledge to avoid exposure to pathogens

Related Factors (r/t)
See risk factors

Client Outcomes/Goals
✓ Free of symptoms of infection.
✓ States symptoms of infection to be observed.
✓ Demonstrates appropriate care of site prone to infection.
✓ WBC count and differential within normal limits.
✓ Demonstrates appropriate hygienic measures, such as handwashing, oral care, and perineal care.

Nursing Interventions
- Observe for symptoms of infection: redness, warmth, discharge, and increased body temperature.
- Note laboratory values (WBC, differential, serum protein, serum albumin, and cultures).
- Encourage intake of balanced diet, especially proteins to feed immune system.
- Encourage adequate rest to bolster immune system.
- Utilize careful sterile technique when utilizing invasive monitoring or other invasive procedures.
- Utilize careful sterile technique at site where loss of skin integrity.
- Ensure appropriate hygienic care with handwashing, bathing, hair care, nail care, and perineal care (either given by nurse or self-care).

Geriatric
- Recognize that geriatric clients may be seriously infected with less obvious symptoms because of depression of immune system from aging or chronic disease.
- Foot care beyond simple toenail cutting should be done by a podiatrist.
- Elderly can have infections with low grade fevers, thus be suspicious of any rise in temperature or sudden confusion—may be only sign of infection.
- Protect the older person from people with obvious infections, such as colds and flu.
- Recommend clients receive influenza immunizations yearly, pneumococcal vaccine once lifetime, and tetanus vaccine every 10 years, especially if client is chronically ill.

Client/Family Teaching
- Instruct in symptoms of infection: redness, warmth, swelling, tenderness/pain, new onset of drainage or change in drainage from wound or increased body temperature.
- Instruct in need for good nutrition, especially protein intake and need for rest to bolster immune function.
- Teach how to care for any area of nonintact skin to prevent infection.
- If person with AIDS, discuss continued need to practice safe sex, need to avoid unsterile needle use, and need to maintain healthy lifestyle to prevent infection.
- Refer to social services/community resources to obtain support in maintaining lifestyle to increase immune function: adequate nutrition, rest, and freedom from excessive stress.

HIGH RISK FOR INJURY

Definition
A state in which the individual is at risk for injury as a result of environmental conditions interacting with the individual's adaptive and defensive resources.

Note: There is overlap of this nursing diagnosis and other diagnoses, such as *High Risk for Trauma, High Risk for Poisoning, High Risk for Suffocation*, and *High Risk for Aspiration*. The reader is referred to these other diagnoses if they are more specific for the client situation.

Defining Characteristics
Presence of risk factors such as:
Evidence of environmental hazards
Lack of knowledge of environmental hazards
Lack of knowledge of safety precautions
History of accidents
Impaired mobility
Sensory deficit
Cerebral dysfunction
(Adapted from Carpenito)

Related Factors (r/t)
See risk factors

Client Outcomes/Goals
✓ Client free of injuries.
✓ Client/family explains actions can take to prevent injury.

Nursing Interventions
- Monitor mental status, if any signs of confusion increase vigilance in protecting client.
- Provide reality orientation every time interact with client if needed.
- Monitor risk of injury to individual.
- Avoid use of restraints, obtain physicians order if necessary to use.
- Request family to stay with client to prevent accidental falls, or pulling out tubes.
- Remove all possible hazards in environment such as razors, medications, or matches.
- Keep environment clear of obstructions.
- If unsteady on feet, utilize walking belt; use two nursing staff when ambulating client.
- Admit client prone to injury near the nurses station.
- Keep client's personal items and call light readily available.
- Answer client's call light promptly.
- Keep siderails up as appropriate.

Geriatric
- Encourage client to wear glasses, hearing aid, and utilize walking aids when ambulating.

Client/Family Teaching
- Teach how to safely ambulate at home, including use of safety measures such as handrails in bathroom.
- Teach to identify significant places in environment that must be easily located by covering with bright colors, such as yellow or red, including stair edges, and stove controls.
- If dizzy when getting up, teach methods to decrease dizziness, such as rising slowly, remaining seated several minutes before arising, flexing feet upward several times, avoiding holding breath, or having someone with you when rising.

KNOWLEDGE DEFICIT (SPECIFY)

Definition
The state in which an individual or group experiences a deficiency in cognitive knowledge or psychomotor skills regarding the condition or treatment plan.

Defining Characteristics
Verbalization of the problem.
Inaccurate follow through of previous instruction.
Inaccurate performance of test.
Inappropriate or exaggerated behaviors, e.g., hysterical, hostile, agitated, or apathetic.

Related Factors (r/t)
Lack of exposure
Lack of recall
Information misinterpretation
Cognitive limitation
Lack of interest in learning
Unfamiliarity with information resources

Client Outcomes/Goals
✓ Explains disease state, recognizes need for medications, and understands treatments.
✓ Explains how to incorporate new health regimen into his lifestyle.
✓ States he is able to deal with health situation and remain in control of his life.
✓ Demonstrates how to perform procedure(s) satisfactorily.
✓ Lists resources that can be utilized if client needs more information or support after discharge.

Nursing Interventions
- Observe client's previous knowledge of subject matter and willingness to learn.
- Observe client's ability to learn: determine if healthy enough to learn, mental acuity, ability to see, hear, and understand language.
- Determine social and cultural background of the client, reading ability, and presence of language barriers.
- Identify support persons/significant others who will require information and support client through illness process.
- Provide quiet, nondistracting environment for teaching.
- Provide written information to take home.
- Provide positive reinforcement for learning as much as possible; avoid negative statements.
- Involve client in own learning with active role promoting sense of control or mastery over situation.
- Establish a written contract with client specifying desired behavior, consequences, and date of evaluation.
- Utilize resources, such as programmed learning, charts, or handouts; use audiovisual aids, such as videotapes, audiotapes, or anatomical models.
- Request order for home health services/community agency to reinforce teaching as needed.
- Help client identify support system to help maintain change in health habits.

Geriatric
- Ensure that client utilizes any reading aids (glasses or magnifying lenses) or hearing aids before educational session.
- Recognize importance of building on client's previous knowledge and client's possible resistance to change in life-long patterns.
- Refer to peer counseling, since it is effective in teaching about age-related changes.

Client/Family Teaching
- Encourage client/family to verbalize concerns about disease or treatment.
- Teach subject content that concerns client first, e.g., how to give injections.
- Teach about disease, including action of medications, dosages, and side effects.
- Teach procedures step-by-step; have client/family demonstrate the procedures.
- Teach stress reduction skills, e.g., relaxation breathing techniques, or visualization-imagery.
- Refer to group teaching sessions as available and appropriate.

IMPAIRED PHYSICAL MOBILITY

Definition
A state in which the individual experiences a limitation of ability for independent physical movement.

Defining Characteristics
Inability to purposefully move within the physical environment, including bed mobility, transfer, and ambulation
Reluctance to attempt movement
Limited range of motion
Decreased muscle strength, control, or mass
Imposed restrictions of movement; including mechanical, or medical protocol
Impaired coordination

Related Factors (r/t)
Intolerance to activity   Perceptual-cognitive impairment
Decreased strength and endurance   Neuromuscular impairment
Depression-severe anxiety   Pain or discomfort
Musculoskeletal impairment

Suggested Functional Level Classification
0 = Completely independent
1 = Requires use of equipment or device
2 = Requires help from another person, for assistance,
    Supervision, or teaching
3 = Requires help from another person and equipment device
4 = Dependent, does not participate in activity

Client Outcomes/Goals
✓ Participates in required physical activity.
✓ Verbalizes feelings of increased strength and ability to move.
✓ Demonstrates use of adaptive equipment (wheelchairs or walkers) to increase mobility.

Nursing Interventions
- Observe cause of impaired mobility; determine if physical or psychological basis.
- Monitor and record client's ability to tolerate activity and use all four extremities; note pulse rate, blood pressure, dyspnea, and skin color before and after activity.
- Observe for pain before activity and treat pain before activity if possible.
- Check to make sure client is in good body alignment, ask the client each time they move, reposition as needed.
- Refer to physical therapy for help to increase mobility of client as needed

- Obtain any assistive devices needed before activity begins such as walking belt, walker, cane, crutches, wheel chair, stretcher chair.
- If client immobile, perform range of motion at least twice a day using gentle, prolonged stretching technique.
- Encourage client to perform strengthening exercises, such as gluteal or quadriceps sitting exercises, as prescribed by physical therapy or physician.

Geriatric
- Consider reduced flexibility, endurance and balance and diminished eyesight and hearing; and slowed response time when planning to increase client's mobility.
- Plan regular consistent regimens for exercise and mobilization.

Client/Family Teaching
- Teach client how to get out of bed slowly, to transfer from the bed to the chair.
- Instruct client in use of relaxation techniques to utilize during activity.
- Teach client how to utilize relevant equipment or medications during activity.
- Contract with client to develop health plan and to set goals for increased activity, include measurable landmarks of progress.

NONCOMPLIANCE (SPECIFY)

Definition
A person's informed decision not to adhere to a therapeutic recommendation.

Defining Characteristics
*Behavior indicative of failure to adhere (by direct observation or by statements of patient or significant others)
Objective tests (physiological measures, detection of markers)
Evidence of development of complications; evidence of exacerbation of symptoms
Failure to keep appointments
Failure to progress.
(*Critical)

Related Factors (r/t)
Patient value system
Health beliefs, cultural influences

Spiritual values
Client-provider relationships

Client Outcomes/Goals
✓ Describes consequence of continuing noncompliance of treatment regimen.
✓ States goals for health and means to obtain them.
✓ Communicates understanding of disease and treatment.
✓ Lists treatment regimen and expectations, including agreement to follow through with them.
✓ Lists alternative ways to meet goals.
✓ Describes family participation to help client achieve goals.

Nursing Interventions
- Observe cause for noncompliance with therapeutic protocol.
- Monitor client's/family's knowledge of illness and treatment.
- Observe cultural influence, educational level, and developmental age.
- Monitor ability to follow directions, solve problems, and concentrate.
- Observe reading and writing ability; provide appropriate educational aids (flip charts or printed materials).
- Observe support system as helping or hindering therapy.
- Monitor sensory deficits: hearing, vision, or tactile sensation.
- Develop therapeutic relationship; spend time with client, and remain nonjudgmental.
- Monitor anxiety as possible cause for noncompliance.
- Listen to client's statements of abilities; encourage use of them in self-care.
- Have client repeat instructions in his own words.
- Accept client's choices, adapt plan accordingly.
- Develop a written contract with client and evaluate the criteria set forth in contract on a regular basis.

- Consult with health care person who has prescribed treatment regimen about possible alterations to encourage compliance.

Geriatric

- Monitor for memory deficits, signs of depression, or dementia.
- Use repetition, verbal clues, and memory aids in teaching health care regimen.

Client/Family Teaching

- Teach importance of following treatment regimen and consequences of noncompliance.
- Share information about appropriate services that may help in compliance; such as dietician, home health agencies, social service, and community educational services.
- Teach medication side effects so that client understands them and feels comfortable in discussing their occurrence, i.e.,. sexual function/dysfunction, mental changes, and so on. (Several medications cause impotence leading to a pattern of noncompliance.)

ALTERED NUTRITION: LESS THAN BODY REQUIREMENTS

Definition

The state in which an individual experiences an intake of nutrients insufficient to meet metabolic needs.

Defining Characteristics

Loss of weight with adequate food intake
Body weight 20% or more under ideal
Reported inadequate food intake less than recommended daily allowance
Weakness of muscles required for swallowing or mastication
Reported or evidence of lack of food
Avesion to eating
Reported altered taste sensation
Satiety immediately after ingesting food
Abdominal pain with or without pathology
Sore, inflamed buccal cavity
Hyperactive bowel sounds
Lack of interest in food
Perceived inability to ingest food
Pale conjunctival and mucous membranes
Poor muscle tone
Excessive loss of hair
Lack of information or misinformation
Misconceptions

Related Factors (r/t)

Inability to ingest or digest food or absorb nutrients because of biological, psychological, or economic factors.

Client Outcomes/Goals

✓ Has progressive weight gain towards desired goal; weight within normal range for height and age.
✓ Describes understanding of factors contributing to low weight if known.
✓ Verbalizes an understanding of nutritional requirements.
✓ Is able to eat foods high in protein and calories.
✓ Is free of signs of malnutrition.

Nursing Interventions

- Observe client's mechanical ability to eat, drink, and swallow; position in high Fowler's for swallowing and safety.
- Observe client's ability to consume foods that vary in texture from liquids to solids.
- Weigh client weekly (calorie gain is slow and daily weights can be discouraging) with client wearing the same clothes, using the same scale at the same time.
- Determine ideal body weight for height and age.
- Monitor food intake, be specific when recording amounts eaten e.g., 25%, 50%; consult with dietician for an actual calorie count.
- Monitor state of oral cavity: gums, tongue, mucosa, or teeth.
- Evaluate laboratory studies: BUN, serum albumin, serum total protein, creatinine, and transferrin.
- Determine relationship of eating or events to onset of nausea, vomiting, diarrhea, or abdominal pain.

- Determine the time of day when the client's appetite is the greatest, and plan the highest calorie meal for that time.
- Administer antiemetics as ordered before mealtimes.
- Recognize that immobility leads to negative nitrogen balance fostering anorexia.
- Work with the client to determine time of meals, likes/dislikes, food temperature, and eating environment.
- Provide for and offer good oral hygiene before and after meals.
- Use behavior modification; if problem is anorexia nervosa, offer positive feedback for food eaten.
- Observe client's relationship with food as part of multidisciplinary plan; fears about food or eating (psychotic symptoms; food not tasting good).
- Provide supervision at mealtime to encourage client to eat and drink.
- Encourage eating by offering small amounts of food at one time; consider six small meals.
- If client paces or is excessively agitated, offer high carbohydrate food and fluids that can be carried as he paces. Finger foods, such as bananas, are helpful.
- If there is lactose intolerance, offer yogurt and ice cream, which cause less flatulence and cramping.
- Offer foods rich in vitamin C, folic acid, and iron if the client suffers from anemia.

Geriatric
- Observe factors that may be interfering with nutrition: no transportation, fixed income, high priced convenience store use.
- Observe fit of dentures (if worn) and insert before meals, provide appropriate food textures for chewing ease.
- Monitor social contact during meals; plan increased social contact; consider serving meals in a group setting.
- Provide assistive devices needed to facilitate eating, e.g., large handle forks and spoons.
- When feeding client allow him to choose order of eating food if he is able and provide adequate time to eat/swallow (minimum 20 minutes); sit at eye level while feeding.
- Ensure that meals are pleasant and nonthreatening, be aware of nonverbal communication.
- Insure adequate intake of calcium and vitamin D.
- Offer fluids shortly before mealtime to stimulate the appetite and moisten the oral mucosa if there is anorexia and dry mouth from medication side effects.
- If there is cognitive or physical impairment, assist in food selection and self-feeding.

Client/Family Teaching
- Explain the need for consumption of carbohydrates, protein, minerals, fats, and fluids.
- Teach the client to rest before meals.
- Provide dietary instructions to the client and family.
- Reinforce dietary instructions with written materials.
- Refer the client to counseling or family therapy if indicated.
- Refer to Meals on Wheels.
- Teach the client/family how to provide the feedings at home, care of hyperalimentation, if ordered.

ALTERED NUTRITION: MORE THAN BODY REQUIREMENTS

Definition
The state in which an individual is experiencing an intake of nutrients that exceeds metabolic needs.

Defining Characteristics
Weight 10% over ideal for height and frame
*Weight 20% over ideal for height and frame
*Triceps skinfold greater than 15 mm in men, 25 mm in women
Sedentary activity level
Reported or observed dysfunctional eating pattern
Pairing food with other activities
Concentrating food intake at the end of day
Eating in response to external cues, such as time of day, or social situation
Eating in response to internal cues other than hunger, e.g., anxiety
(*Critical)

Related Factors (r/t)
Excessive intake in relation to metabolic need

Client Outcomes/Goals
✓ Relates factors that contribute to weight gain.
✓ Identifies behaviors that remain under his/her control.
✓ Explains current eating patterns.
✓ Complies with dietary modifications to promote balanced nutritional intake.
✓ Accomplishes desired weight loss over a reasonable length of time, e.g., one pound/week.

Nursing Interventions
- Observe behavior indicative of nutritional intake more than body requirements.
- Determine client's prehospital eating patterns; ask them what they usually ate in a 24-hour period.
- Determine client's knowledge of nutritional diet.
- Have client keep a "food diary" stating what is eaten and when; identify patterns, e.g., eating when under stress.
- Review current exercise level and work with client to develop an exercise plan that client is willing to follow.
- Consult with dietician to develop a diet that is reasonable and nutritious to accomplish client's desired weight loss.
- Set attainable goals for weekly weight loss; only weigh once a week.
- Discuss importance of adequate intake; allow occasional treat.

- Use behavior modification techniques:
    -eat only in specific location (e.g., dining table)
    -avoid other activities (TV, reading, and so on) while eating
    -drink full glass of liquid before eating
    -use smaller plate
    -plan eating splurges by saving portion of calories and having treat once a week
- Establish client contract that involves rewards for attaining progressive goals with reinforcing reward for maintenance of desired weight.

Geriatric
- Observe socioeconomic factors influencing food choices, i.e., carbohydrates are less expensive; plan a menu for client on a fixed income.
- Increase client's activity within physiological limits.
- Experiment with a variety of flavorings since taste sensation decreases in the elderly and they crave sweets.
- Involve client in senior citizen groups to occupy time with activities other than eating.

Client/Family Teaching
- Provide information regarding the nutritional plan for both the client and family.
- Inform the client of health risks associated with obesity.
- Refer to community resource, e.g., Weight Watchers or Overeaters Anonymous.
- Teach the importance of exercise.
- Teach stress reduction techniques other than eating.

231

ALTERED NUTRITION: HIGH RISK FOR MORE THAN BODY REQUIREMENTS

Definition
The state in which an individual is at risk of experiencing an intake of nutrients that exceeds metabolic needs.

Defining Characteristics
Presence of risk factors such as:
Reported or observed obesity in one or both parents
Rapid transition across growth percentiles in infants or children
Reported use of solid food as major food source before 5 months of age
Observed use of food as reward or comfort measure
Reported or observed higher baseline weight at beginning of each pregnancy
Dysfunctional eating patterns
Pairing food with other activities
Concentrating food intake at end of day
Eating in response to external cues, such as time of day or social situation
Eating in response to internal cues other than hunger such as anxiety

Related Factors (r/t)
See risk factors

Client Outcomes/Goals
✓ Demonstrates an understanding of nutritional concepts for balanced nutritional intake.
✓ Explains current eating patterns.
✓ Complies with dietary modifications to promote balanced nutritional intake.

Nursing Interventions
Refer to care plan: *Altered Nutrition: More than Body Requirements.*
- Observe for presence of risk factors.
- Increase client's knowledge and awareness of actions that contribute to excessive food intake.
- Observe eating patterns.
- Increase client's activity level to increase calorie utilization.
- Consult dietician to develop client appropriate diet plan.
- Provide alternate rest and moderate activity periods.
- Provide diversional activities.
- Refer the client to counseling or a support group.
- Identify the client's reinforcers for maintaining reduced weight.
- Encourage decision making regarding change in eating patterns.
- Encourage the client to strive toward realistic goals.

Geriatric
Plan to decrease calories in the least painful way, e.g., decrease fat in meals rather than eliminating the cookie after dinner that client has had for years.

Client/Family Teaching

* Educate client about actions that contribute to excess food intake.
* Teach client behavior modification techniques to decrease calorie intake, e.g., eat slowly and chew food thoroughly, eat only at a specific spot at home, prepare enough small portions for one meal, and do not eat while doing other activities, such as watching television, substitute low calorie snacks for high calorie snacks and have them conveniently available, do not keep high calorie food in house.
* If dietician not available, educate client about proper nutrition; clarify misconceptions; and discuss breakdown of protein/fat/carbohydrates in diet.
* Instruct client to read nutritional analysis section of food labels; advise clients to overlook cholesterol free claims and read actual label for fat content from vegetable oil sources; teach to observe "natural food" products' labels for sugar/honey/concentrated fruit juice content versus sugar-free.

ALTERED ORAL MUCOUS MEMBRANE

Definition
The state in which an individual experiences [or is at risk of experiencing] disruptions in the tissue layers of the oral cavity.

Defining Characteristics
Oral pain/discomfort

Coated tongue

Xerostoma (dry mouth)

Stomatitis

Oral lesions or ulcers

Lack of or decreased salivation

Leukoplakia

Edema

Hyperemia

Oral plaque

Desquamation

Vesicles

Hemorrhagic gingivitis, carious teeth, or halitosis

Related Factors (r/t)
Pathological conditions of oral cavity (radiation to head or neck)

Dehydration

Trauma (chemical, e.g., acidic foods, drugs, noxious agents, or alcohol; mechanical, e.g., ill-fitting dentures, Braces, or tubes such as endotracheal/nasogastric)

Surgery in oral cavity

NPO for more than 24 hours

Ineffective oral hygiene; mouth breathing

Malnutrition

Infection

Lack of or decreased salivation

Medication

Client Outcomes/Goals
✓ Lips, oral mucosa, gums, and tongue are intact and without lesions.

✓ States measures to take to maintain oral mucous membranes.

✓ Experiences decreased pain and discomfort.

✓ Maintains adequate oral intake.

✓ Describes/demonstrates measures to maintain/regain intact mucous membranes.

Nursing Interventions
- Inspect oral cavity at least twice a day, noting any lesions, edema, bleeding, exudate, or dryness.
- Observe for mechanical/chemical agents that could cause trauma (refer to Related Factors above).
- Monitor client's nutritional and fluid status to determine if adequate; recognize that dehydration and malnutrition are a predispositions to altered mucous membranes.

- Determine client's mental status, if client unable to do own oral care, care must be provided by nursing personnel.
- Determine client's usual method of doing oral care, also any concerns about oral hygiene.
- Encourage client to brush teeth after every meal and floss teeth daily, if he/she is free of bleeding disorders.
- If whitish patches with reddened base appear in mouth and on tongue, consider fungal infection and consult with physician.
- If mouth is extremely inflamed and it is painful to swallow, consult with physician for order for numbing agent to be used before meals.
- Keep inside of mouth moist with frequent sips of water, rinse mouth with salt water rinse (1/2 tsp salt in 1 cup warm water), or use artificial saliva.
- If mouth severely inflamed, establish a schedule of frequent mouth care every 2 hours while awake, if needed.
- Keep lips well lubricated.
- If platelets decrease or client is unable to swallow, use moistened toothettes to give oral care; use dilute solution of hydrogen peroxide to moisten toothette if there is a large amount of crusting and debri present in mouth.
- If client unable to swallow, keep suction nearby when providing oral care.

Geriatric
- Observe oral cavity for lesions; malignant lesions are more common in elderly especially if there is a history of smoking or alcohol use.
- Ensure that dentures are removed and cleaned preferably after every meal and before bedtime; dentures left in the mouth at night impede circulation to the palate and predispose client to lesions.

Client/Family Teaching
- Teach client/family how to inspect oral cavities.
- Teach client/family how to provide oral care, including appropriate schedule to administer care.

PAIN

Definition
A state in which an individual experiences and reports the presence of severe discomfort or an uncomfortable sensation.

Defining Characteristics
Subjective: Communication (verbal or coded) of pain descriptions.
Objective: Guarding behavior, protective
Self-focusing
Narrowed focus (altered time perception, withdrawal from social contact, impaired thought process)
Distraction behavior (moaning, crying, pacing, seeking out other people, or activities, such as restlessness)
Facial mask of pain (eyes lack luster, "beaten look," fixed or scattered movement, or grimace)
Alteration in muscle tone (may span from listless to rigid)
Autonomic responses not seen in chronic stable pain (diaphoresis, blood pressure and pulse change, pupillary dilation, increased, or decreased respiratory rate).

Related Factors (r/t)
Injury agents (biological, chemical, physical, psychological)

Client Outcomes/Goals
✓ States free from pain, or pain controlled and tolerable; comfortable facial expression.
✓ States able to obtain sufficient amount of sleep.

Nursing Interventions
- Monitor the severity (scale of 1-10) of the pain, location, quality, associated manifestations, aggravating factors that increase pain, and factors that alleviate pain.
- Encourage client to talk about pain experience and validate reality of experience.
- Provide massage, heat applications, or application of cold as ordered and as therapeutic to client.
- Help client utilize distraction techniques during times of increased pain: music, television, counting to self, reading, stroking, and controlled breathing.
- Provide ordered pain medication on a schedule to prevent onset of pain if possible.
- Provide information to decrease anxiety, and allow client to have as much control over the management of pain as possible.
- Schedule activities to correspond with times of less pain.

Geriatric
- Handle client's body gently; allow client to move at own speed.
- Use variety of pain relief measures; include what the client believes will be effective.

Client/Family Teaching

- Teach client/family distraction techniques for pain management: relaxation breathing, visualization, rocking, stroking, music, or television.
- Teach client/family how to effectively utilize pain medication.
- Teach client to use pain relief measures before the pain becomes severe.

CHRONIC PAIN

Definition
A state in which the individual experiences pain that continues for more than 6 months.

Defining Characteristics
Major: Verbal report or observed evidence of pain experienced for more than 6 months
Minor: Fear of reinjury
Physical and social withdrawal
Altered ability to continue previous activities
Anorexia
Weight changes
Changes in sleep patterns
Facial mask
Guarded movement

Related Factors (r/t)
Chronic physical/psychosocial disability

Client Outcomes/Goals
✓ Reports pain controlled by pain management regimen.
✓ Has a comfortable facial expression.
✓ Explains three methods that can be utilized to distract self when in pain.
✓ Explains how to safely and effectively take ordered pain medication.
✓ States able to obtain sufficient amount of sleep.

Nursing Interventions
- Observe the severity (scale of 1-10) of the pain, location, quality, associated manifestations, common precipitating and alleviating events, and current pain relief regimen.
- Encourage client to talk about pain experience and validate reality of experience.
- Determine client's usual way to deal with stressful events.
- Encourage use of oral medications if possible, start with loading dose, then maintenance dose given PRN or routinely. Add aspirin, acetaminophen, or nonsteroidal antiinflammatory drug (NSAID) to potentiate drug effect with physician's input.
- Have client keep written record of pain, including timing, precipitating events, schedule of pain medication, and relief obtained from pain medication.
- If receiving large doses of narcotics, observe for toxicity: decreased respiratory rate, decreased blood pressure, constipation, or change in level of consciousness.
- Provide massage treatments, heat applications, or application of cold as ordered and therapeutic to client.
- Develop an exercise program to meet client's needs, and plan exercise in times of decreased pain.
- Set up bowel routine to avoid constipation associated with inactivity or narcotic use.

- If prolonged-release morphine sulfate tabs ordered, be sure to have client swallow whole, do not crush or allow client to chew.
- Help client utilize distraction techniques during times of increased pain: music, television, counting to self, reading, stroking, or controlled breathing.
- Encourage client to utilize support persons, such as family or spiritual advisor.
- Provide information to decrease anxiety and allow client to have as much control over the management of pain as possible.
- Schedule activities to correspond with times of less pain.
- Help client displace the pain to a smaller, less vulnerable area of the body, e.g., as you continue to be aware of the discomfort in your lower back, move it ever so slowly down your leg to the back of your thigh . . . feel it throbbing in your thigh muscle . . .
- Refer client to a pain specialist or center for pain treatment.

Geriatric
- Address own guilt about inability to relieve client's pain so that avoidance of client or minimization of pain does not occur.
- Teach use of medications prophylactically (i.e., nitroglycerin).

Client/Family Teaching
- Teach the client/family about the nature of pain and responses to presence of pain.
- Teach client/family distraction-coping techniques for pain management: relaxation breathing, visualization, hobbies, yoga, meditation, massage, ice, exercise, or cutaneous stimulation (touch).
- Discuss the need for exercise to maintain strength, decrease stress, and promote sleep.
- Teach client/family how to effectively utilize pain medication.
- Teach client use of transcutaneous energy nerve stimulator (TENS) if ordered.

PARENTAL ROLE CONFLICT

Definition
The state in which a parent experiences role confusion and conflict in response to crisis.

Defining Characteristics
Major: Parent(s) expresses concerns/feelings of inadequacy to provide for child's physical and emotional needs during hospitalization or in the home
Demonstrated disruption in care taking routines
Parent(s) express concerns about changes in parental role, family functioning, family communication, or family health
Minor: Parent(s) expresses concern about perceived loss of control over decisions relating to child
Parent reluctant to participate in usual caretaking activities even with encouragement and support
Parent verbalize and demonstrate feelings of guilt, anger, fear, anxiety, or frustrations about effect of child's illness on family processes

Related Factors (r/t)
Separation from child due to chronic illness
Intimidation with invasive or restrictive modalities (e.g., isolation or intubation), specialized care centers, or policies
Home care of child with special needs (e.g., apnea monitoring, postural drainage, or hyperalimentation)
Change in marital status.
Interruptions of family life due to home care regimen (treatments, caregivers, or lack of respite)

Client Outcomes/Goals
✓ Parents state positive feelings in regard to care of child's physical and emotional needs during hospitalization.
✓ Parents able to carry out caretaking routines or describe alternate plan to use during child's hospitalization.
✓ Parents participate in care of child.

Nursing Interventions
- Explain all procedures/equipment used in caring for child.
- Provide facilities so parent may stay with sick child (cot or chair that reclines).
- Demonstrate safe places where parent may touch or stroke child.
- Encourage parent to talk to child, if they are comfortable they may sing to the child.
- Adjust equipment so that parent is able to hold child; provide comfortable chair, preferably a rocking chair.
- Provide time for parent to share feelings regarding child's illness.
- Encourage parent to share feelings with peer support groups.

- Demonstrate care that parent may give sick child; provide opportunities for successful caregiving and offer praise when it is done.
- Allow parents to bring in familiar items to make health setting homelike (favorite toys, pictures, and clothing).
- Encourage visiting and caregiving by siblings, if possible.
- Encourage respite from caregiving duties.

Client/Family Teaching
- Teach parents/family skills needed to care for child/equipment at home; allow them to practice skills until they are comfortable doing them.
- Refer to home health agencies that specialize in the care needed by the child.
- Refer to social service agencies (i.e., crippled children) for financial support to modify home to meet health care needs of the child.
- Refer to counseling, or support groups for coping with chronically ill.

ALTERED PARENTING

Definition
The state in which a nurturing figure(s) experiences an inability to create an environment that promotes the optimum growth and development of another human being.

Defining Characteristics
Abandonment
Runaway
Verbalization of being unable to control child
Incidence of physical and psychological trauma
Lack of parental attachment behaviors
Inappropriate visual, tactile, or auditory stimulation
Negative identification of infant/child's characteristics
Negative attachment of meanings to infant/child's characteristics
Constant verbalization of disappointment in gender or physical characteristics of the infant/child
Verbalization of resentment toward the infant/child
Verbalization of role inadequacy
*Inattentive to infant/child needs
Verbal disgust at body functions of infant/child
Noncompliance with health appointments for self or infant/child
*Inappropriate caretaking behavior (toilet training, sleep/rest, or feeding)
Inappropriate or inconsistent discipline practices
Frequent accidents
Frequent illness
Growth and development lag in the child
*History of child abuse or abandonment by primary caretaker
Verbalization of desire to have child call him/herself by first name versus traditional cultural tendencies
Child receives care from multiple caretakers without consideration for the needs of the infant/child
Compulsively seeking role approval from others
(*Critical)

Related Factors (r/t)
Lack of available role model
Ineffective role model
Physical and psychosocial abuse of nurturing figure
Lack of support between/from significant other(s); unmet social/emotional maturation needs of parenting figures
Interruption in bonding process, i.e., maternal, paternal, or other
Unrealistic expectation for self, infant, or partner
Perceived threat to own survival, physical and emotional

Mental or physical illness
Presence of stress (financial, legal, recent crisis, cultural move)
Lack of knowledge
Limited cognitive functioning
Lack of role identity
Lack or inappropriate response of child to relationship
Multiple pregnancies

Client Outcomes/Goals
✓ Initiates bonding process.
✓ Verbalizes the need for providing a nurturing environment for child/infant.
✓ Provides a nurturing environment that will promote the optimum growth and development of the infant/child.

Nursing Interventions
- Observe client's readiness to bond with infant.
- Provide early and repeated parent/infant contact.
- Model appropriate parenting activities.
- Encourage and reinforce parenting behaviors.
- Demonstrate infant's positive behaviors and characteristics.
- Document parent/child interaction.
- Observe parent's comprehension of the need for a nurturing environment.
- Encourage verbalization of perception of child.
- Encourage verbalization of feelings about parenting.
- Refer to support services as needed (community health nurse, social services, counseling, or child protective agencies).
- Refer to support group.

Client/Family Teaching
- Teach parents unique characteristics of child emphasizing strengths.
- Teach parenting skills.
- Teach stress management.

HIGH RISK FOR ALTERED PARENTING

Definition
The state in which a nurturing figure(s) is at risk to experience an inability to create an environment that promotes the optimum growth and development of another human being.

Defining Characteristics
Presence of risk factors such as:
Lack of parental attachment behaviors
Inappropriate visual, tactile, auditory stimulation
Negative identification of infant/child's characteristics
Negative attachment of meanings to infant/child's characteristics
Constant verbalization of disappointment in gender or physical characteristics of the infant/child
Verbalization of resentment toward the infant/child
Verbalization of role inadequacy
*Inattentive to infant/child's needs
Verbal disgust at body functions of infant/child
Noncompliance with health appointments for self or infant/child
*Inappropriate caretaking behaviors (toilet training, sleep/rest, or feeding)
Inappropriate or inconsistent discipline practices
Frequent accidents
Frequent illness
Growth and development lag in the child
History of child abuse or abandonment by primary caretaker
Verbalization of desire to have child call him/herself by first name versus traditional cultural tendencies
Child receives care from multiple caretakers without consideration for the needs of the infant/child
Compulsively seeking role approval from others
(*Critical)

Related Factors (r/t)
Lack of available role model
Ineffective role model
Physical and psychosocial abuse of nurturing figure
Lack of support between/from significant other(s)
Unmet social/emotional maturation needs of parenting figures
Interruption in bonding process, i.e., maternal, paternal, or other: unrealistic expectation for self, infant, partner
Perceive threat to own survival, physical and emotional
Mental or physical illness
Presence of stress (financial, legal, recent crisis, cultural, move)
Lack of knowledge

Limited cognitive functioning
Lack of role identity
Lack of appropriate response of child to relationship
Multiple pregnancies

Client Outcomes/Goals, Nursing Interventions and Client/Family Teaching
✓ Refer to *Altered Parenting*.

HIGH RISK FOR
PERIPHERAL NEUROVASCULAR DYSFUNCTION

Definition
A state in which an individual is at risk of experiencing a disruption in circulation, sensation, or motion of an extremity.

Risk Factors
Fractures

Mechanical compression, e.g., tourniquet, cast, brace, dressing or restraint, orthopedic surgery, trauma, immobilization, burns, or vascular obstruction.

Client Outcomes/Goals
✓ Circulation, sensation, and motion of extremity within normal limits for individual.

Nursing Interventions
- Monitor affected extremity for circulation, sensation and movement, edema, and change in color every _____ hours or minutes.
- Ask client to move toes/fingers, have client close his/her eyes and tell the nurse which extremities are being touched.
- Monitor for pain; neurovascular compromise does not respond to usual pain relief measures.
- Monitor appropriate application/function of corrective device every _____ hours or minutes.
- Position extremity in correct alignment with each position change.
- If extremity is to be elevated, elevate entire extremity to prevent venous pooling and stasis of dependent portion of extremity.
- Monitor temperature of extremity if heat or cold are applied and remove if circulation is being compromised.
- Use strict aseptic technique when changing dressings.
- Monitor for any signs of infection: edema, warmth, elevated temperature, or white blood cell count.
- Assist client to perform prescribed exercises every _____ hour(s).
- Proved adequate nutrition and fluid replacement to promote healing and maintain normal circulation.

Geriatric
- Use heat/cold therapies cautiously due to decreased sensation.

Client/Family Teaching
- Teach signs of neurovascular dysfunction and to report signs immediately to health careworker.
- Teach proper body alignment.
- Emphasize good nutrition to promote healing.
- Refer to rehabilitation facility if necessary for proper use of assistive devices and measures to improve mobility without compromising neurovascular function.

PERSONAL IDENTITY DISTURBANCE

Definition
Inability to distinguish between self and nonself.

Defining Characteristics
Withdrawal from social contact
Change in ability to determine relationship of body to environment
Inappropriate, grandiose behavior (adapted from Carpenito)

Related Factors (r/t)
Situational crisis, psychological impairment, chronic illness, or pain.

Client Outcomes/Goals
✓ Shows interest in surroundings.
✓ Responds to stimuli with appropriate affect.
✓ Able to perform self-care and self-control activities appropriate to age.
✓ Acknowledges personal strengths.
✓ Is able to engage in interpersonal relationships.
✓ Verbalizes willingness to change lifestyle, including willingness to use appropriate community resources.

Nursing Interventions
- Have all team members approach client in a consistent manner.
- Provide time for one-to-one interaction to establish a therapeutic relationship.
- Encourage client to talk about his feelings about self and his body image; have client make a list of positive strengths.
- Hold client responsible for age-appropriate behavior; involve client in planning self-care.
- Give positive feedback when appropriate self-control is used.
- Encourage participation in group therapy to receive feedback from others regarding behavior and build skills for relationships.
- Use a daily diary to set goals and monitor successes.
- Work with client to set achievable realistic goals.

Geriatric
- Monitor for signs of depression, grief and withdrawal.
- Address the client by his full name, preceded by the proper title: Mr, Ms, or Miss; only use nickname or first names if suggested by the client; do not use terms of endearment, i.e., honey.
- Practice reality orientation principles; ask specifically how the client feels about events that are happening.
- Ask about important past experiences that have been meaningful and what plans are being made for the future.

247

Client/Family Teaching

- Teach stress reduction, relaxation techniques, and guided imagery.
- Refer to community resources or Adult Children of Alcoholics, Parent-Effectiveness group or other self-help groups appropriate to client's underlying problem.

HIGH RISK FOR POISONING

Definition

Accentuated risk of accidental exposure to or ingestion of drugs or dangerous products in doses sufficient to cause poisoning.

Defining Characteristics

Presence of risk factors such as:
Internal (individual): reduced vision
Verbalization of occupational setting without adequate safeguards
Lack of safety or drug education
Lack of proper precaution
Cognitive or emotional difficulties
Insufficient finances
External (environmental)
Large supplies of drugs in house
Medicines or dangerous products placed or stored within the reach of confused persons
Availability of illicit drugs potentially contaminated by poisonous additives
Chemical contamination of food and water
Unprotected ventilated areas or without effective protection
Presence of poisonous vegetation
Presence of atmospheric pollutants

Related factors (r/t)

See risk factors

Client Outcomes/Goals

✓ States and uses safety measures to prevent accidental exposure or ingestion of drugs or dangerous products.
✓ Evidence of accidental poisoning.
✓ Locks drugs and harmful substances out of reach of children and clients with cognitive and emotional difficulties.
✓ Labels all poisonous substances.

Nursing Interventions

- Keep all medicines and dangerous products out of reach of children and confused persons.
- Provide labels with large print for visually impaired.
- Provide caregiver to be in charge of medications for client's with emotional and cognitive difficulties.
- Provide "Mr. Yuk" labels for families with children.
- If poisoning occurs:
  - Place victim with head turned to the side.

- Monitor respiratory, circulatory, and mental status.
- Attempt to identify the type and amount of substance ingested.
- Before doing any other intervention call the poison control center.
- If an acid substance has been ingested, the parent may be instructed to give milk; if it was an alkaline substance, lemon juice or vinegar may be used.
- Follow poison control centers direction, such as induce vomiting, save vomitus, or bring person to the emergency room.

Geriatric
- Instruct not to store medications with similar common items, i.e., nitroglycerine ointment tube near toothpaste tube.

Client/Family Teaching
- Teach family to always call medicine by name when giving to children; do not refer to it as candy.
- Teach family to keep potentially dangerous substances out of reach of children and confused persons, locked cupboards may be required.
- Teach family to always store potentially harmful substances in their original containers; poisonous substances by law must have antidotes on the label.
- Teach family never to store medication or substances in food containers.
- Teach family to keep poisonous house plants out of the reach of children.
- Teach children to avoid eating out of containers with "Mr. Yuk" label.
- Teach client/family for each person to only take medicine prescribed specifically for them.
- Teach family to read and follow labels on all products before use, being careful to adjust doses for age.
- Instruct family with young children to keep syrup of ipecac on hand at all times; instruct to use only after contacting physician or poison control center.
- Inform the family of the number of the local poison control center; instruct to place near phone for all caregivers.
- Refer client's with substance abuse problems to appropriate community agency.

POST-TRAUMA RESPONSE

Definition
The state of an individual experiencing a sustained painful response to an overwhelming traumatic event(s).

Defining Characteristics
Major: Reexperience of the traumatic event that may be identified in cognitive, affective, or sensory motor activities (flashbacks, intrusive thoughts, repetitive dreams or nightmares, excessive verbalization of the traumatic event, verbalization of survival guilt, or guilt about behavior required for survival)

Minor: Psychic/emotional numbness (impaired interpretation of reality, confusion, dissociation or amnesia, vagueness about traumatic event, or constricted affect)

Altered lifestyle (self-destructiveness, such as substance abuse, suicide attempt or other acting out behavior, difficulty with interpersonal relationship, development of phobia regarding trauma, poor impulse control/irritability, and explosiveness)

Related Factors (r/t)
Disaster

Wars

Epidemics

Rape

Assault

Torture

Catastrophic illness or accident

Client Outcomes/Goals
✓ Acknowledges the traumatic event and begins to work with the trauma by talking over the experience and expressing feelings, such as fear, anger, and guilt.

✓ Directs anger at event as opposed to significant other.

✓ Acknowledges that feelings are personal, real, and individual.

✓ Identifies and makes connection with support persons/resources.

✓ Assimilates the experience into a meaningful whole and goes on to pursue his/her life as evidenced by goal setting.

Nursing Interventions
- Observe the client's response, its severity, and its effect on his/her current functioning.
- Provide a safe, therapeutic environment where client can regain control.
- Stay with client and offer support during episodes of high anxiety.
- Use touch with client's permission (hand on shoulder, or holding hand).
- Provide a safe/structured environment for person to describe the traumatic experience and express feelings.
- Help client ventilate feelings; spend one-to-one time with client.
- Explore available support systems.
- Provide or arrange follow-up treatment.

Geriatric
- Observe client for concurrent losses that may affect client's coping skills.

251

- Allow client more time to establish trust and express anger, guilt, or shame about the trauma.
- Review past coping skills and give positive reinforcement for successfully dealing with other life crisis.
- Monitor client for clinical signs of depression, anxiety, and refer to physician for medication if appropriate.

Client/Family Teaching
- Teach client and family the signs and symptoms that may reoccur periodically after traumatic event.
- Teach relaxation skills to decrease anxiety when flashbacks and intrusive thoughts occur.
- Refer to peer support groups.

POWERLESSNESS

Definition

Perception that one's own action will not significantly affect an outcome; a perceived lack of control over a current situation or immediate happening.

Defining Characteristics

Severe: Verbal expressions of having no control or influence over situation

Verbal expressions of having no control over self-care

Depression over physical deterioration that occurs despite patient compliance with regimens

Apathy

Moderate: Nonparticipation in care or decisionmaking when opportunities are provided

Expressions of dissatisfaction over inability to perform previous tasks or activities

Does not monitor progress

Expression of doubt regarding role performance

Reluctance to express true feelings

Fearing alienation from caregivers

Passivity

Inability to seek information regarding care

Dependence on others that may result in irritability, resentment, anger, and guilt

Does not defend self-care practice when challenged

Related Factors (r/t)

Health care environment

Interpersonal interaction

Lifestyle of helplessness

Illness-related regimen

Client Outcomes/Goals

✓ States feelings of powerlessness and other feelings related to powerlessness (anger, sadness, or hopelessness).

✓ Identifies things that he/she has control over.

✓ Participates in planning care; makes decisions over care and treatment when possible.

✓ Asks questions about care and treatment.

✓ Verbalizes a hopeful future.

Nursing Interventions

▪ Observe factors contributing to powerlessness: immobility, hospitalization, unfavorable prognosis, no support system, misinformation about situation, inflexible routine.

▪ Establish therapeutic relationship with client: spend time one-to-one; assign same caregiver; keep commitments; "I will be back to answer your questions in the next hour."

253

- Allow client to express hope (may be only that "I hope my coffee will be hot"; or more serious "I hope I will die with my significant other here"); listen to client's priorities.
- Allow time for questions (15 to 20 minutes every shift); have client write questions down.
- Have client assist in planning care if possible (what time to bathe, pain medication before uncomfortable procedures, and food and fluid preferences) document specifics in care plan.
- Keep items client uses and needs within reach to allow control: urinal, tissues, phone, and TV control.
- Work with client to set achievable short-term goals, such as walk to window to wave to children by end of week.
- Have client write goals and plans to achieve them (dangle at bedside 10 minutes for 2 days, then sit in chair 10 minutes for 2 days, then walk to window).
- Give praise for accomplishments.
- Help client identify those things over which they do have power.
- Keep interactions with client focused on client (not family or physician focused).
- Acknowledge subjective concerns, and fears.
- Allow client to take control of as many ADLS as possible and keep client informed of all care that will be given.
- Assist client to develop realistic goals within the limitations of illness, do not emphasize limitations.
- Develop contract with client stating client's and nurses responsibilities and privileges.

Client/Family Teaching
- Explain all procedures, treatments, and expected outcomes.
- Provide written instructions for treatment and procedures for which client will be responsible.
- Help client practice assertive communication techniques; use role-playing ("Tell me what you are going to ask your doctor").
- Refer to support groups, pastoral care, or social services.

ALTERED PROTECTION

Definition
The state in which an individual experiences a decrease in the ability to guard the self from internal or external threats, such as illness or injury.

Defining Characteristics
Major: Deficient immunity
Impaired healing
Altered clotting
Maladaptive stress response
Neurosensory alteration
Minor: Chilling
Perspiring
Dyspnea
Cough

Itching
Restlessness
Insomnia
Fatigue
Anorexia
Weakness
Immobility
Disorientation
Pressure sores

Related Factors (r/t)
Extremes of age
Inadequate nutrition
Alcohol abuse
Abnormal blood profiles (leukopenia, thrombocytopenia, anemia, or coagulation)
Drug therapies (antineoplastic, corticosteroid, immune, anticoagulant, or thrombolytic)
Treatments (surgery or radiation) and diseases, such as cancer and immune disorders

Client Outcomes/Goals
✓ Displays no signs of infection/injury/bleeding.
✓ Explains precautions and actions that should be taken to prevent infection/injury/bleeding.
✓ Explains precautions and or actions needed to protect self (e.g., changes in physical environment, avoidance of ill persons, maintenance of balanced diet, and adequate rest).
✓ Nourished and well-rested.
✓ Experiences adequate rest.
✓ Demonstrates personal cleanliness and maintains a sanitary and safe environment.

Nursing Interventions
- Take temperature, pulse, and respiration and blood pressure every _____ hours.
- Observe nutritional status; weight, serum protein and albumin, and muscle mass size.
- Refer to dietician if malnourished.
- Observe sleep pattern, if altered, refer to nursing interventions for *Sleep Pattern Disturbance*.
- Evaluate amount of stress in client's life.

Prevention of Infection

- ▸ Monitor for signs of infection: fever, chills, flushed skin, or edema or redness in traumatized area.
- ▸ If white blood count severely decreased, initiate protective isolation.
- ▸ Refer to *High Risk for Infection* for more interventions on prevention of infection.

Prevention of Injury

- ▸ Refer to *High Risk for Injury* for intervention on preventing injury.

Prevention of Bleeding

- ▸ Monitor client's bleeding risk, evaluate clotting studies, and amount of trauma.
- ▸ Initiate bleeding precautions: use toothette only for mouth care, smaller needles for injections or avoid injections, and watch for bruising and bleeding.
- ▸ Avoid salicylates to decrease risk of bleeding.
- ▸ Apply pressure for 5 minutes over venipuncture sites.

Client/Family Teaching

- • Teach client to wear medic-alert bracelet and notify all health care personnel of bleeding disorder.
- • Teach client/family signs of bleeding and precautions to take to prevent bleeding.
- • Teach client/family methods to decrease stress, such as relaxation therapy, imagery, and exercise.
- • Teach client/family (especially neonates and persons with depressed bone marrows) to avoid crowds and contact with persons who have infections.
- • Teach client/family about protection-enhancing effects of adequate nutrition, rest, and conservation of energy.
- • Teach client/family methods to decrease spread of infection.

RAPE-TRAUMA SYNDROME

Definition
Forced violent sexual penetration against the victim's will and consent. The trauma syndrome that develops from this attack or attempted attacks includes an acute phase of disorganization of the victim's life-style and a long-term process of reorganization of lifestyle.

Note: This syndrome includes the following three subcomponents: *Rape-Trauma, Compound Reaction*, and *Silent Reaction*. There are additional nursing care plans for each of these diagnoses).

Defining Characteristics
Acute phase: Emotional reactions (anger, embarrassment, fear of physical violence and death, humiliation, revenge, or self-blame)

Irritability, easily triggered crying

Multiple physical symptoms (gastrointestinal irritability, genitourinary discomfort, muscle tension, and sleep pattern disturbance).

Long-term phase: Changes in lifestyle (change in residence, dealing with repetitive nightmare and phobias, seeking family support, seeking social network support).

Client Outcomes/Goals
✓ Shares feelings, concerns, and fears.
✓ Recognizes that rape or attempt was not client's fault.
✓ States that no matter what the situation no one has the right to assault you.
✓ Identifies behaviors/situations within own control to prevent or reduce risk or recurrence.
✓ Describes treatment procedures and reasons for treatment.
✓ Reports absence of physical complications, or pain.
✓ Identifies support systems and is able to ask them for help in dealing with this trauma.
✓ Functions at same level as before crisis.
✓ Recognizes that full recovery may often take a year and that this is normal.

Nursing Interventions
- Observe responses: anger, fear, self-blame, sleep pattern disturbance, or phobias.
- Monitor psychological state: verbal and nonverbal, crying, wringing of hands, or avoiding interaction and/or eye contact with staff.
- Stay with client initially or have a trusted person stay with client.
- Explain each part of treatment.
- Observe for signs of physical injury.
- Encourage verbalization of feelings.
- Provide privacy for client to express feelings.
- Enlist help of supportive counselors experienced with rape trauma.
- Discuss importance of pelvic examination, if first examination, explain instruments and let client know when you will touch them and where.

- Explain collection of specimens for evidence; provide for self-care needs after examination (personal hygiene).
- Discuss possible pregnancy and sexually transmitted disease and treatments available.
- Explain choice of client whether or not to report rape.
- If interview by law enforcement personnel is permitted, stay with the client, and offer nonverbal support by presence.
- Discuss support system; involve support system if appropriate and if client grants permission.
- Refer to psychotherapist, mental health clinic, or rape crisis counselor.
- Explain you may need to keep client's undergarments for evidence, instruct client when they go home to put other clothing in a paper bag and not to wash it until it is known if clothing will be needed for evidence.
- Obtain blood alcohol level if indicated.

Geriatric
- Embarrassment may prevent reporting.
- Observe for psychosocial distress, e.g., memory impairment, sleep disturbances, regression, changes in bodily functions.
- Build trusting relationship.
- Allow for expression of anger.

Client/Family Teaching
- Explain possible physical discomfort; pruritis; side effects of diethylstilbestrol (DES); nausea and vomiting; when medication discontinued, possible spotting.
- Teach relaxation techniques.
- Discuss practical lifestyle changes within clients control to reduce future risk of attack, e.g., keeping doors locked, checking car before getting in, not walking alone at night, keeping someone informed of whereabouts, someone to check if client has not arrived within reasonable amount of time, keep lights on in entry way, and have keys in hand when approaching car or house.
- Refer to self-defense classes.
- Teach new appropriate outlets for anger.
- Encourage significant other to direct anger at event and attacker, not at victim.
- Emphasize vulnerability of victim and that her reactions are appropriate.

RAPE-TRAUMA SYNDROME: COMPOUND REACTION

Definition
Refer to *Rape-Trauma Syndrome*.

Defining Characteristics
Refer to *Rape-Trauma Syndrome*
Additional characteristics: reactivated symptoms of such previous conditions, i.e., physical illness, psychiatric illness; reliance on alcohol or drugs.

Related Factors (r/t)
Rape

Client Outcomes/Goals
Refer to *Rape-Trauma Syndrome*.

Nursing Interventions
Refer to *Rape-Trauma Syndrome, Powerlessness, Ineffective Individual Coping, Dysunfctional Grieving, Anxiety, Fear, Violence: Self-Directed, Sexual Dysfunction.*
Geriatric
Refer to *Rape-Trauma Syndrome*.

Client/Family Teaching
- Teach client what reactions to expect during acute and long-term phase; say "that you may or may not have the following reactions: *acute phase*: anger, fear, self-blame, embarrassment, revenge; physical symptoms, muscle tension, sleeplessness, stomach upset, genitourinary discomfort; *long-term phase*: changes in lifestyle, residence, nightmares, phobias, and seeking family and social network support.
- Encourage psychiatric consultation if client is suicidal, violent, or is not able to continue activities of daily living.

RAPE-TRAUMA SYNDROME: SILENT REACTION

Definition
Refer to *Rape-Trauma Syndrome*.

Defining Characteristics
Abrupt changes in relationships with men
Increase in nightmares
Increased anxiety during interview, i.e., blocking of associations, long periods of silence, minor stuttering, physical distress
Pronounced changes in sexual behavior
No verbalization of the occurrence of rape
Sudden onset of phobic reactions

Related Factors (r/t)
Rape

Client Outcomes/Goals
✓ Resumes previous level of relationships with significant other.
✓ States improvement in sleep without nightmares.
✓ Able to express feelings and to discuss the rape.
✓ Return to usual pattern of sexual behavior.
✓ Free of phobic reactions.

Nursing Interventions
Refer to Nursing Diagnosis *Rape-Trauma Syndrome, Powerlessness, Ineffective Individual Coping, Dysfunctional Grieving, Anxiety, Fear, Violence; Self-Directed, Sexual Dysfunction, Impaired Communication*
- Observe disruptions in relationships with significant other.
- Monitor signs of increased anxiety: silence, stuttering, physical distress, irritability, unexplained crying spells.
- Observe changes in sexual behavior.
- Identify phobic reactions to objects in environment: strangers, doorbell ringing, being with groups of people, knives.
- Provide support by listening when client is ready to talk.
- Be nonjudgmental when feelings are expressed; explain normalcy of anger and need to verbalize.
- Remain with client while anxious even if client is silent.
- Evaluate somatic complaints.

Geriatric
Refer to *Rape-Trauma Syndrome.*

Client/Family Teaching
Refer to *Rape Trauma Syndrome.*
- Reassure client that they are not "bad;" it was not her fault.
- Teach procedure for pelvic exam.
- Refer to sexual-assault counselor.

RELOCATION STRESS SYNDROME

Definition
Physiological and/or psychosocial disturbances as a result of transfer from one environment to another.

Defining Characteristics
Major: Anxiety
Apprehension
Increased confusion (elderly)
Depression
Loneliness
Minor: Verbalization of unwillingness to relocate
Sleep disturbance
Change in eating habits
Dependency
Gastrointestinal disturbances
Increased verbalization of needs

Insecurity
Lack of trust
Restlessness
Sad affect
Unfavorable comparison of post/pre-transfer staff
Verbalization of being concerned /upset about transfer
Vigilance
Weight change
Withdrawal

Related Factors (r/t)
Past, concurrent, and recent losses, losses involved with decision to move, feeling of powerlessness
Lack of adequate support system
Little or no preparation for the impending move
Moderate to high degree of environmental change
History and types of previous transfers
Impaired psychosocial health status
Decreased physical health status

Client Outcomes/Goals
✓ States feels less anxious.
✓ Oriented to person, place, and time.
✓ Able to share feelings of sadness, loneliness.
✓ Seeks out staff or one identified person daily for 30 minutes.
✓ States benefits of new living situation.
✓ Able to carry out activities of daily living in usual manner.
✓ Maintains previous health status (elimination, nutrition, sleep, social interaction).

Nursing Interventions
▪ Establish how the client would like to be addressed e.g. Mr. Mrs., Miss. or by first name.
▪ Give a thorough explanation of all new situations, treatments; take time to answer questions; encourage client to write out a list of questions to ask Doctor/Caregiver.

- Use reality orientation if needed; today is _____, the date is _____, you are at _____ facility, repeat information as needed; provide clock/calendar.
- Spend one-to-one time with client allowing them to express their feelings; convey acceptance of feelings and emphasize that feelings are real and individual; it's OK to be sad or angry about moving.
- Assign the same staff to clients who are anxious and express fears of being alone.
- Assist client to identify staff or significant other that he can share his feelings with; specify time length so client does not ruminate (continued repetitive thoughts) over events one cannot control.
- Have client state one positive aspect of new living situation daily.
- Monitor client's health status and provide appropriate interventions for problems with elimination, nutrition, sleep and social interaction.
- If client is being transferred within an agency have staff from new unit visit client prior to transfer.
- Once client is transferred, have previous staff make occasional visits until client is comfortable in new surroundings.
- Orient client to new surroundings and make sure they know how to call for staff assistance when needed.
- If client is being transferred to a nursing home or adult foster care try and arrange a visit beforehand; if this is not possible see, if new staff will visit; if neither can be done, try and arrange a phone interview and obtain pictures of new care facility.
- Have a familiar person accompany the client to the new facility.
- Allow client to grieve old situation, explaining it is normal to feel sadness over change and loss.
- Allow client to participate in care as much as possible and to make decisions when possible e.g. "I prefer the bed by the window"; choice of roommate; make an effort to accommodate the client.

Geriatric
- Monitor need for transfer and use only when necessary, recognizing that some client's adapt poorly and often lose areas of function as a result.
- Protect from injury as falls are common with relocation.

Client/Family Teaching
- Teach about the grief process associated with change and loss
- Refer to the Department on Aging for support services that are available in the community
- Teach relaxation techniques e.g. breathe in say "re" breathe out say "lax", use this technique when the client starts to have feelings of anxiety

ALTERED ROLE PERFORMANCE

Definition
Disruption in the way one perceives one's role performance.

Defining Characteristics
Change in self-perception of role
Change in others perception of role
Conflict in roles
Change in physical capacity to resume role
Lack of knowledge of role
Change in usual patterns of responsibility

Related Factors (r/t)
To be developed

Client Outcomes/Goals
✓ Identifies realistic perception of role.
✓ States personal strengths.
✓ Acknowledges problems contributing to inability to carry out usual role.
✓ Accepts physical limitations regarding role responsibility and considers ways to change lifestyle to accomplish goal associated with role performance.
✓ Demonstrates knowledge of appropriate behaviors associated with new or changed role.
✓ States knowledge of change in responsibility and new behaviors associated with new responsibility.
✓ Verbalizes acceptance of new responsibility.

Nursing Interventions
- Observe client's knowledge of behaviors associated with role.
- Have client make a list of strengths that are needed for the role; acknowledge which strengths client has and which strengths need to be developed.
- Have client list problems associated with role and look at ways of overcoming problems; if pain is worse late in day have client get necessary role tasks done early in day.
- Look at ways to compensate for physical disability; have a ramp built to provide access to house; put household objects within client's reach from wheelchair.
- Help client identify resources for assistance in caring for disabled/aging parent (adult day care).

Geriatric
- Explore community needs after assessing client's strengths: suggest functional activities e.g. foster grandparent, mentors for small businesses.
- Refer to family counseling as needed for adjustment to role changes.

Client/Family Teaching

- Refer to appropriate community agency to learn skills for functioning in new or changed role; vocational rehabilitation, parenting classes, hospice, respite care.

BATHING/HYGIENE SELF-CARE DEFICIT

Definition
A state in which the individual experiences an impaired ability to perform or complete bathing/hygiene activities for oneself.

Defining Characteristics
*Inability to wash body or body parts
Inability to obtain or get to water source
Inability to regulate temperature or flow
(*Critical)

Functional level classification (*Impaired Physical Mobility*)
0=Completely independent
1=Requires use of equipment or device
2=Requires help from another person, for assistance, supervision, or teaching
3=Requires help from another person and equipment device
4=Dependent, does not participate in activity

Related Factors (r/t)
Intolerance to activity
Decreased strength and endurance
Pain, discomfort
Perceptual or cognitive impairment
Neuromuscular impairment
Musculoskeletal impairment
Depression, severe anxiety

Client Outcomes/Goals
✓ Skin intact, free of body odor.
✓ States and uses methods to bathe with minimal difficulty.
✓ Sets realistic levels of self care to be achieved.

Nursing Interventions
- Observe cause of inability to bathe (see related factors).
- Ask client for ideas on how to provide better bathing methods.
- If client acutely ill, provide bed bath.
- Provide adaptive equipment as needed to assist with bathing, e.g. bar on wall to assist getting into tub, stool in tub, chair or commode chair with pan removed in shower, washcloth mitt, long handled brush, and so on.
- Provide all bathing supplies within easy reach.
- If needed, medicate for pain before bathing activity.
- Observe condition of skin during bathing, provide lotion for additional lubrication if needed.
- Avoid excessive use of soap; rinse off soap thoroughly.

- Have client bathe any portion of body as able and provide praise for accomplishment; increase body portion bathed as client's tolerance increases.
- Keep call light readily available if client bathing alone.
- Monitor for fatigue, frustration, inability to tolerate bathing activity.
- Supervise until you determine the client's ability to carry out bathing independently.

Geriatric
- Divide the bathing/hygiene tasks into small, easy to manage steps.
- Use verbal and physical prompting to teach.
- Use privacy; bath blankets for warmth and dignity.

Client Family Teaching
- Teach client/family use of adaptive devices to utilize when bathing.
- Teach family how to bath client including appropriate schedule, use of soap, maintaining privacy, preventing chilling, inspecting skin, keeping skin well lubricated.
- Teach client the basics of personal hygiene, including how to use soap.

DRESSING/GROOMING SELF-CARE DEFICIT

Definition
A state in which the individual experiences an impaired ability to perform or complete dressing and grooming activities for oneself.

Defining Characteristics
*Impaired ability to put on or take off necessary items of clothing
Impaired ability to obtain or replace articles of clothing
Impaired ability to fasten clothing
Inability to maintain appearance at a satisfactory level
*(Critical)

Related Factors (r/t)
Intolerance to activity
Decreased strength and endurance
Pain, discomfort
Perceptual or cognitive impairment

Neuromuscular impairment
Musculoskeletal impairment
Depression, severe anxiety

Client Outcomes/Goals
✓ Dressed appropriately.
✓ Able to utilize adaptive devices to dress.
✓ Able to dress self and fasten clothing or if not able tasks are done or assistance is provided by caregiver.

Nursing Interventions
- Observe cause of inability to dress self (refer to related factors).
- Ask client for input on how to increase the ease of dressing self.
- Provide adaptive equipment as needed to help dress self, e.g. velcro closures on front of clothing, long handled grasping devices, zipper pull, button hook.
- Encourage client to wear regular clothing instead of sleeping apparel.
- Lay clothing out in order that it will be put on by client.
- If needed, medicate for pain before dressing activity.
- Choose clothing that is easy to put on with wide sleeves, large pant legs, elastic waist band, velcro closing.
- Help client decide on easiest place to keep appropriate clothing.
- Refer to occupational therapy for further help.
- Plan activities to avoid fatigue before dressing.

Geriatric
- Use verbal and physical prompting to encourage dressing self.
- Allow caregiver latitude to provide adequate supervision for dressing, e.g., do not insist that clients be finished with dressing at an early hour.

Client/Family Teaching

- If client has lack of use or weakness of one side of the body, teach the client to dress the affected side first, than the unaffected side.
- Teach techniques to simplify dressing; help client establish a routine for dressing behavior.
- Teach client which clothes are appropriate for season, temperature, weather.
- Teach client/family use of adaptive device for dressing/grooming.

FEEDING SELF-CARE DEFICIT

Definition
A state in which the individual experiences an impaired ability to perform or complete feeding activities for oneself.

Defining Characteristics
Inability to bring food from a receptacle to the mouth

Related Factors (r/t)
Intolerance to activity, decreased strength and endurance
Pain, discomfort
Perceptual or cognitive impairment

Neuromuscular impairment
Musculoskeletal impairment
Depression, severe anxiety

Client Outcomes/Goals
✓ Feeds self.
✓ Demonstrates use of adaptive devices to assist in feeding.
✓ Caregiver provides assistance with feeding when necessary.

Nursing Interventions
- Observe client's ability to feed self including ability to utilize hands, motivation (refer to related factors above).
- Test gag reflex bilaterally, also give small sips of water and determine ability to swallow if appropriate.
- Place food on unaffected side of mouth and instruct client to chew and swallow on that side.
- Obtain adaptive devices to help with feeding including cup with large handle, built up spoon, plate guard, suction device to immobilize plate, rocker knife, hand splints.
- Have suction machine readily available, if needed.
- Provide oral hygiene before or after meals as preferred by client, if one sided involvement, always provide oral care after meal.
- Provide pleasant mealtime environment: sitting up, free of pain, free of odors, avoid noxious or painful procedures before meals.
- Avoid overwhelming client with food; place a few foods in front of client at one time, place food on one plate if possible.
- Praise all feeding attempts.
- Refer to Occupational Therapy, Physical Therapy for further help in relearning feeding behavior.
- Plan activities to avoid fatigue before mealtime.

Note: If dysphagia present, refer to Nursing Diagnosis: *Impaired Swallowing*.

Geriatric
- Provide "finger foods" for clients with coordination problems.
- Use verbal and physical prompting to eat a meal.

Client/Family Teaching

- Teach client how to utilize adaptive devices to assist in feeding.
- Teach visually impaired client how to eat by naming foods according to numbers on a clock.

CHRONIC LOW SELF-ESTEEM

Definition
Long-standing negative self-evaluation/feelings about self or self capabilities.

Defining Characteristics
Major: Self-negating verbalization
Expressions of shame or guilt
Evaluates self as unable to deal with events
Rationalizes away or rejects positive feedback and exaggerates negative feedback about self
Hesitant to try new things or situations
Minor: Frequent lack of success in work or other life events
Overly conforming or dependent on other's opinions
Lack of eye contact
Nonassertive or passive
Indecisive
Excessively seeks reassurance

Client Outcomes/Goals
✓ Identifies personal strengths and is able to accept compliments.
✓ Recognizes feelings of guilt and works through them.
✓ States accurate perception of events and ways to deal with them.
✓ Tries one new thing (set time frame; weekly or monthly).
✓ Attempts to set small achievable goals.
✓ Able to make own decisions without consulting others.
✓ Makes eye contact.

Nursing Interventions
▪ Actively involve client in plan of care.
▪ Give positive feedback when tasks are accomplished or goals are attained.
▪ Involve client in diversional activity so thoughts are focused outside of self, such as reading, crafts, radio, television, or visiting with others.
▪ Set limits for negative expressions (10 minutes/hour) and gradually decrease time—replace with positive expressions; make a list of positive traits (refer to *Self-Esteem Disturbance*).
Geriatric
▪ Give positive reinforcement for participation in senior activities.
▪ Use reminiscent therapy, identifying strengths and accomplishments.

Client/Family Teaching
*Refer to community agencies for individual counseling; group therapy.

SELF-ESTEEM DISTURBANCE

Definition
Negative self-evaluation/feelings about self or self-capabilities, which may be directly or indirectly expressed.

Defining Characteristics
Self negating verbalization
Expressions of shame or guilt
Evaluates self as unable to deal with events
Rationalizes away or rejects positive feedback and exaggerates negative feedback about self
Rationalizing personal failures
Hesitant to try new things or situations
Denial of problems obvious to others
Projection of blame or responsibility for problems
Hypersensitive to slight or criticism
Grandiosity

Client Outcomes/Goals
✓ Identifies personal strengths.
✓ States accurate perception of events and ways to deal with them.
✓ Able to accept compliments.
✓ Tries new things/situations.
✓ Accepts responsibility for own actions.
✓ Accepts criticism and attempts to correct problems.

Nursing Interventions
- Treat client in a nonjudgmental way, realizing each person has own personal values and beliefs.
- Assist client to identify origins of self-esteem; it is learned behavior so it can be changed.
- Assist client to recognize that negative self-esteem can change.
- Have client make a list of positive personal strengths.
- Have client participate in daily grooming routine.
- Spend time with client and allow him to express feelings about treatment and any change illness or treatment may have had on his body image.
- Have client practice making positive statements about self and responding in a positive way when compliments are given, role play may be used.

Geriatric
- Promote positive self-image; compliment on appearance; assist client to look his or her best.
- Do not appear rushed; encourage verbalization of client's fears about illness or dysfunction.
- Assist client in life review, identifying successes.
- Encourage participation in support-reminiscence group.
- Assist in planning schedule for family/significant others to visit regularly.

Client/Family Teaching

*Teach that self-esteem is a learned behavior; any learned behavior can be changed.

*Refer to community agencies; self-help groups, counseling as needed.

SITUATIONAL LOW SELF-ESTEEM

Definition
Negative self-evaluation/feelings about self that develop in response to a loss or change in an individual who previously had a positive self-evaluation.

Defining Characteristics
Major: Episodic occurrence of negative self-appraisal in response to life events in a person with a previous positive self-evaluation

Minor:
Verbalization of negative feelings about the self (helplessness or uselessness)
Self negating verbalizations
Expressions of shame or guilt
Evaluates self as unable to handle situations or events
Difficulty making decisions

Related Factors (r/t)
Situational crisis

Client Outcomes/Goals
✓ States effect of life events in relationship to feelings about self.
✓ States positive personal strengths.
✓ Acknowledges presence of guilt and does not blame self if action was related to another person's appraisal.
✓ Seeks help for situations feels cannot handle independently.

Nursing Interventions
- Observe cause of situational low self-esteem.
- Ask client to state his perception of events that may be causing negative feelings toward self.
- Assist client to recognize that the only one he has control over is himself "No one can make you feel guilty without your consent."
- Discuss how client handled difficult situations in the past.
- Reinforce positive coping behaviors.
- Have client write out his strengths. (Refer to *Self-Esteem Disturbance* and *Chronic Low Self-Esteem*.)

Client/Family Teaching
- Refer to appropriate community resources; crisis intervention center

HIGH RISK FOR SELF-MUTILATION

Definition

A state in which an individual is at high risk to perform a deliberate act on the self with the intent to injure, not kill, which produces immediate tissue damage to the body.

Risk Factors

Groups at risk: Clients with borderline personality disorder, especially females 16 to 25 years of age
Clients in psychotic state—frequently males in young adulthood
Emotionally disturbed or battered children
Mentally retarded and autistic children
Clients with a history of self-injury

Related Factors

Inability to cope with increased psychological/physiological tension in a healthy manner
Feelings of depression, rejection, self-hatred, separation anxiety, guilt and depersonalization, or fluctuating
   emotions
Command hallucinations
Need for sensory stimuli
Parental emotional deprivation
Dysfunctional family

Client Outcomes/Goals

✓ States appropriate ways to cope with increased psychological/physiological tension.
✓ Able to express feelings.
✓ Seeks help when hallucinations are present.
✓ Uses appropriate community agencies when caregivers are unable to attend to emotional needs.

Nursing Interventions

- Monitor the client's behavior; stagger 15 minute checks so client does not observe a pattern.
- Secure a written or verbal contract from client that he will notify staff when he experiences feelings of self-mutilation.
- Monitor for presence of hallucinations, ask specifically, "Do you hear voices that other people do not hear?"
- Tell client that you will stay with him when he hears voices and that he will be safe, provide referrals for medication.
- If self-mutilation occurs, care for the wounds in a matter-of-fact way so as not to support inappropriate attention getting.
- When client is experiencing extreme anxiety, provide one-to-one staff.
- Reinforce alternate ways of dealing with anxiety, e.g., exercise, engaging in unit activities, or talking about feelings.

- Keep environment safe; remove all harmful objects from the area.
- If client is unable to control behavior, time-out in a quiet room may be necessary; ensure safety by providing staff observation.
- Give positive reinforcement when client makes appropriate choices for behavior; confront inappropriate behavior.
- Involve client in careplan and emphasize that he can make choices.
- Emphasize that client must comply with the rules on the unit; give positive reinforcement when he does this; minimize attention to disruptive behavior.
- Concentrate on client's strengths; have him make a list of strengths and carry it on a 3 x 5 card, have the client refer to the list when he has negative thoughts about himself.
- Refer to protective services if there is evidence of abuse.

Client/Family Teaching
- Teach stress reduction techniques, such as imagery; controlled breathing (breath in on "re" and breath out on "lax"), teaching client to sustain the breathing out phase.
- Provide client/family with phone numbers of appropriate community agencies for therapy or counseling.
- Refer to appropriate agencies for job training skills or education to give positive things on which to focus.

SENSORY/PERCEPTURAL ALTERATIONS (SPECIFY) (VISUAL, AUDITORY, KINESTHETIC, GUSTATORY, TACTILE, OLFACTORY)

Definition

A state in which an individual experiences a change in the amount or patterning of oncoming stimuli accompanied by a diminished, exaggerated, distorted or impaired response to such stimuli.

Defining Characteristics

Disoriented to time or place, or with persons
Altered abstraction
Altered conceptualization
Change in problem-solving abilities
Reported or measured change in sensory acuity
Change in behavior pattern
Anxiety
Apathy
Change in usual response to stimuli
Indication of body image alteration
Restlessness
Irritability
Altered communication patterns

Other Possible Characteristics

Complaints of fatigue
Alterations in posture
Change in muscular tension
Inappropriate responses
Hallucinations

Related Factors (r/t)

Altered environmental stimuli, excessive or insufficient
Altered sensory reception, transmission or integration
Chemical alterations, endogenous (electrolyte) or exogenous (drugs)
Psychological stress

Client Outcomes/Goals

✓ Demonstrates understanding by verbal, written, or signed response.
✓ Demonstrates relaxed body movements or facial expression.
✓ Explains plan to modify lifestyle to accommodate vision/hearing impairment.

✓ Remains free of physical harm from loss of vision, hearing, loss of tactile sensation, or decreased balance.

✓ Has contact with appropriate community resources.

Nursing Interventions (Sensory Deprivation/Overload)

- Observe for factors that can cause sensory-perceptual alterations, such as insufficient sleep, sensory deprivation, sensory overload with excessive noise and stimuli, substance abuse, medication effect, electrolyte imbalance, or normal aging process.

Sensory Deprivation

- Orient to time, place and person with each contact if possible; inform of current weather, and news items.
- Explain all activities.
- Help client get out of bed and into environment with other people.
- Provide radio or TV, clocks, or calendars to encourage orientation.
- Encourage visits from significant others, keep pictures of family and friends at bedside.

Visual (photophobia): keep room darkened.

Sensory Overload

- Reduce amount of stimuli the client receives, move client away from sources of noise.
- Have essential personnel only care for client.
- Limit TV viewing of roommates and turn off nonessential alarms.

Nursing Interventions-Auditory

- Observe emotional needs; encourage expression of feelings.
- Keep background noise to minimum, turn off TV or radio when communicating with client.
- Stand or sit directly in front of client if possible, make sure adequate light is on nurse's face, establish eye contact, and use nonverbal gestures.
- Speak distinctly in lower voice tones if possible.
- Provide communication board if needed, or personnel who know sign language.
- Refer to appropriate resources such as speech therapy, hearing testing, and hearing aid evaluation as needed.
- Be aware that hearing loss may cause frustration, anger, fear and self-imposed isolation.
- Assist with placement of hearing aid if necessary and check battery.

Nursing Interventions-Visual

- Observe emotional needs and encourage expression of feelings.
- Identify name and purpose when entering client's room.
- Orient to time, place, person, or surroundings; provide radio, or talking books.
- If decreased vision, keep environment well lighted, but reduce glare (waxed floors, or blinding sunlight into room).
- Keep doors completely open or closed; keep furniture out of way to bathroom; do not rearrange furniture.
- Feed client at mealtimes if temporary blindness.
- Keep siderails up for clients safety, explain precaution.
- Converse with and touch client frequently during care to decrease social isolation; tell him you are going to touch him before you do, ask permission if necessary.
- Walk client by having client grasp nurse's elbow and nurse walk partly in front of client.

- If client frightened or confused, walk by having client put both hands on nurse's shoulders; nurse back up in desired direction while holding client around the waist.
- Keep call light within client's reach, check location of call light before leaving the room.
- Ensure access to eyeglasses or magnifying glass if used.
- Plan for eye examination if prescription seems inadequate.

Note: For *Sensory Perceptual Alterations: Kinesthetic and Tactile*, refer to *Potential for Injury*. For *Sensory Perceptual Alteration: Olfactory and Gustatory* refer to *Altered Nutrition, Less than Body Requirements*.

Geriatric

- Recognize that geriatric client may become more agitated in late afternoon and evening and wander; keep environment quiet, soothing, and familiar.
- Describe where client's body parts are when moving client.
- Avoid use of extremes of hot and cold in foods, and bath water.
- If sensory deprivation, encourage family to give sensory stimulation by providing familiar smells, music, voices, photographs, touch, and changes in light.

Client/Family Teaching

- Teach family how to provide appropriate stimuli in home environment to prevent sensory/perceptual alterations.
- Teach blind client how to feed self; identify food placement as the hours on a clock.
- Teach client/family actions that can be taken to deal with vision or hearing loss.
- Refer to community agencies for help in dealing with sensory/perceptual losses.

SEXUAL DYSFUNCTION

Definition
The state in which an individual experiences a change in sexual function that is unsatisfying, unrewarding, or inadequate.

Defining Characteristics
Verbalization of problem
Alterations in achieving perceived sex role
Actual or perceived limitation imposed by disease or therapy
Conflicts involving values
Alteration in achieving sexual satisfaction
Inability to achieve desired satisfaction
Seeking confirmation of desirability
Alteration in relationship with significant other
Change of interest in self and others

Related Factors (r/t)
Biopsychosocial alteration of sexuality
Ineffectual or absent role models
Physical abuse
Psychosocial abuse, e.g., harmful relationships
Vulnerability
Values conflict
Lack of privacy
Lack of significant other
Altered body structure or function (pregnancy, recent childbirth, drugs, surgery, anomalies, disease process, trauma, or radiation)
Misinformation or lack of knowledge

Client Outcomes/Goals
✓ Identifies individual cause of sexual dysfunction.
✓ Identifies stresses that contribute to dysfunction.
✓ Discusses alternative/satisfying/acceptable sexual practices for self or partner.
✓ Able to discuss with partner concerns about body image, sex role.

Nursing Interventions
- Perform sexual history: normal pattern of function, use client's vocabulary.
- Determine client's/partner's current knowledge.
- Observe for stress, anxiety, or depression as possible cause of dysfunction.
- Observe grief related to loss: amputation, mastectomy, or ostomy.

- Explore physical causes: diabetes, arteriosclerotic heart disease, drugs/medication side-effects, or smoking in males.
- Provide privacy, be nonjudgmental verbally and nonverbally.
- Provide privacy to allow sexual expression for client and partner.
- Explain need for client to share concerns with partner.
- Validate normalcy of client's feelings, correct wrong information.

Geriatric
- Discuss with client and partner their present role adjustments.
- Explore with client and partner various sexual gratification alternatives (e.g., caressing or sharing feelings).
- Discuss the difference between sexual functioning and sexuality.
- Teach to use nitroglycerine, if prescribed, before sexual activity.

Client/Family Teaching
- Teach importance of resting before sexual activity (mornings are the best time for some clients).
- Teach that usual or previous types of activity may be resumed when client can climb two flights of stairs without symptoms (change in breathing pattern, heart rate or pain).
- Teach client to take prescribed pain medications before sexual activity.
- Teach possible need for modifying positions (side to side; limit time resting on arms; heavier person on bottom).
- Refer to appropriate literature on sexuality and function.
- Refer to appropriate community resources: clinical specialist, family counseling, or sexual counselor.
- Teach how drug therapy effects sexual response, such as possible side effects and the need to report them.

ALTERED SEXUALITY PATTERN

Definition
The state in which an individual expresses concern regarding his/her sexuality.

Defining Characteristics
Reported difficulties, limitations, or changes in sexual behaviors or activities.

Related Factors (r/t)
Knowledge/skill deficit about alternative responses to health-related transitions
Altered body function or structure, illness or medical cause
Lack of privacy
Lack of significant other
Ineffective or absent role models
Conflicts with sexual orientation or variant preferences
Fear of pregnancy or of acquiring a sexually transmitted disease
Impaired relationship with a significant other

Client Outcomes/Goals
✓ States knowledge of difficulties, limitations, or changes in sexual behaviors or activities.
✓ States knowledge of sexual anatomy and functioning.
✓ States acceptance of altered body structure or function.
✓ Describes acceptable alternative sexual practices.
✓ Identifies importance of discussing sexual issues with significant other.
✓ Describes practice of "safe sex" in regard to pregnancy and avoidance of sexually transmitted diseases.

Nursing Interventions
- Give client permission to discuss issues dealing with sexuality (after you have established rapport or a therapeutic relationship); "Have you or are you concerned about functioning sexually because of your health status?"
- Observe client's perception of normal function, and what client feels are cause of difficulties, limitations, or changes.
- Teach normal anatomy and function if needed.
- Discuss alternative sexual expressions for altered body function or structure; closeness and touching are other forms of expression, some client's choose masturbation for sexual release.
- Discuss modifying positions because of altered physical state; instruct in the use of pillows to provide comfort.
- Encourage client to discuss concerns with significant other.
- Provide the client privacy for sexual expressions of his choice; close the door when significant other visits and put a Do Not Disturb sign on the door.

Geriatric
- Discuss the difference between sexual functioning and sexuality.
- Allow client to verbalize feelings regarding loss of sexual partner or significant other.

Client/Family Teaching
- Refer to appropriate community agency; certified sex counselor, Reach to Recovery, Ostomy Association.
- Discuss contraceptive choices; refer to appropriate health professional: gynecologist, nurse practitioner.
- Teach "safe sex': use a condom for intercourse, wash with soap immediately after sexual contact, do not ingest semen, avoid oral contact with the penis or rectum, do not exchange saliva, avoid multiple partners, abstain from sexual activity when ill, avoid recreational drugs and alcohol when engaging in sexual activity.

IMPAIRED SKIN INTEGRITY

Definition
A state in which the individual's skin is adversely altered.

Defining Characteristics
Disruption of skin surface
Destruction of skin layers
Invasion of body structures

Related Factors (r/t)
External (environmental): hyper- or hypothermia
Chemical substance
Mechanical factors (shearing forces, pressure, or restraint)
Radiation
Physical immobilization
Humidity
Internal (somatic): medication
Altered nutritional state (obesity, emaciation)

Altered metabolic state
Altered circulation
Altered sensation
Altered pigmentation
Skeletal prominence
Developmental factors
Immunological deficit
Alterations in turgor (change in elasticity)

Client Outcomes/Goals
✓ Skin surface will maintain/regain intactness.
✓ Indicates measures that will protect skin, including care of any skin lesions.

Nursing Interventions
- Observe skin condition thoroughly on admission and at least every 2 hours noting presence of any redness, swelling, or lesions.
- Inspect areas at high risk of developing skin ulcers every 8 hours including ears, elbows, sacrum, occiput, scapula, trochanter, scrotum, or heels.
- Note presence of any systemic disorders predisposing to skin breakdown such as diabetes mellitus, renal failure, or compromised immune system.
- Observe for bowel and urinary incontinence or diarrhea; if present, clean promptly and apply protective lotion to skin.
- Monitor client's nutritional status and fluid status; recognize that good hydration and nutrition is necessary to maintain skin condition.
- If skin broken and no signs of infection, apply hydrocolloid dressing, such as Duo-derm or semipermeable transparent dressing according to agency protocol to protect skin and allow healing to take place.
- Reduce the pressure on skin by use of devices such as air mattresses, low air loss beds
- Reposition frequently, at least every 2 hours if immobile.
- Keep skin clean and well lubricated; rub bony prominences gently with lotion with every position change.

- Keep linens clean and wrinkle free.
- Keep turning sheet under immobile client; use to avoid shearing force when turning or pulling client up in bed.
- Consult with enterstomal therapist for further help in healing skin lesions.

Geriatric
- Do not use tape on skin if avoidable.
- Avoid use of soap on skin, use bath oil in water to cleanse; utilize nondrying soap only.

Client/Family Teaching
- Teach client/family need for turning schedule, and good skin care, including need for inspection of skin.
- Teach client/family appropriate care of skin lesions.
- Teach family how to prevent burns.

HIGH RISK FOR IMPAIRED SKIN INTEGRITY

Definition
The state in which an individual's skin is at risk of being adversely altered.

Defining Characteristics
Presence of risk factors such as:
External (environmental): Hypothermia or
  hyperthermia
Chemical substance
Mechanical factors such as shearing forces,
  pressure, or restraint
Radiation
Physical immobilization
Humidity
Internal (somatic): Medication
Altered nutritional state (obesity or emaciation)

Altered metabolic state
Altered circulation
Altered sensation
Altered pigmentation
Skeletal prominence
Developmental factors
Immunological deficit
Alterations in skin turgor (change in elasticity)
Psychogenic
Immunological

Related Factors (r/t)
See risk factors

Client Outcomes/Goals, Nursing Interventions and Client/Family Teaching
Refer to Nursing Diagnosis *Impaired Skin Integrity*.

SLEEP PATTERN DISTURBANCE

Definition
Disruption of sleep time causes discomfort or interferes with desired lifestyle.

Defining Characteristics
Verbal complaints of difficulty falling asleep
*Awakening earlier/later than desired
Interrupted sleep
*Verbal complaints of not feeling wellrested
Changes in behavior and performance (increasing irritability, restlessness, disorientation, or lethargy listlessness)
Physical signs (mild fleeting nystagmus, slight hand tremor, ptosis of eyelid, expressionless face, dark circles under eyes, frequent yawning, or changes in posture)
Thick speech with mispronunciation and incorrect words
(*Critical)

Related Factors (r/t)
Sensory alterations: internal (illness or psychological stress)
External (environmental changes or social cues)

Client Outcomes/Goals
✓ Wakes up less during night.
✓ Awakens refreshed and has less fatigue during day.
✓ Falls asleep without difficulty.
✓ Verbalizes plan to implement bedtime routines.

Nursing Interventions
- Identifies presence of internal/external factors interfering with sleep, e.g., chronic pain, depression, metabolic diseases, such as hyperthyroidism, and diabetes.
- Treat anxiety or depression psychiatrically/medically.
- Observe medication, diet, or caffeine intake.
- Monitor presence of sleep apnea; if obstructive, treat accordingly with reducing diet.
- Position with pillows for increased air flow.
- Plan pain relief measures shortly before bedtime.

Geriatric
- Observe underlying illnesses, e.g., nocturia occurring with benign hypertrophic prostatitis.
- Teach management techniques as appropriate for chronic illness.
- Observe elimination patterns; initiate bladder training if appropriate.
- Note boredom; provide changes as necessary, e.g., change in decorations or new social activities may allay boredom.

- Provide measures to assist with sleep: warm bath before bedtime, warm milk, or back massage.
- Suggest light reading, or nonexcitable TV as evening activity.
- Increase daytime physical activity.
- Reduce daytime napping, if the client must nap limit naps to short intervals as early in the day as possible.

Client/Family Teaching
- Encourage avoidance of coffee, food, and liquid products with caffeine.
- Refer for sleep apnea studies.
- If client lives with family member, teach him/her to monitor sleep apnea.
- Teach relaxation techniques, pain relief measures, and or use of imagery before sleep.
- Encourage daytime exercise and activities as tolerated.

IMPAIRED SOCIAL INTERACTION

Definition
The state in which an individual participates in an insufficient or excessive quantity or ineffective quality of social exchange.

Defining Characteristics
Major:
Verbalized or observed discomfort in social situations
Verbalized or observed inability to receive or communicate a satisfying sense of belonging, caring, interest, or shared history
Observed use of unsuccessful social interaction behaviors
Dysfunctional interactions with peers, family or others
Minor:
Family report of change of style of pattern of interaction

Related Factors (r/t)
Knowledge/skill deficit about ways to enhance mutuality
Communication barriers
Self-concept disturbance
Absence of available significant others or peers

Limited physical mobility
Therapeutic isolation
Sociocultural dissonance
Environmental barriers
Altered thought processes

Client Outcomes/Goals
✓ Identifies barriers causing impaired social interactions.
✓ Discusses feelings that accompany impaired social interactions.
✓ States comfort in social situations.
✓ Able to communicate; states feelings of belonging and demonstrates caring and interest in others.
✓ Family states effective interaction with client.

Nursing Interventions
- Observe cause for discomfort in social situations; ask client if they can relate when discomfort began, any losses they may have experienced, e.g., loss of health, job, significant other, or aging; also any changes that may have occurred; marriage, birth, or adoption of a child; change in body appearance.
- Ask client to state any feelings of discomfort they may have in social situations and if they can identify any precipitating or causative factors.
- Monitor client's use of defense mechanisms and support healthy defenses, e.g., client is able to focus on here and now and avoids placing blame on others for his own behavior.

- Have client list behaviors that cause discomfort and discuss alternate ways to react to alleviate discomfort, e.g., focus on others and their interests and practice making caring statements: "I understand you are feeling sad."
- Encourage client to express his own feelings to others, e.g., "I feel sad also."
- Identify strengths of client; have client make a list of his own strengths and refer to it when he is experiencing negative feelings (client may find it helpful to put list on a 3x5 card to carry at all times).
- In a group have the group identify each other's strengths .
- Role play positive and negative social interactions and ways to respond; instead of ignoring a friendly greeting acknowledge it; if someone makes a rude remark respond with an "I" statement: "I understand you may feel that way, but this is how I feel."
- Model appropriate social interactions; give positive feedback for appropriate behavior; verbal and nonverbal; "I'm proud you were able to make it to work on time and that you did all the tasks assigned to you without telling your supervisor they were picking on you"; If not contraindicated touch the person's arm or hand when speaking to them and make eye contact.

Geriatric
- Use behavior modification techniques to teach social skills; stay with client during initial interaction to provide security, and reinforcement.
- Act as a role model through appropriate interactions with him/her and other clients.
- Provide group situations for the client.

Client/Family Teaching
- Help the client accept responsibility for his own behavior; you may have client use a journal and then review it with him at prescheduled intervals, giving him positive feedback for appropriate behavior and suggesting alternate approaches for behavior that did not enhance social interaction.
- Teach and practice with client how to approach others and how to ask them for what he needs.
- Practice social skills one-to-one and when client is ready in group sessions.
- Refer to appropriate social agencies for assistance; family therapy, self-help groups, and crisis intervention.

SOCIAL ISOLATION

Definition
Aloneness experienced by the individual and perceived as imposed by others and as a negative or threatened state.

Defining Characteristics
Objective: *Absence of supportive significant other(s) (family, friends, or group)
    sad, dull affect
Inappropriate or immature interests/activities for developmental age/stage
Uncommunicative, withdrawn, or no eye contact
Preoccupation with own thoughts, repetitive meaningless actions
Projects hostility in voice, behavior
Seeks to be alone or exists in a limited subculture
Evidence of physical/mental handicap or altered state of wellness
Shows behavior unaccepted by dominant cultural group
Subjective: *Expresses feelings of aloneness imposed by others
Expresses feelings of rejection
Experiences feelings of difference from others
Inadequacy in or absence of significant purpose in life
Inability to meet expectations of others
Insecurity in public
Expresses values acceptable to the subculture but unacceptable to the dominant cultural group
Expresses interests inappropriate to the developmental age/state
(*Critical)

Related Factors (r/t)
Factors contributing to the absence of satisfying personal relationships, such as:
Delay in accomplishing developmental tasks
Immature interests
Alterations in mental status
Unacceptable social behavior
Unaccepted social values
Altered state of wellness
Inadequate personal resources
Inability to engage in satisfying personal relationships

Client Outcomes/Goals
✓ Identifies the reasons for feelings of isolation.
✓ Practices social and communication skills needed to interact with others.
✓ Initiates interactions with others; sets and meets goals.

✓ Participates in activities and programs at level of ability and desire.

✓ Describes feelings of self-worth.

Nursing Interventions

- Observe barriers: limitations, and decreasing ability to form relationships, lack of transportation, money, support system, or knowledge.
- Note risk factors: age, ethnic/racial minority, environment, physical and or mental altered states of wellness.
- Discuss causes of perceived or actual isolation.
- Promote social interaction; support grieving, and verbalization of feelings.
- Establish trust through one-to-one, then introduce to others gradually.
- Use active listening skills; establish therapeutic relationship, and spend time with the client.
- Work with client to establish goals that are easy to reach to experience success, e.g., spends 10 minutes with peer and is able to converse with peer.
- Provide positive reinforcement when client seeks out others.
- Help client identify appropriate diversional activities to encourage socialization when ready.
- Encourage physical closeness (touch) if possible.
- Identify support systems available and involve in care.
- Encourage liberal visitation for hospitalized clients.
- Help client identify role models and others with similar interests.

Geriatric

- In health care facility schedule nurse-client visits every 2 to 3 hours for at least 10 minutes.
- Engage client in dialogue on topics of interest.
- Assist client in contacting community agencies that provide social services/activities.

Client/Family Teaching

- Teach skills for problem-solving, communication, social interaction, activities of daily living, and positive self-esteem.
- Encourage to initiate contacts to self-help groups, counseling, and therapy.
- Provide information to client about senior citizen services, house sharing, pets, day care centers, and church and community resources.

SPIRITUAL DISTRESS
(DISTRESS OF THE HUMAN SPIRIT)

Definition
Disruption in the life principle that pervades a person's being and that integrates and transcends one's biological and psychosocial nature.

Defining Characteristics
*Expresses concern with meaning of life/death or belief systems
Anger toward God
Questions meaning of suffering
Verbalizes inner conflict about beliefs
Verbalizes concern about relationship with deity
Questions meaning of own existence
Unable to participate in usual religious practices
Seeks spiritual assistance
Questions moral/ethical implications of therapeutic regimen
Gallows humor
Displacement of anger toward religious representatives
Description of nightmares/sleep disturbances
Alteration in behavior/mood evidenced by anger, crying withdrawal, preoccupation, anxiety, hostility, apathy, and so on
(*Critical)

Related Factors (r/t)
Separation from religious/cultural ties
Challenged belief and value system, e.g., due to moral/ethical implications of therapy, or intense suffering

Client Outcomes/Goals
✓ Able to state conflicts or disturbances related to practice of belief system.
✓ Discusses beliefs about spiritual issues.
✓ States feelings of trust in self, God, or other belief systems.
✓ Continues spiritual practices not detrimental to health.
✓ Discusses feelings about death.
✓ Displays appropriate mood for the situation.

Nursing Interventions
▪ Observe self-esteem, self-worth, feelings of futility, or hopelessness.
▪ Monitor support systems, be aware of own belief systems, and accept client's spirituality.
▪ Be physically present, available, and help client determine religious, or spiritual choices.

- Provide quiet time for meditation, prayer, or relaxation.
- Assist client to make list of important/nonimportant values.
- Ask how you can be most helpful, actively listen and reflect; seek clarification.
- Hold client's hand or place hand gently on client's arm if client is comfortable with touch.
- Assist client in developing short-term goals and tasks; help client to accomplish goals.
- Help client find reason for living and be available for support.
- Listen to client's feelings about death; be nonjudgmental; allow time for grieving.
- Assist in developing coping skills to deal with illness and changes in lifestyle; include client in planning for care.
- Provide appropriate religious materials and artifacts as requested.
- Provide privacy to pray with others or to be read to by members of own faith.

Geriatric
- Assist in life review and identify experiences that are noteworthy.
- Join with client in discussing personal definitions of spiritual wellness.
- Discuss with the client his perception of God in relation to his illness.
- Offer to pray with client or caregivers.
- Offer to read from *Bible* or other book chosen by client.

Client/Family Teaching
- Refer client to spiritual advisor of choice; prepare for religious rituals chosen.
- Refer to counseling, therapy, support groups, hospice, and so on.

HIGH RISK FOR SUFFOCATION

Definition
Accentuated risk of accidental suffocation (inadequate air available for inhalation).

Defining Characteristics
Presence of risk factors such as:
Internal (Individual):
Reduced olfactory sensation
Reduced motor abilities
Lack of safety education
Lack of safety precautions
Cognitive or emotional difficulties
Disease or injury process
External (environmental)
Pillow placed in infant's crib
Propped bottle in infant's crib
Vehicle warming in closed garage
Children playing with plastic bags or inserting small objects into their mouths or noses
Discarded or unused refrigerators or freezers without removed doors
Children left unattended in or near bathtubs/pools/hot tubs
Household gas leaks
Smoking in bed
Use of fuel-burning heaters not vented to outside
Low-strung clotheslines
Pacifier hung around infant's head
Person who eats large mouthfuls of food

Related factors (r/t)
See risk factors

Client Outcomes/Goals
✓ States knowledge of safety measures.
✓ Demonstrates appropriate knowledge of care based on the chronological/developmental age of the client.
✓ Demonstrates appropriate measures for physically/emotionally challenged clients.
✓ Identifies potential hazards and means to correct them.
✓ Demonstrates CPR.

Nursing Interventions
- Position client with altered mental status so that tongue is not including airway, provide artificial airway if necessary.

- Observe presence of gag-reflex before feeding client.
- If the client experiences difficulty swallowing use semisolid foods instead of liquids.
- Feed only small amounts of food at a time.
- Do not use pillows in infant's crib.
- Hold infant for feeding or place at least in 45 degree angle in an infant seat.
- Stay with infant/child or developmentally/emotionally delayed client when they are near water (bathing or recreational).
- Do not hang objects around infant's head.
- Keep infants crib away from any environmental hazards they could become entangled in.
- Do not leave plastic bags or small objects where infant or developmentally/emotionally delayed client could reach them.
- Avoid foods that can be aspirated, such as peanuts, popcorn, hard candy, or gum.
- Do not use powder or lint-containing dressings around clients with tracheostomies; teach to use creme/razor (not electric) if shaving is indicated.
- Refer to *Airway Clearance; Sleep Pattern Disturbance.*

Geriatric
- Observe client for pocketing of food in side of mouth and remove food as needed.
- Position in high Fowler's position when eating and for a half hour after.

Client/Family Teaching

- Teach safety measures appropriate for chronological/developmental age of the client (review nursing interventions).
- Teach overall safety: disposal of used refrigerators or freezers or removal of doors; no smoking in bed or if tired; keep garage door open when warming car; have heating systems checked and make sure there is proper ventilation; have working smoke detectors installed in residence.
- Instruct on the importance of knowing CPR and refer to classes.

IMPAIRED SWALLOWING

Definition
The state in which an individual has decreased ability to voluntarily pass fluids or solids from the mouth to the stomach.

Defining Characteristics
Major: Observed evidence of difficulty in swallowing, e.g., stasis of food in oral cavity or coughing/choking
Evidence of aspiration

Related Factors (r/t)
Neuromuscular impairment, e.g., decreased or absent gag reflex, decreased strength or excursion of muscles involved in mastication, perceptual impairment, or facial paralysis
Mechanical obstruction, e.g., edema, tracheostomy tube, or tumor
Fatigue
Limited awareness
Reddened, irritated oropharyngeal cavity

Client Outcomes/Goals
✓ Demonstrates effective swallowing and eating without choking.
✓ Free from aspiration: lungs clear and temperature within normal range,

Nursing Interventions
- Determine cause of swallowing difficulty (refer to Related Factors).
- Consult with physician to determine if any medical treatment is available to increase swallowing ability.
- Observe if client has sensation in tonsillar arch and soft palate; stroke area with a wet cotton swab to determine ability to sense; must have at least some feeling in this area to swallow properly.
- Ask client to touch his palate with his tongue; client will need to relearn this movement to push food back in throat.
- If client has a swallowing reflex, attempt to feed client.
- Position client upright with a pillow propped behind head to bring head forward forcing the trachea to close and esophagus to open.
- Start feeding with small servings of pudding or strained baby food.
- As you feed client, give directions "Open your mouth, feel the spoon in your mouth, taste the pudding, lift the food to the roof of your mouth with your tongue, put your chin down, swallow."
- Avoid giving liquids until client is able to swallow effectively; give liquids and food separately
- If client tolerates pudding and strained baby food, advance to soft diet.
- Keep suction equipment on hand during feeding.
- Check oral cavity for emptying after client swallows and before client finishes meal, nurse may need to manually remove food from mouth (use gloves and keep teeth apart with padded tongue blade).
- Praise client for successfully eating food.

- Consult with dietician for diet to nourish client and assist swallowing, may need thickening agent to put in food.

Client/Family Teaching
- Teach client need to practice touching palate with tongue; stimulate tonsillar arch and soft palate with cotton swab.
- Teach client how to swallow effectively in a step-by-step fashion.
- Educate client/family in rationale for food consistency and choices, appropriate feeding technqiues.

HIGH RISK FOR ALTERED BODY TEMPERATURE

Definition

The state in which the individual is at risk for failure to maintain body temperature within normal range.

Defining Characteristics

Presence of risk factors such as:
Extremes of age
Extremes of weight
Exposure to cold/cool or warm/hot environments
Dehydration
Inactivity or vigorous activity
Medications causing vasoconstriction/vasodilitation
Altered metabolic rate
Sedation
Inappropriate clothing for environmental temperature
Illness or trauma affecting body temperature regulation

Related Factors (r/t)

See risk factors

Client Outcomes/Goals

✓ Temperature within normal range.
✓ Explains measures needed to maintain normal temperature.
✓ Explains symptoms of hypothermia/hyperthermia.

Nursing Interventions

- Check temperature every _____ hour(s).
- Take vital signs every _____ hour(s) noting signs of hypothermia: decreased pulse, respiration, and blood pressure, or hyperthermia: rapid bounding pulse, and increased respiratory rate.
- Monitor for signs of hypothermia: shivering, cool skin, piloerection, pallor, slow capillary refill, cyanotic nail beds, decreased mentation, or comatose
- Monitor for signs of hyperthermia: visual disturbances, headache, nausea-vomiting, muscle flaccidity, absence of sweating, delirious, or comatose. (Refer to Nursing Interventions for *Hypothermia* or *Hyperthermia* as appropriate.)

Geriatric

- Recognize that elderly have decreased ability to adapt to temperature extremes and need protection for extremes: cold, need extra clothing/bedding and heat; hot, need extra fluids and air conditioning

Client/Family Teaching
- Teach client/family signs of hypothermia/hyperthermia.
- Teach client/family how to take temperature.

INEFFECTIVE MANAGEMENT OF THERAPEUTIC REGIMEN (INDIVIDUALS)

Definition

A pattern of regulating and integrating into daily living a program for treatment of illness and the sequelae of illness that is unsatisfactory for meeting specific health goals.

Defining Characteristics

Major: Inappropriate choices of daily living for meeting the goals of a treatment or prevention program
Minor: Acceleration (expected or unexpected) of illness symptoms
Verbalized desire to manage the treatment of illness and prevention of sequelae
Verbalized difficulty with regulation/integration of one or more prescribed regimens for treatment of illness and its effects or prevention of complications
Verbalized that did not take action to include treatment regimens in daily routines
Verbalized that did not take action to reduce risk factors for progression of illness and sequelae

Related Factors

Complexity of health care system
Complexity of therapeutic regimen
Decisional conflicts
Economic difficulties
Excessive demands made on individual or family
Family conflict
Family patterns of health care
Inadequate number and types of cues to action

Knowledge deficits
Mistrust of regimen and or health care personnel
Perceived seriousness
Perceived susceptibility
Perceived barriers
Perceived benefits
Powerlessness
Social support deficits

Client Outcomes/Goals

✓ Follows treatment plan as prescribed.
✓ States understands and will follow treatment plan.
✓ Verbalizes possible reasons for not following treatment plan, e.g., financial, lack of understanding.
✓ States or writes a schedule that includes treatment plan in activities of daily living.
✓ States knowledge of risk factors.

Nursing Interventions

- Observe cause for ineffective management of therapeutic protocol.
- Monitor client's/family's knowledge of illness and treatment.
- Observe cultural influence, educational level, and developmental age.
- Monitor ability to follow directions, solve problems, and concentrate.

- Observe reading and writing ability; provide appropriate teaching aids such as pictures if they are unable to read.
- Observe support system as helping or hindering therapy.
- Monitor sensory deficits, such as hearing or vision.
- Develop therapeutic relationship; spend time with client and remain nonjudgmental.
- Encourage to verbalize feelings about health alteration (disease state); encourage expressions of anger and loss as appropriate.
- Monitor anxiety as possible cause for noncompliance.
- Listen to client's statements of abilities; encourage use of them in self-care.
- Have client repeat instructions in his own words.
- Accept client's choices and adapt plan accordingly: use educational aids (flip charts, printed materials, and computer programs) to enhance individual learning style.
- Incorporate exercise into current lifestyle, e. g., parking the car a distance from the doorway and walking at a brisk pace (plan extra time for this type of exercise).
- Develop a written contract with client and evaluate the criteria set forth in the contract on a regular basis.
- Consult with health care person who has prescribed treatment regimen about possible alterations to encourage compliance.

Geriatric
- Monitor for memory deficits, signs of depression, and dementia.
- Use repetition, verbal clues, and memory aids in teaching health care regimen.

Client/Family Teaching
- Teach importance of following treatment regimen and consequences of noncompliance.
- Share information about appropriate services that may help with compliance: dietician, home health agencies, social services, community educational services, or peer support groups.

303

INEFFECTIVE THERMOREGULATION

Definition

The state in which the individual's temperature fluctuates between hypothermia and hyperthermia.

Defining Characteristics

Major: Fluctuations in body temperature above or below the normal range. See also major and minor characteristics present in *Hypothermia* and *Hyperthermia*.

Related Factors (r/t)

Trauma or illness
Immaturity
Aging
Fluctuating environmental temperature

Client Outcomes/Goals

✓ Temperature within normal range.
✓ Explains measures needed to maintain normal temperature.
✓ Explains symptoms of hypothermia/hyperthermia.

Nursing Interventions

- Check temperature every _____ hour(s).
- Take vital signs every _____ hour(s) noting signs of hypothermia: decreased pulse, respiration, and blood pressure, or hyperthermia: rapid bounding pulse and increased respiratory rate.
- Monitor for signs of hypothermia: shivering, cool skin, piloerection, pallor, slow capillary refill, cyanotic nail beds, decreased mentation, comatose.
- Assess for signs of hyperthermia: visual disturbances, headache, nausea-vomiting, muscle flaccidity, absence of sweating, delirious, comatose. (Refer to nursing diagnoses *Hypothermia* and *Hyperthermia* for further nursing interventions.)

Client/Family Teaching

- Teach client/family how to take temperature.
- Teach client/family signs of, prevention of, and treatment of hypothermia/hyperthermia.

ALTERED THOUGHT PROCESSES

Definition
A state in which an individual experiences a disruption in cognitive operations and activities.

Defining Characteristics
Inaccurate interpretation of environment
Cognitive dissonance
Distractibility

Memory deficit/problems
Hypervigilance or hypovigilance
Inappropriate nonreality-based thinking

Related Factors (r/t)
Factors to consider: Head injury
Mental disorder
Personality disorder
Organic mental disorder

Substance abuse
Severe interpersonal conflict
Sleep deprivation
Sensory deprivation or overload
Impaired cerebral perfusion

Client Outcomes/Goals
✓ Oriented to time, place or person; improved cognitive function.
✓ Free from physical harm and activities of daily living maintained.
✓ Performs activities of daily living appropriately and independently.
✓ Identifies community resources for help after discharge.

Nursing Interventions
- Observe causes of altered thought processes (Refer to Related Factors above).
- Monitor mental status: level of orientation, ability to follow commands, cognitive function.
- Report any new onset or sudden increase in confusion.
- Provide safety measures: bed in low position, side-rails, ambulate with assistance, or use soft restraints judiciously with physician's order (restraints may exacerbate confused behavior).
- Orient client to time, date, place, and person with each nursing contact, include the names of significant others into the conversation.
- Request family to bring in familiar pictures and articles from home; stay with client if appropriate.
- Place clock and calendar in prominent place in the room and refer to them.
- Set predictable routines for care and maintain continuity of staff caring for client.
- Check on client often and have brief interactions to prevent sensory deprivation.
- Keep environment quiet and calm to avoid excessive stimuli.
- Assist with daily hygiene as needed and encourage self-care.
- Provide support to family during client's period of disorientation.
- Initiate social service referral to find help for client following discharge.
- Limit use of sedatives and CNS depressants.

- Observe for presence of hallucinations, such as inappropriate laughter, slow verbal response, moving lips with no sound, smiling when not appropriate, or grimacing.
- Ask direct questions "Are you seeing or hearing something now?" or "Do you sometimes hear or see things that other people don't hear or see?"
- Accept that client is seeing or hearing things that are not there but tactfully let them know you do not hear or see the same things.
- Focus on reality: encourage expression of feelings over delusions, e.g., "Tell me how you feel when someone on TV tells you what to do."
- Set limits on delusional conversation: "We discussed that, let's talk about what is happening now on the unit."
- Ask for clarification if you do not understand client and state you do not understand.
- Assist client to state needs and to ask for assistance.
- Involve in activities for short periods of time.
- Refer to nursing diagnosis *High Risk for Violence* for further interventions.

Geriatric
- Introduce yourself each time you interact with client as needed.
- Keep all instructions simple and allow time for repetition.
- Do one thing at a time.
- Tell client everything that is happening even if they do not seem alert.
- Tuning into the disoriented client's feelings is more important than rigidly insisting he share nurse's reality; give comfort and understanding when client has processing difficulties.

Client/Family Teaching
- Teach family reorientation techniques; need to repeat instructions often.
- Assist family to identify coping skills, supports in the environment, and community services for dealing with clients with chronic mental illnesses.

IMPAIRED TISSUE INTEGRITY

Definition
The state in which an individual experiences damage to mucous membranes, corneal, integumentary, or subcutaneous tissues.

Defining Characteristics
Major: Damaged or destroyed tissue (cornea, mucous membrane, integumentary, or subcutaneous)

Related Factors (r/t)
Altered circulation
Nutritional deficit/excess
Fluid deficit/excess
Knowledge deficit
Impaired physical mobility

Irritants, chemical (including body excretions, secretions, medications)
Thermal (temperature extremes)
Mechanical (pressure, shear, or friction)
Radiation (including therapeutic radiation)

Client Outcomes/Goals
✓ Maintains intact tissue over body.
✓ Indicates measures that will protect tissue integrity of affected body area/part.

Nursing Interventions
- Observe skin condition for lesions and circulation quality.
- Inspect areas at high risk of developing skin ulcers, e.g., ears, elbows, sacrum, occiput, scapula, trochanter, scrotum, and heels.
- Inspect oral cavity, eyes and other mucous membranes.
- Assess for systemic disorders, such as diabetes mellitus.
- Monitor for bowel and urinary incontinence and frequency.
- Evaluate for mechanical trauma or irritation.
- Determine client's level of consciousness.
- Observe client's ability to move in and out of bed.
- Observe for signs and symptoms of tissue ischemia.
- Palpate tissues for consistency beneath the skin.
- Encourage range of motion exercises.
- Reduce the pressure on the client's skin by use of devices, such as air mattresses, low air loss beds.
- Reposition frequently.
- Give frequent skin care; wash and dry skin, especially areas in high moisture areas.
- Use nondrying soap and apply lotion to avoid dryness.
- Keep bedclothes dry and free of wrinkles.
- Encourage good nutrition and hydration with adequate protein to promote growth of healthy tissue .
- Check correct placement of footboards, restraints, traction/casts every 2 hours and assess intactness of skin.

- Assess for compartment syndrome in orthopedic patients.
- Check correct placement of nasogastric, gastrostomy, and endotracheal tubes and catheters and intactness of skin/tissue affected by tape securing placement.
- Assure adequate restraint as necessary to prevent self-extubation or removal of tubes/catheters with inflated balloons.
- Initiate safety measures to protect from excessive heat/cold, burns.

Geriatric
- Turn client gently and more frequently (elderly have decreased tissue perfusion and reduced amounts of subcutaneous fat).
- Maintain safe environment if vision is affected.
- If heat/cold therapies are used, monitor carefully.

Client/Family Teaching
- Educate why tissues over body prominences are especially vulnerable to skin breakdown from excessive pressure.
- Teach client and family how to inspect skin, as well as underlying tissues.
- Educate client and family about methods that can be used to reduce or prevent vulnerability of skin and protect tissue integrity of affected body area/part.
- Educate family about prevention of burns (thermal, chemical, or ultraviolet).

ALTERED TISSUE PERFUSION (SPECIFY TYPE) (CEREBRAL, RENAL, CARDIOPULMONARY, GASTROINTESTINAL, PERIPHERAL)

Definition
The state in which an individual experiences decrease in nutrition and oxygenation at the cellular level due to a deficit in capillary blood supply.

Defining Characteristics
Skin temperature: cold extremities
Skin color
  Dependent, blue or purple
*Pale on elevation, and color does not return on
  lowering leg
*Diminished arterial pulsations
Skin quality: shining
Lack of lanugo

Round scars covered with atrophied skin
Gangrene
Slow-growing, dry, thick, brittle nails
Claudication
Blood pressure changes in extremities
Bruits
Slow healing of lesions
(*Critical)

Related Factors (r/t)
Interruption of arterial flow
Interruption of venous flow
Exchange problems
Hypovolemia
Hypervolemia

Client Outcomes/Goals
✓ Demonstrates adequate tissue perfusion as evidenced by palpable peripheral pulses, warm and dry skin, adequate urinary output and absence of respiratory distress.
✓ Verbalizes knowledge of treatment regime; including medications, actions, and possible side effects.
✓ Lists any suggested lifestyle changes.
✓ Identifies factors causing decreased tissue perfusion.

Nursing Interventions
- Monitor vital signs, respiratory pattern, and peripheral pulses for presence and quality.
- Monitor lung fields for clarity.
- Monitor intake and output.
- Determine level of consciousness.
- Monitor for confusion, as well as complaints of dizziness and syncope.
- Note skin color and temperature.
- Inspect for pallor, cyanosis, mottling, cool, or clammy skin.

- Monitor for Homan's sign.
- Monitor bowel sounds; note any nausea or abdominal distention or discomfort.
- Monitor Laboratory values such as blood urea nitrogen, creatinine, liver function studies, or coagulation studies.
- Encourage active and passive leg exercises; unless clot formation is present.
- Elevate entire leg if venous insufficiency, use pillows lengthwise under entire leg; do not use knee gatch on bed.
- Use paper tape not adhesive.
- Change positions every 1 to 2 hours.
- Encourage ambulation if possible.
- Encourage rest after meals.
- Provide small meals of easily digested food and fluids.
- Elevate head of the bed and keep head neck in midline position.
- Keep room quiet.
- Avoid activities that increase cardiac workload (Valsalva maneuver).

Geriatric
- Monitor for irregular pulse (elderly have more irritable myocardium).
- Change positions slowly when getting out of bed (elderly have decrease in barorecptor sensitivity).

Client/Family Teaching
- Inform client and family of monitoring parameters.
- Explain pathophysiological state as appropriate.
- Explain importance of proper foot care.
- Stress importance of not smoking.
- Teach to avoid exposure to cold, to use warm clothing and limit exposure to brief periods if going out is necessary.
- Teach signs and symptoms that need to be reported to physician: change in skin temperature, color, or sensation.
- Teach to avoid Valsalva maneuver (bending at waist, holding breath while moving), teach to exhale when moving, avoid straining to have a bowel movement.

TOILETING SELF-CARE DEFICIT

Definition
A state in which the individual experiences an impaired ability to perform or complete toileting activities for oneself.

Defining Characteristics
*Unable to get to toilet or commode
*Unable to sit on or rise from toilet or commode
*Unable to manipulate clothing for toileting
*Unable to carry out proper toilet hygiene
Unable to flush toilet or commode
*(Critical)

Related Factors (r/t)
Impaired transfer ability
Impaired mobility status
Intolerance to activity, decreased strength and endurance
Pain, discomfort/perceptual or cognitive impairment
Neuromuscular impairment
Musculoskeletal impairment
Depression, severe anxiety

Client Outcomes/Goals
✓ Free of impaction, no urine or stool on skin.
✓ Explains methods that can be utilized to be independent in toileting.

Nursing Interventions
- Observe cause of inability to toilet independently (see related factors).
- Ask client for ideas on how to better provide toileting activities.
- Determine usual pattern for toileting and usual terminology for toileting activity.
- If client acutely ill, provide bed pan at appropriate intervals (see next intervention).
- Assist client with toileting every 2 hours, including first thing in morning, after meals, and before bedtime until self-care ability increases.
- Provide a commode next to the bed if necessary if client is able to get out of bed.
- Obtain assistive devices as needed, such as raised toilet seat, fracture bedpan, spill-proof urinal, or support rail next to toilet.
- Work with client to aim towards independence in toileting, praise independent toileting activity.
- Keep call light readily available and answer it promptly so client has rapid access to toileting facilities to decrease incontinence.

- Refer to Physical Therapy for help in working with client to transfer from bed to commode.

Geriatric

- Avoid use of indwelling or condom catheters, if possible, because they are a source of infection, and decrease the chance that the client will become independent.
- Help client develop a regular toileting schedule; use verbal prompting to impart awareness of need.

Client/Family Teaching

- Teach family how to help client toilet, including use of bedpan, commode, or appropriate toileting schedule.

HIGH RISK FOR TRAUMA

Definition
Accentuated risk of accidental tissue injury, e.g., wound, burn, or fracture.

Defining Characteristics
Presence of risk factors such as:
Internal (individual)
Weakness
Balancing difficulties
Reduced temperature or tactile sensation
Reduced large or small muscle coordination
Reduced hand-eye coordination
Lack of safety education
Lack of safety precautions
Insufficient finances to purchase safety equipment or effect repairs
Cognitive or emotional difficulties
History of previous trauma
External (environmental)
Slippery floors, e.g. wet or highly waxed
Snow or ice collected on stairs, walkways
Unanchored rugs
Bathtub without hand grip or anti-slip equipment
Use of unsteady ladders or unanchored electric wires
Litter or liquid spills on floors or stairways
High beds
Children playing without gates at the top of the stairs
Obstructed passageways
Unsafe window protection in homes with young children
Inappropriate call-for-aid mechanisms for bedresting client
Pot handles facing toward front of stove
Bathing in very hot water, e.g., unsupervised bathing of young children
Potential igniting gas leaks
Delayed lighting of gas burner or oven, experimenting with chemical or gasoline
Unscreened fires or heaters
Wearing plastic apron or flowing clothes around open flame
Children playing with matches, candles, cigarettes
Inadequately stored combustible or corrosives, e.g., matches, oily rags, lye
Contact with rapidly moving machinery, industrial belts, or pulleys, sliding on coarse bed linen or struggling within bed restraints
Faulty electrical plugs, frayed wires, or defective appliances

Contact with acids or alkalis

Playing with fireworks or gun powder

Use of cracked dishware or glasses

Knives stored uncovered

Guns or ammunition stored unlocked

Large icicles hanging from the roof

Exposure to dangerous machinery

Children playing with sharp-edged toys

High crime neighborhood and vulnerable clients

Driving a mechanically unsafe vehicle

Driving after partaking of alcoholic beverages or drugs

Driving at excessive speeds

Driving without necessary visual aids

Children riding in the front seat in car

Smoking in bed or near oxygen

Overloaded electrical outlets

Grease waste collected on stoves

Use of thin or worn potholders

Misuse of necessary headgear for motorized cyclists or young children carried on adult bicycles

Unsafe road or road-crossing conditions

Play or work near vehicle pathways, e.g. driveways, laneways, railroad tracks

Nonuse or misuse of seat restraints

Related Factors (r/t)

See risk factors

Client Outcomes/Goals

✓ Free from trauma.

✓ Explains actions that can be taken to prevent trauma.

Nursing Interventions

- Provide vision aids for clients with vision problems.
- Assist clients with ambulation.
- Have family member evaluate water temperature for client.
- Use reality orientation to improve cognition.
- Make social service referral for financial assistance.
- Keep walkways clear of snow, debri, and household goods.
- Provide assistive devices in bathrooms: handrails, or nonslip decals on floor of shower and bathtub.
- Ensure that call-light systems are functioning and that client is able to use them.
- Never leave young children unsupervised around water or cooking areas.
- Keep flammable and potentially flammable articles out of the reach of young children.
- Keep harmful objects, such as guns, locked up.

- Observe safety in high-crime neighborhoods: lock doors, do not leave home at night without a companion, and keep entry ways well lighted.
- Refer to appropriate resources regarding drug/alcohol education.
- Refer to interventions for *High Risk for Injury*.
- Refer to interventions for *Impaired Home Maintenance Management, High Risk for Poisoning, High Risk for Aspiration*, and *High Risk for Suffocation*.

Geriatric
- Perform a home safety assessment.
- Mark stove knobs with bright colored markings; outline step borders.

Client/Family Teaching
- Educate family regarding age appropriate child safety, environmental safety precautions, and how to intervene in an emergency.
- Educate family to assess day-care center, baby-sitters knowledge regarding child safety, environmental safety precautions, and ability to assist child in an emergency.
- Discuss various ways adolescent can protect self from trauma while maintaining relationships with peers. (Refer to Care Plans for *High Risk for Poisoning, High Risk for Aspiration, High Risk for Suffocation, High Risk for Injury*, and *Impaired Home Maintenance Management*)

UNILATERAL NEGLECT

Definition
The state in which an individual is perceptually unaware of and inattentive to one side of the body.

Defining Characteristics
Major: Consistent inattention to stimuli on an affected side
Minor: Inadequate self care
Positioning and/or safety precautions in regard to the affected side
Does not look toward affected side
Leaves food on plate on the affected side

Related Factors (r/t)
Effects of disturbed perceptual abilities, e.g., hemianopsia
One-sided blindness
Neurological illness or trauma

Client Outcomes/Goals
✓ Demonstrates techniques that can be used to minimize unilateral neglect.
✓ Both sides of the body are cared for appropriately and the affected side is free from harm.
✓ No injury, skin breakdown, or contractures of the affected body parts.

Nursing Interventions
- Monitor for signs of unilateral neglect: one side not washed or shaved, client found sitting or lying inappropriately on affected extremity, and eating food on only one side of plate, and so on.
- Recognize that unilateral neglect is more common if neurological pathology is in right nondominant side of brain with resultant left side affected.
- Turn and position every 2 hours to minimize pressure on skin, keep the involved arm on a pillow to decrease dependent edema.
- Place in bed positioned so unaffected side is closest to the doorway.
- Position bed so client approaches on the side where his vision is intact.
- Place call light, overbed table, TV, personal supplies, and telephone on unaffected side.
- Encourage the client to touch the affected side, encourage verbalization of what the affected side feels like.
- When client is up in the chair have the client bring his arm into the midline, and check for position of the arm at intervals.
- Use a sling for the affected arm when the client is up walking.
- Refer to a rehabilitation nurse speciaiist for continued help in dealing with unilateral neglect.

Client/Family Teaching
- Explain the pathology and symptoms of unilateral neglect.
- Teach the client to check the position of his body parts with his eyes at intervals and to turn his head from side to side when ambulating for safety.
- Teach the client to turn his plate around half way through the meal or to move the plate within his field of vision.
- Teach the client/family how to perform range of motion and position the affected side.
- Teach the family techniques to prevent injury, skin breakdown, and contractures of the affected side.

ALTERED URINARY ELIMINATION

Definition
The state in which the individual experiences a disturbance in urine elimination.

Note: This is a general diagnosis that is relevant when the pattern or source of the problem has not been identified. Please refer to more specific nursing diagnoses on urinary elimination (*Stress Incontinence, Urge Incontinence, Relfex Incontinence, Functional Incontinence, Urinary Retention*, or *Total Incontinence*) as appropriate.

Defining Characteristics
Dysuria

Frequency

Hesitancy

Incontinence

Nocturia

Retention

Urgency

Related Factors (r/t)
Multiple causality, including: anatomical obstruction, sensory motor impairment, or urinary tract infection.

Client Outcomes/Goals
✓ Voids clear amber urine without difficulty in appropriate receptacle, 1200-1500 cc/day.
✓ Explains measures that should be taken to prevent urinary tract infection.

Nursing Interventions
- Monitor pattern of voiding and characteristics of urine and keep intake and output.
- If there is dysuria or other signs of urinary tract infection monitor temperature, blood pressure, and pulse every 4 hours watching for signs of sepsis and shock.
- Provide fluids (offer fluids every 2 hours while the client is awake) and encourage intake of 2000-2400 cc within the clients cardiac reserve, avoid citrus juices, tomato juices, and fluids containing caffeine.
- Provide fluids that the client prefers.
- Provide unobstructed access to bathroom or toilet.
- Help client plan a voiding schedule that will fit into his lifestyle so that he voids approximately 300 ml per voiding.
- Ensure that pericare is done daily and prn.
- Encourage verbalization of feelings about problems with urination.

Geriatric
- For toileting problems, determine factors that interfere with self care and remove any barriers that exist.
- Gear interventions toward maintaining continence, functional independence, and self-care.

Client/Family Teaching

- Teach the need to take all of the medication ordered for the urinary tract infection until the medication is gone.
- Teach need for follow-up urine specimens.
- Teach symptoms of urinary tract infections: burning on urination, frequency of urination, or urgency to urinate.
- Instruct to call health care provider when symptoms are present so the infection can be treated.
- Teach methods to prevent urinary tract infections: frequent voiding, increased fluid intake, take showers not tub baths, void after intercourse, and wipe perineum from front to back.
- Teach client how to perform Kegel exercise and fit exercise into client's lifestyle.

URINARY RETENTION

Definition
The state in which the individual experiences incomplete emptying of the bladder.

Defining Characteristics
Major: Bladder distention, small frequent voiding, or absence of urine output

Minor: Sensation of bladder fullness

Dribbling

Residual urine

Dysuria

Overflow incontinence

Related Factors (r/t)
High urethral pressure caused by weak detrusor

Inhibition of reflex arc

Strong sphincter

Blockage

Client Outcomes/Goals
✓ Urinates 1200 to 1500 cc clear straw-colored urine in 24 hours and has less than 50 cc residual urine.

✓ States relief from pain of full bladder and suprapubic area is free of bladder distension.

✓ Describes measures needed to prevent, or treat urinary retention.

Nursing Interventions
- Evaluate medications that might cause urinary retention; especially tricyclic antidepressants, phenothiazines, anticholinergics, antihistamines, antihypertensives, drugs for parkinsonism, and some analgesics.
- Keep accurate intake and output, note color, clarity, and specific gravity of urine.
- Monitor for dystonia, urgency, and frequency.
- Monitor for bladder distension; request order for catheterization prn.
- Provide privacy for voiding.
- Assist male to stand to void, assist female up on the commode or toilet to void.
- Run water in the sink and pour measured amount of warm water over the perineum.
- Increase fluid intake to 2000 ml/day within cardiac and renal reserve.
- Use Crede's method prn, if not contraindicated by surgery or other condition.
- Play tape recorded sounds of waterfall or ocean prn to encourage voiding.
- Offer pain medication prn for pain that can interfere with voiding.
- Trigger reflex arc by having client lightly touch the perineal area.

Geriatric
- Assist elderly man to sit on commode to void.
- Assess for fecal impaction, if present, treat according to protocol.

Client/Family Teaching

- Teach use of relaxation techniques, such as deep breathing and visualization, e.g., visualize a waterfall.
- Teach methods to increase voiding: valsalva maneuver or Crede's method if no contraindications.
- Teach intermittent self catheterization if retention continues, and ordered by physician.
- Instruct in plan for home care: voiding routine, fluid intake, symptoms of retention, symptoms of urinary tract infection, when to notify physician, and available community resources.
- Teach client to respond to voiding urge.

INABILITY TO SUSTAIN SPONTANEOUS VENTILATION

Definition
A state in which the response pattern of decreased energy reserves results in an individual's ability to maintain breathing adequate to support life.

Defining Characteristics
Major: Dyspnea
Increased metabolic rate
Minor: Increased restlessness
Apprehension
Increased use of accessory muscles
Decreased tidal volume

Increased heart rate
Decreased pO_2
Increased pCO_2
Decreased cooperation
Decreased SaO_2

Related Factors (r/t)
Metabolic factors
Respiratory muscle fatigue

Client Outcomes/Goals
✓ Arterial blood gasses within safe parameters for client.
✓ Free of dyspnea, restlessness and is cooperative.

Nursing Interventions
- Monitor client for dyspnea, including respiratory rate, use of accessory muscles, intercostal retractions, and flaring of nostrils.
- Recognize that somnolence may be an ominous sign of respiratory failure with carbon dioxide narcosis.
- If signs of dyspnea, panic, deteriorating ABGs, collaborate with physician to place client on ventilator.
Note: The remaining nursing interventions are written for the client on a ventilatory.
- Ensure that bilateral breath sounds heard and chest x-ray done after intubation to ensure proper placement of ET tube.
- Retape ET tube every 24 hours, or according to protocol carefully noting gum/teeth line on ET tube with each taping.
- Provide oral care every 4 hours, noting gum/teeth line, condition of the oral cavity, possible pressure damage from position of the ET tube.
- Auscultate breath sounds every _____ hour(s), listen both anteriorly and posteriorly, note bilateral ventilation.
- Count respiratory rate for one minute and compare with rate of ventilator.
- Assess for symmetry of chest movement, ease of respiration, watching for synchronization of client's breaths with ventilator, note any "bucking" with the ventilator.
- Obtain ABGs and interpret after any ventilator adjustments.

- Coach client to increase strength of respiratory muscles: "Feel the difference between the machine's breaths and your own. Work to make your own breaths as deep and full as the machine's."
- Mediate for pain and anxiety as ordered.
- Ensure client is well-nourished; recognize need for increased fats in client with respiratory failure.
- Position client in semi-Fowler's position, change position at least every 2 hours.
- Suction PRN, hyperoxygenate, and hyperventilate client before and after suctioning.
- Check to ensure all alarms are on; never disable an alarm.

If Low Pressure Alarm On:

▶ Make sure client not disconnected from ventilator.
▶ Consult with respiratory therapist regarding ventilator malfunction; "bag" client if necessary until problem is resolved.
▶ Check to make sure tubing intact.
▶ Auscultate neck for possible leak around ET cuff.

If High Pressure Alarm On:

▶ Suction client if indicated.
▶ Note if client is "bucking" the ventilator; medicate as ordered.
▶ Consult with respiratory therapist regarding ventilator malfunction; "bag" client if necessary until problem is resolved.
▶ Check to ensure ventilator tubing not compressed.
▶ Empty water out of tubing PRN (not necessary with newer ventilators).
▶ Assess for possible cause of decreased lung compliance: fluid overload, hypoxia, atelectasis.

Note: For interventions on oral care, refer to *Impaired Oral Mucous Membranes*; for interventions on anxiety, refer to *Anxiety*; for interventions on communication, refer to *Impaired Verbal Communications*; for interventions on weaning, refer to *Dysfunctional Ventilatory Weaning Response*.

DYSFUNCTIONAL VENTILATORY WEANING RESPONSE (DVWR)

Definition
A state in which a patient cannot adjust to lowered levels of mechanical ventilator support, which interrupts and prolongs the weaning process.

Defining Characteristics
Mild DVWR
Major: Restlessness
Slight increased respiratory rate from baseline
Minor: Responds to lowered levels of mechanical ventilator support with: expressed feelings of increased
Need for oxygen
Breathing discomfort
Fatigue, warmth
Queries about possible machine malfunction
Increased concentration on breathing

Moderate DVWR
Major: Responds to lowered levels of mechanical ventilator support with: slight increase from baseline blood pressure <20 mm Hg
Slight increase from baseline heart rate <20 beats/minute
Baseline increase in respiratory rate <5 breaths/minute
Minor: Hypervigilance to activities
Inability to respond to coaching
Inability to cooperate
Apprehension
Diaphoresis
Eyes widening: "wide-eyed look"
Decreased air entry on auscultation
Color changes: pale, slight cyanosis
Slight respiratory accessory muscle use

Severe DVWR
Major: Responds to lowered levels of mechanical ventilator support with: agitation, deterioration in Arterial blood gases from current baseline, increase from baseline blood pressure >20 beats/minute, respiratory rate increases significantly from baseline
Minor: Profuse diaphoresis
Full respiratory accessory muscle use
Shallow, gasping breaths
Paradoxical abdominal breathing
Discoordinated breathing with the ventilator
Decreased level of consciousness, adventitious breath sounds, audible airway secretions, or cyanosis

Related Factors

Physical: Ineffective airway clearance

Sleep pattern disturbance

Inadequate nutrition

Uncontrolled pain or discomfort

Psychological: Knowledge deficit of the weaning process, patient role

Patient perceived inefficacy about the ability to wean

Decreased motivation

Decreased self-esteem

Anxiety: moderate or severe

Fear

Hopelessness

Powerlessness

Insufficient trust in the nurse

Situational: Uncontrolled episodic energy demands or problems

Inappropriate pacing of diminished ventilator support

Inadequate social support

Adverse environment, such as noisy, active environment, negative events in the room, low nurse-patient ratio, extended nurse absence from bedside, or unfamiliar nursing staff)

History of ventilator dependence >1 week

History of multiple unsuccessful weaning attempts

Client Outcomes/Goals

✓ Weaned from the ventilator with adequate arterial blood gases, return of blood pressure, pulse and respiration to baseline, and free of dyspnea and restlessness.

Nursing Interventions

- While on the ventilator, coach to increase strength of respiratory muscles: "Feel the difference between the machine's breaths and your own. Work to make your own breaths as deep and full as the machine's."
- Have the client well nourished before starting the weaning process; add extra calories and fats.
- Schedule rest periods at intervals.
- Normalize situation: assist client to be well-groomed; shave male, and provide female with make-up.
- Provide diversional activities, such as TV; use humor and sharing by nurse to make environment less frightening.
- Determine readiness to wean: awake/alert, psychologically ready, vital signs stable, inspiratory force >20 cm, and airway free of secretions.
- Negotiate to set goals for weaning; push the client to accomplish more within capabilities.
- If weaning goal not accomplished, reframe event as a practice session, not a failure; maintain self-esteem and self-efficacy.
- Have client free of pain before weaning; teach relaxation and imagery as alternatives to narcotic use.
- Do not give narcotic right before weaning; schedule pain medication/weaning carefully, weaning after narcotic's sedative but not analgesic effect has worn off.

325

- Schedule weaning periods in morning when client is rested; avoid doing other procedures during weaning, and keep environment quiet.
- Position client in semi-Fowler's position.
- Limit visitors (close supportive person only) during weaning, have visitor leave if they are having a negative affect on the weaning process.
- Have nurse who has positive relationship with client stay during weaning; coach client through ineffective breathing pattern and anxiety, give positive reinforcement, use touch and hold client's hand with permission.
- Avoid pharmacological sedation if possible; consult with physician in selecting a sedative drug with minimal muscle relaxant effects.
- Terminate weaning with physician collaboration when: blood pressure or pulse > or < 20 mm Hg; respiration >25 or <8; dysrhythmias, especially PVCs; oxygen saturation levels drop; panic; dyspnea, use of accessory muscles, intercostal retraction, flaring of nostrils, somnolence.
- If severe DVWR, slow down the weaning process, consider weaning in 5 minute periods only.

HIGH RISK FOR VIOLENCE: SELF-DIRECTED OR DIRECTED AT OTHERS

Definition
A state in which an individual experiences behaviors that can be physically harmful either to the self or others.

Defining Characteristics
Presence of risk factors such as:
Body language: Clenched fists, tense facial expression, rigid posture, or tautness indicating effort to control
Hostile threatening verbalizations: boasting of or prior abuse of others
Increased motor activity: pacing, excitement, irritability, or agitation
Overt and aggressive acts: goal-directed destruction of objects in environment
Possession of destructive weapon: gun or knife
Rage
Self-destructive behavior, such as active aggressive suicidal acts
Suspicion of others, paranoid ideation, delusions, hallucinations
Substance abuse/withdrawal

Other Possible Characteristics
Increasing anxiety levels: fear of self or others
Inability to verbalize feelings
Repetition of verbalizations: continued complaints, requests, and demands
Anger
Provocative behavior: argumentative, dissatisfied, overreactive, hypersensitive
Vulnerable self-esteem
Depression: specifically active, aggressive, or suicidal acts

Related Factors (r/t)
Antisocial character
Battered women
Catatonic excitement
Child abuse
Manic excitement
Organic brain syndrome
Panic states
Rage reactions
Suicidal behavior
Temporal lobe epilepsy
Toxic reactions to medications

Client Outcomes/Goals
✓ Does not harm self or others.
✓ Relaxed body language, decreased motor activity.
✓ No aggressive activity.
✓ States feelings of trust.

✓ Expresses decreased anxiety, or control of hallucinations.
✓ Able to talk about feelings, expresses anger appropriately.
✓ No access to harmful objects.

Nursing Interventions

- Monitor and document client's potential for suicide.
- Identify behaviors that indicate impending violence against self or others.
- Monitor suicidal behaviors; verbal statements; giving away of possessions, statements: "I'm going to kill myself," "My parents won't have to worry about having me around anymore."
- Monitor seriousness of intent: "Do you have a plan?" "How will you do it?" "Do you have the means?"
- Identify stimuli that instigate violence.
- Allow and encourage client to verbalize anger.
- Assist client to identify when anger occurs; have client keep an anger diary and discuss alternative responses.
- Maintain a calm attitude (anxiety is contagious).
- Provide low level of stimuli in client's environment.
- Observe client's behavior every 15 minutes; stagger times so client does not memorize pattern.
- Remove all dangerous objects from client's environment.
- Use suicide precautions if indicated: one-to-one staffing (constant attendance) and removal of all dangerous objects.
- Make a verbal or written contract with client: have client state or write "I will notify staff if I have suicidal or violent thoughts." I will not act on my thoughts."
- Redirect possible violent behavior; physical activity, e.g., punching bags, hitting pillows, walking, or jogging (if client is physically able).
- Provide sufficient staff if show of force is necessary to demonstrate control over situation to client.
- Use chemical restraints as ordered.
- Follow institutions protocol for releasing restraints; observe client closely; remain calm; provide positive feedback as behavior becomes controlled.
- Use mechanical restraints if indicated as ordered.

Geriatric

- Monitor for suicidal risk.
- Observe for dementia and depression.
- Monitor for paradoxical drug reactions; violent behavior can be stimulated when the desired action was to calm the client.
- Decrease environmental stimuli if violence is directed at others.

Client/Family Teaching

- Teach relaxation and exercise as ways to release angry feelings.
- Refer for individual or group therapy.
- Instruct family how to recognize an increase in risk for suicide; change in behavior, change in communication: verbal and nonverbal, withdrawal, evidence of depression (or depression lifting—client is at peace because plan is made and he has the energy to carry out plan).

APPENDIXES

NURSING DIAGNOSES ARRANGED BY MASLOW'S HIERARCHY OF NEEDS

Because human beings adapt in many ways to establish and maintain the self, health problems are much more than simple physical matters. Maslow's hierarchy of needs (see diagram) is a system of classifying human needs. Maslow's hierarchy is based on the idea that lower-level physiologic needs must be met before higher-level abstract needs can be met.

For nurses, Maslow's hierarch has special significance in decision making and planning for care. By considering need categories as you identify patient problems, you will be able to provide more holistic care. For example, a patient who demands frequent attention for a seemingly trivial matter may require help with self-esteem needs. Need levels vary from patient to patient. If a patient is short of breath, he is probably not interested in or capable of discussing his spirituality. In addition, a patient's need level ma change throughout planning and intervention, so you will need to be vigilant in your assessment.

Read the descriptions of each category in the diagram, and then see how you would relate them to nursing diagnoses. Compare your evaluation with how the authors categorized the nursing diagnoses according to this hierarchy. Be sure to assess patients for potential problems at all levels of the pyramid, no matter what their initial complaint.

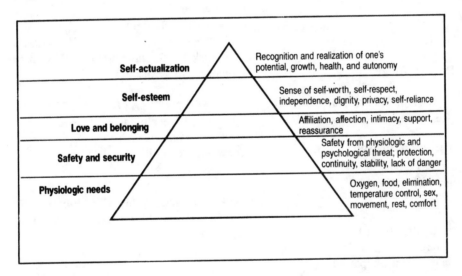

PHYSIOLOGIC NEEDS
Activity Intolerance
Airway Clearance, Ineffective
Aspiration, High Risk for
Breastfeeding, (Effective, Ineffective,
Interrupted)
Breathing Pattern, Ineffective
Cardiac Output, Decreased
Constipation (Colonic, Perceived)
Diarrhea

Fatigue
Fluid Volume Deficit
Fluid Volume Excess
Gas Exchange, Impaired
Hyperthermia
Hypothermia
Incontinence (Bowel, Functional, Reflex, Stress,
    Total, Urge)
Infant Feeding Pattern, Ineffective
Mobility Impairment
Nutrition, Altered
Oral Mucous Membrane, Altered
Pain (Chronic)
Protection, Altered
Self-Care Deficit (Specify)
Sensory-Perceptual Alteration
Sexual Dysfunction
Sexuality Pattern, Altered
Sleep Pattern Disturbance
Swallowing Impairment
Temperature, High Risk for
Altered Body
Thermoregulation, Impaired
Thought Process, Altered
Tissue Integrity, Impaired
Urinary Elimination Pattern, Altered
Urinary Retention
Ventilation, Inability to Sustain Spontaneous
Ventilatory Weaning Response, Dysfunctional

SAFETY AND SECURITY NEEDS
Communication, Impaired Verbal
Disuse Syndrome, High Risk for
Dysreflexia
Fear
Grieving (Anticipatory, Dysfunctional)
Health Maintenance, Altered
Home Maintenance Management, Impaired
Infection, High Risk for
Injury, High Risk for
Knowledge Deficit
Peripheral Neurovascular Dysfunction, High
    Risk for
Therapeutic Regimen, Ineffective Management
Unilateral Neglect

LOVE AND BELONGING NEEDS
Care Giver Role Strain
Coping, Ineffective Family
Parental Role Conflict
Parenting, Altered
Relocation Stress Syndrome
Social Interaction, Impaired
Social isolation

SELF ESTEEM
Adjustment, Impaired
Body Image Disturbance
Coping (Defensive, Ineffective Family,
    Ineffective Individual)
Decisional Conflict
Denial
Diversional Activity Deficit
Hopelessness
Noncompliance
Personal Identity Disturbance
Post-Trauma Response
Powerlessness
Rape-Trauma Syndrome
Self-Esteem (Chronic Low, Self Mutilation,
High Risk for Situational Low, Disturbance)
Violence, High Risk for

SELF ACTUALIZATION NEEDS
Growth and Development, Altered
Health Seeking Behavior
Knowledge Deficit
Spiritual Distress

Sparks, SM and Taylor, CM: *Nursing Diagnosis
Reference Manual,* Springhouse, PA, 1991,
Springhouse Corp.

NURSING DIAGNOSES ARRANGED BY GORDON'S FUNCTIONAL HEALTH PATTERNS

I. Health Perception - Health Management Pattern

Altered Health Maintenance
Altered Protection
Noncompliance
High Risk for Infection
High Risk for Injury
High Risk for Trauma
High Risk for Poisoning
High Risk for Suffocation
Health Seeking Behaviors
Ineffective Management of Therapeutic Regimen (Individuals)

II. Nutritional - Metabolic Pattern

Altered Nutrition: High Risk for More than Body Requirements
Altered Nutrition: More than Body Requirements
Altered Nutrition: Less than Body Requirements
Effective Breastfeeding
Ineffective Breastfeeding
Interrupted Breastfeeding
Ineffective Infant Feeding Pattern
High Risk for Aspiration
Impaired Swallowing
Altered Oral Mucous Membrane
High Risk for Fluid Volume Deficit
Fluid Volume Deficit
Fluid Volume Excess
High Risk for Impaired Skin Integrity
Impaired Skin Integrity
Impaired Tissue Integrity
High Risk for Altered Body Temperature
Ineffective Thermoregulation
Hyperthermia
Hypothermia

III. Elimination Pattern

Constipation
Perceived Constipation
Colonic Constipation
Diarrhea
Bowel Incontinence
Altered Patterns of Urinary Elimination
Functional Incontinence
Reflex Incontinence
Stress Incontinence
Urge Incontinence
Total Incontinence
Urinary Retention

IV. Activity - Exercise Pattern

High Risk for Activity Intolerance
Activity Intolerance
Impaired Physical Mobility
High Risk for Disuse Syndrome
Fatigue
Bathing/Hygiene Self-Care Deficit
Dressing/Grooming Self-Care Deficit
Feeding Self-Care Deficit
Toileting Self-Care Deficit
Diversional Activity Deficit
Impaired Home Maintenance Management
Ineffective Airway Clearance
Ineffective Breathing Pattern
Impaired Gas Exchange
Decreased Cardiac Output
Altered Tissue Perfusion: (Specify) Renal, Cerebral, Cardiopulmonary, Gastrointestinal, Peripheral
Dysreflexia
High Risk for Peripheral Neurovascular Dysfunction
Dysfunctional Ventilatory Weaning Response (DVWR)
Inability to Sustain Spontaneous Ventilation
Altered Growth and Development

V. Sleep - Rest Pattern

Sleep Pattern Disturbance

VI. Cognitive - Perceptual Pattern

Pain
Chronic Pain
Sensory Perceptual Alterations (Specify) Visual,
    Auditory, Kinesthetic, Gustatory, Tactile,
    Olfactory
Unilateral Neglect
Knowledge Deficit
Altered Thought Processes
Decisional Conflict

VII. Self-perception - Self-concept Pattern

Fear
Anxiety
Hopelessness
Powerlessness
Body Image Disturbance
Personal Identity Disturbance
Self-Esteem Disturbance
Chronic Low Self-Esteem
Situational Low Self-Esteem

VIII. Role - Relationship Pattern

Anticipatory Grieving
Dysfunctional Grieving
Altered Role Performance
Care Giver Role Strain
High Risk for Care Giver Role Strain
Social Isolation
Impaired Social Interaction
Altered Family Processes
High Risk for Altered Parenting
Altered Parenting
Parental Role Conflict
Impaired Verbal Communication
High Risk for Violence: Self-Directed or Directed
    at Others

IX. Sexuality - Reproductive Pattern

Sexual Dysfunction
Altered Sexuality Patterns
Rape-Trauma Syndrome
Rape-Trauma Syndrome: Compound Reaction
Rape-Trauma Syndrome: Silent Reaction

X. Coping - Stress Tolerance Pattern

Ineffective Individual Coping
Defensive Coping
Ineffective Denial
Impaired Adjustment
Post-Trauma Response
High Risk for Self-Mutilation
Relocation Stress Syndrome

XI. Value - Belief Pattern

Spiritual Distress

Based on Gordon M: *Manual of nursing diagnosis 1993-1994*, St. Louis, 1993, Mosby.

Nursing Diagnoses Arranged by Taxonomy I, Revised of the North American Nursing Diagnosis Association

EXCHANGING

Altered Nutrition: More than Body Requirements
Altered Nutrition: Less than Body Requirements
Altered Nutrition: High Risk for More than Body
Requirements High Risk for Infection
High Risk for Altered Body Temperature
Hypothermia
Hyperthermia
Ineffective Thermoregulation
Dysreflexia
Constipation
Perceived Constipation
Colonic Constipation
Diarrhea
Bowel Incontinence
Altered Urinary Elimination
Stress Incontinence
Reflex Incontinence
Urge Incontinence
Functional Incontinence
Total Incontinence
Urinary Retention
Altered (Specify) Tissue Perfusion (Renal,
   Cerebral, Cardiopulmonary)
Fluid Volume Excess
Fluid Volume Deficit
High Risk for Fluid Volume Deficit
Decreased Cardiac Output
Impaired Gas Exchange
Ineffective Airway Clearance
Ineffective Breathing Pattern
Inability to Sustain Spontaneous Ventilation
Dysfunctional Ventilatory Weaning Response
   (DVWR)
High Risk for Injury
High Risk for Suffocation
High Risk for Poisoning
High Risk for Trauma
High Risk for Aspiration
High Risk for Disuse Syndrome

Altered Protection
Impaired Tissue Integrity
Altered Oral Mucous Membrane
Impaired Skin Integrity
High Risk for Impaired Skin Integrity

COMMUNICATING
Impaired Verbal Communication

RELATING
Impaired Social Interaction
Social Isolation
Altered Role Performance
Altered Parenting
High Risk for Altered Parenting
Sexual Dysfunction
Altered Family Processes
Caregiver Role Strain
High Risk for Caregiver Role Strain
Parental Role Conflict
Altered Sexuality Patterns

VALUING
Spiritual Distress

CHOOSING
Ineffective Individual Coping
Impaired Adjustment
Defensive Coping
Ineffective Denial
Ineffective Family Coping: Disabling
Ineffective Family Coping: Compromised
Family Coping: Potential for Growth
Ineffective Management of Therapeutic Regimen
   (Individuals)
Noncompliance
Decisional Conflict
Health Seeking Behaviors

335

MOVING

Impaired Physical Mobility

High Risk for Peripheral Neurovascular
Dysfunction

Activity Intolerance

Sleep Pattern Disturbance

Diversional Activity Deficit

Impaired Home Maintenance Management

Altered Health Maintenance Feeding Self-Care
Deficit Impaired Swallowing

Ineffective Breastfeeding

Interrupted Breastfeeding

Effective Breastfeeding

Ineffective Infant Feeding Pattern

Bathing/Hygiene Self-Care Deficit

Dressing/Grooming Self-Care Deficit

Toileting Self-Care Deficit

Altered Growth and Development

Relocation Stress Syndrome

PERCEIVING

Body Image Disturbance

Self-Esteem Disturbance

Chronic Low Self-Esteem Situational Low Self-
Esteem Personal Identity Disturbance

Sensory/Perceptual Alterations (Specify) (Visual,
auditory, kinesthetic, gustatory, tactile,
olfactory)

Unilateral Neglect

Hopelessness

KNOWING

Knowledge Deficit

Altered Thought Processes

FEELING

Pain

Chronic Pain

Dysfunctional Grieving

Anticipatory Grieving

High Risk for Violence: Self-Directed or Directed
at Others

High Risk for Self-Mutilation

Post-Trauma Response

Rape-Trauma Syndrome

Rape-Trauma Syndrome: Compound Reaction

Rape-Trauma Syndrome: Silent Reaction

Anxiety

Fear

336

REFERENCES

Ackley E and Valentine S: Smoking cessation by patients with coronary artery disease, *Focus On Crit Care* 12(2):50-56, 1985

American Psychiatric Association: *Diagnostic and statistical manual of mental disorders*, ed 3, revised Washington DC, 1987, The Association.

Auerbach KG: The effect of nipple shields on maternal milk volume, *J Obste, Gynecol, and Neonat Nurs* 19:419-427, 1990.

Axton SE, Fugate T: *Neonatal and pediatric critical care plans*, Baltimore, 1989, Williams & Wilkins.

Bernard-Bonnin A, Stachtchenko, S, Girard G, et al: Hospital practices and breastfeeding duration: a meta-analysis of controlled clinical trials, Birth 16:64-66, 1989.

Bobak IM, Jensen MD, Zalar MK: *Maternity and gynecologic care*, ed 4, St. Louis, 1989, Mosby.

Bulechek GM, McCloskey JC: *Nursing interventions: treatments for nursing diagnoses*, Philadelphia, 1985, Saunders.

Carpenito LJ: *Handbook of nursing diagnosis*, ed 4, Philadelphia, 1991, JB Lippincott.

Carpenito LJ: *Nursing care plans and documentation: nursing diagnoses and collaborative problems*, Philadelphia, 1991, JB Lippincott.

Carpenito, LJ: *Nursing diagnosis: application to clinical practice*, Philadelphia, 1989, JB Lippincott.

Carroll-Johnson, M: *Classification of nursing diagnoses: proceedings of the ninth conference*, Philadelphia, 1991, JB Lippincott Co.

Cox HC, Hinz MD, Lubno MA, et al: *Clinical applications of nursing diagnosis: adult health, child health, women's health, mental health, and home health*, Baltimore, 1989, Williams & Wilkins.

Coyle N: Analgesics and pain, *Nurs Clin North Am* 22(3):727-741, 1987.

Doenges ME, Kenty JR, Moorhouse MF: *Maternal/newborn care plans*, Philadelphia, 1988, FA Davis.

Doenges M, et al: *Nursing care plans: guidelines for planning patient care*, ed 2, Philadelphia, 1989, FA Davis.

Doenges M , Moorhouse M: *Nurse's pocket guide: nursing diagnosis with interventions*, Philadelphia, 1991, FA Davis.

Doenges ME, Townsend MC, Moorhouse MF: *Psychiatric care plans: guidelines for client care*, Philadelphia, 1989, FA Davis.

Frank DA, Wirtz SJ, Sorenson JR, et al: Commercial discharge packs and breast-feeding counseling: effects on infant-feeding practices in a randomized trial, *Pediatrics* 80:845-854, 1987.

Gallagher M, Kahn C: Lasers: scalpels of light, *RN*, 46-52, 1990.

Hudak CM, Gallo BM, Benz, JJ: *Critical care nursing: a holistic approach*, Philadelphia, 1990, JB Lippincott.

Hufler DR: Helping your dysphagic patient eat, *RN*, 36-39, Sept 1987.

Jakovac-Smith D: Continence restoration in the homebound patient, *Nurs Clin of North Am* 23(1):207, 1988.

Jaffe MS, Melson KA: *Maternal unfant health care plans*, Springhouse, Penn, 1989, Springhouse.

Jones L, Brooks J: The ABCs of PCA, *RN*, 54-56, 1990.

Jurf J, Clements L, Llorente J: Cholecystectomy made easier, *Am J of Nurs* 90(12):38-39, 1990.

Keefe MR: The impact of infant rooming-in on maternal sleep at night, *J of Obste, Gynecol, Neonat Nurs* 17:122-126, 1990.

Kim MJ, McFarland GK, McLane AM: *Pocket guide to nursing diagnoses*, ed 5, St Louis, 1993, Mosby.

Knebel AR: When weaning from mechanical ventilation fails, *Am J Crit Care* 1(3):19-29, 1992.

Kozier B, Erb G, Liverti R: *Fundamentals of nursing concept, process and practice*, ed 4, Redwood City, Calif, 1991, Addison-Wesley.

Ladwig G, Anderson M: Substance abuse in women: relationship between chemical dependency of women and past reports of physical and/or sexual abuse, *Int J Addict* 24(8):00, 1989.

Lederer M, Mocnik S: *Care planning pocket guide, a nursing diagnosis approach*, ed 4, New York, 1991, Springhouse.

Lewis SM, Collier IC: *Medical-surgical nursing assessment and management of clinical problems*, ed 2, New York, 1987, McGraw Hill.

338

Lincoln R, Roberts R: Continence issues in acute care, *Nurs Clin of North Am* 24(3):741-754, 1989.

Luckmann J, Sorensen K: *Medical-surgical nursing*, Philadelphia, 1987, WB Saunders.

Matteson MA, McConnell ES: *Gerontological nursing: concepts and practice*, Philadelphia, 1988, WB Saunders.

McLane AM (ed): *Classification of nursing diagnosis: proceedings of the seventh conference, North American Nursing Diagnosis Association*, St. Louis, 1987, Mosby.

Milliken ME: *Understanding human behavior: a guide for health care providers*, ed 4, New York, 1987, Delmar.

Moore JB, Loxley CM, Cress SS, *The Pocket guide to clinical nursing process for the pediatric client*, New York, 1984, Miller Press.

Moorhouse MF, Doenges ME: *Nurse's clinical pocket manual: nursing diagnoses, care planning, and documentation*, Philadelphia, 1990, FA Davis.

Moorhouse MF, Geissler AC, Doenges ME: *Critical care plans: guidelines for patient care*, Philadelphia, 1987, FA Davis.

Murray RB, Huelskoetter MW: *Psychiatric/nental health nursing giving emotional care*, ed 3, Englewood Cliffs, NJ, 1991, Appleton & Lange.

NANDA Taxonomy I with Official Nursing Diagnoses: North American Nursing Diagnosis Association, St. Louis, 1990, The Association.

Neal MC, Paquette M, Mirch M: *Nursing diagnosis care plans for diagnosis-related groups*, Boston, 1990, Jones & Bartlett.

Nelson N, Beckel J: *Nursing care plans for the pediatric patient*, St. Louis, 1987, Mosby.

Newman D, Lynch K, Smith D, Cell P: Restoring urinary continence, *AJN* 23(1):28-34, 1991.

Pallett P, O'Brien M: *Textbook of neurological nursing*, Boston, 1985, Little Brown.

Paquette M, Neal M, Rodemich C: *Psychiatric nursing diagnosis care plans for DSMIII-R*, Boston, 1991, Jones & Bartlett.

Patrick ML, Woods SL, Craven RF, Rokosky J, Bruno PM: *Medical-surgical nursing: pathophysiological concepts*, Philadelphia, 1991, JB Lippincott.

Phipps WJ, Long BC, Woods N, Cassmeyer VL: *Medical-surgical nursing: concepts and clinical practice,* ed 4, St. Louis, 1991, Mosby.

Porth CM: *Pathophysiology: concepts of altered health states,* ed 3, Philadelphia, 1990. JB Lippincott.

Rasin J: Confusion, *Nurs Clin North Am* 25(4):909-916, 1990.

Roberts SL: *Nursing diagnosis and the critically ill patient,* Philadelphia, 1987, FA Davis.

Rousseau P: Hearing loss in the elderly, *Family Pract* 36(3):108-113, 1990.

Schonlau VLC: *The client's perspective of advocacy by nurses: implications for nurse clinicians, educators, and nanagers.* Paper presented at the meeting of the Iota Eta Chapter, Sigma Theta Tau, Long Beach, Calif, March 1991.

Schultz JM, Dark SL: *Manual of psychiatric nursing care plans,* ed 3, Glenview, Ill, 1990, Scott, Foresman/Little Brown.

Scordo K: Helping your patient cope with mitral valve prolapse, *Nurs '92* 22(10):34-39, 1992.

Servonsky J, Opas SR: *Nursing management of children,* Boston, 1987, Jones & Bartlett.

Sparks SM, Taylor CM: *Nursing diagnosis reference manual,* Springhouse, Penn, 1991, Springhouse.

Spyr J, Preach MA: Pulse oximetry, understanding the concept, knowing the limits, *RN,* 38-44, 1990.

Stutte PC, Bowles BC, Morman GY: The effects of breast massage on volume and fat content of human milk, *Genesis,* 10:22-24, 1990.

Swearingen P: *Manual of nursing therapeutics: applying nursing diagnoses to medical disorders,* St. Louis, 1990, Mosby.

Taylor C, Lillis C, LeMone P: *Fundamentals of nursing: the art and science of nursing care,* Philadelphia, 1989, JB Lippincott.

Thelan LK, Davie JK, Urden LD: *Textbook of critical care nursing: diagnosis and nanagement,* St. Louis, 1990, Mosby.

Thompson JM, et al: *Clinical nursing,* ed 2, St. Louis, 1989, Mosby.

Townsend MC: *Nursing diagnoses in psychiatric nursing: a pocket guide for care plan construction,* Philadelphia, 1988, FA Davis.

Wadle K: Diarrhea, *Nurs Clin of North Am* 25(4):901-908, 1990.

Wesorick B: *Standards of nursing care: a model for clinical practice*, Philadelphia, 1990, JB Lippincott.

Whaley LF, Wong DL: *Essentials of Pediatric Nursing* ed 2, St. Louis, 1985, Mosby.

Wong DL, Whaley LF: *Clinical manual of pediatric nursing*, St. Louis, 1990, Mosby.

Wyman J: Nursing assessment of incontinent geriatric outpatients, *Nurs Clin North Am* 23(1): 173-187, 1990.

INDEX

B

Back Pain, 19

Bathing/Hygiene Self Care Deficit, 19, 266

Battered Child Syndrome, 19

Battered Person; see Abuse—Parent, Significant Other, Caregiver

Bedsores; see Pressure Ulcers

Bedwetting; see Enuresis

Benign Prostatic Hypertrophy; see Prostatic Enlargement

Biliary Atresia, 19-20

Bipolar Disorder: Depression-Mania, 20

Bladder Distension, 20

Bladder Training, 20

Bladder Tumor, 20

Blindness, 20

Blood Pressure, Decrease; see Hypotension

Blood Pressure, Increase; see Hypertension

Body Image Disturbance, 128

Body Temperature, High Risk for Altered, 300

Bone Marrow Biopsy, 20

Borderline Personality, 20

Boredom, 20

Bowel Incontinence, 20, 206

Bowel Obstruction, 20

Bowel Sounds, Absent/Diminished, 21

Bowel Sounds, Hyperactive, 21

BPH, 21

Bradycardia, 21

Bradypnea, 21

Brain Injury; see Intracranial Pressure, Increased

Brain Surgery; see Craniotomy/Craniectomy

Brain Tumor, 21

Breast Feeding, Effective, 21, 130

Breast Feeding, Ineffective, 21, 132

Breast Feeding, Interrupted, 22, 134

Breast Cancer, 22

Breast Lumps, 22

Breath Sounds, Decreased or Absent; see Atelectasis; Pneumothorax

Breathing Pattern, Ineffective, 22, 135

Bronchitis, 22

Bronchopulmonary Dysplasia, 22

Bruits, Carotid, 22

Bulimia, 22

Burns, 22-23

Bursitis, 23

C

CABG; see Coronary Artery Bypass Grafting

Cachexia, 24

Calcium Decrease; see Hypocalcemia

Calcium Increase; see Hypercalcemia

Cancer, 24

Capillary Refill Time, Prolonged, 24

Cardiac Catheterization, 24-25

Cardiac Disorders in Pregnancy, 25

Cardiac Dysrhythmias; see Dysrhythmias

Cardiac Output, Decreased, 25, 137

Caregiver Role Strain, 25, 139, 142

Carious Teeth; see Cavities in Teeth

Carotid Endarterectomy, 25

Carpal Tunnel Syndrome, 25

Carpopedal Spasm, 25

Casts, 26

Cataract Extraction, 26

Catatonic Schizophrenia, 26

Catheterization, 26

Cavities in Teeth, 26

Cellulitis, 26

Cellulitis, Periorbital, 26

Central Line Insertion, 26

Cerebral Palsy, 26

Cerebrovascular Accident; see CVA

Cesarean Delivery, 27

Chemical Dependency; see Alcohol Abuse; Drug Abuse

Chemotherapy, 27

Chest Pain, 27

Chest Tubes, 27

Cheyne-Stokes Respirations, 27

Chicken Pox; see Communicable Diseases, Childhood

Child Abuse, 28

Child with Chronic Condition, 28-29

Chills, 29

Chlamydia Infection; see Sexually Transmitted Disease

Choking/Coughing with Feeding, 29

Cholecystectomy, 29

Discharge Planning, 39
Discomforts in Pregnancy, 39-40
Dissociative Disorder, 40
Disuse Syndrome, High Risk for, 40, 162
Diversional Activity Deficit, 40, 164
Diverticulitis, 40
Dizziness, 41
Down's Syndrome; see Mental Retardation; Child
   with Chronic Illness
Dressing Self, Inability to Do, 41, 268
Dribbling of Urine, 41
Drooling, 41
Drug Abuse, 41
Drug Withdrawal, 41
DVT; see Alcohol Withdrawal
Dysfunctional Eating Pattern, 41
Dysfunctional Grieving, 41
Dysfunctional Family; see Family Problems
Dysmenorrhea, 41
Dyspareunia, 42
Dyspepsia, 42
Dysphagia, 42
Dysphasia, 42
Dyspnea, 42
Dysreflexia, 42, 166
Dysrhythmia, 42
Dysthymia, 42
Dysuria, 42

E

Earache, 43
Ear Surgery, 43
Eclampsia, 43
Ectopic Pregnancy, 43
Eczema, 43
Edema, 43
Elderly Abuse; see Battered Person
Emaciated Person, 43
Emesis; see Vomiting
Emotional Problems; see Coping Problems
Emphysema; see COPD
Encephalitis; see Meningitis/Encephalitis
Endocardial Cushion Defect; see Congenital Heart
Disease/Cardiac Anomalies
Endocarditis, 44

Endometriosis, 44
Endometritis, 44
Endoscopic Laser Cholecystectomy; see
   Cholecystectomy
Enuresis, 44
Epididymitis, 44
Epiglotitis, 44
Epilepsy, 44
Episiotomy, 44
Epistaxis, 45
Esophageal Varices, 45
Esophagitis, 45
Evisceration; see Dehiscence
Exposure to Hot or Cold Environment, 45
Eye Surgery, 45

F

Failure to Thrive, 46
Family Processes, Altered, 46, 174
Fatigue, 46, 176
Fear, 46, 176
Febrile Seizure; see Seizure Disorders, Childhood
Fecal Impaction; see Impaction of Stool
Fecal Incontinence, 46
Femoral Popliteal Bypass, 46
Fetal Alcohol Syndrome; see Infant Substance
Abusing Mother
Fetal Distress, 47
Fever, 47
Filthy Home Environment, 47
Financial Crisis in the Home Environment, 47
Flashbacks, 47
Fluid Volume Deficit, 47, 180, 182
Fluid Volume Excess, 47, 183
Foreign Body Aspiration, 47
Formula Feeding, 47
Fractured Hip; see Hip Fracture
Fractures, 47
Frequency of Urination, 48
Frostbite, 48
Functional Incontinence, 208
Fusion, Lumbar, 48

P

Pacemaker, 80
Pain, 80, 236
Pain, Chronic, 80, 238
Painful Breasts—Cracked Nipples, 80
Painful Breasts—Engorgement, 80
Pallor of Extremities, 80
Pancreatitis, 80
Panic Attacks, 80
Paralysis, 80-81
Paralytic Ileus, 81
Paranoid Disorder, 81
Paraplegia; see Spinal Cord Injury
Parent Role Conflict, 81, 240
Parenthood, Adjustment to New, 81
Parenting, Altered, 81, 242
Parenting, High Risk for Altered, 81, 244
Paresthesia, 81
Parkinson's Disease, 82
Paroxysmal Nocturnal Dyspnea, 82
Patent Ductus Arteriosus; see Congenital Heart Disease/Cardiac Anomalies
Patient Controlled Analgesia; see PCA
Patient Education, 82
PCA, 82
Pelvic Inflammatory Disease; see PID
Pericardial Friction Rub, 82
Pericarditis, 82
Peripheral Neurovascular Dysfunction, High Risk for, 82, 246
Peripheral Vascular Disease, 82
Peritoneal Dialysis, 83
Peritonitis, 83
Persistent Fetal Circulation; see Congenital Heart Disease/Cardiac Anomalies
Personal Identity Disturbance, 83, 247
Personality Disorder, 83
Pertussis; see Respiratory Infections, Acute Childhood
Petechiae; see Clotting Disorder
Phobia, 83
PID, 83-84
PIH, 84
Piloerection, 84
Placenta Previa, 84

Pleural Effusion, 84
Pleural Friction Rub, 84
Pleurisy, 84-85
PMS, 85
Pneumonia, 85
Pneumothorax, 85
Poisoning, High Risk for, 85, 249
Polydipsia; see Diabetes Mellitus
Polyphagia; see Diabetes Mellitus
Polyuria; see Diabetes Mellitus
Postoperative Care; see Surgery, Postoperative
Postpartum Hemorrhage, 86
Postpartum, Normal Care, 86
Post Trauma Response, 86, 251
Potassium Decrease; see Hypokalemia
Potassium Increase; see Hyperkalemia
Powerlessness, 86, 253
Pregnancy—Cardiac Disorders; see Cardiac Disorders in Pregnancy
Pregnancy Induced Hypertension; see PIH
Pregnancy Loss, 86-87
Pregnancy—Normal, 87
Premature Dilation of the Cervix, 87
Premature Infant (Child), 87
Premature Infant (Parent), 88
Premature Rupture of Membranes, 88
Premenstrual Tension Syndrome; see PMS
Prenatal Care—Normal, 88
Prenatal Testing, 88
Preoperative Teaching, 88
Pressure Ulcer, 88
Preterm Labor, 89
Projection, 89
Prolapsed Umbilical Cord, 89
Prolonged Gestation, 89
Prostatectomy; see Transurethral Prostatectomy (TURP)
Prostatic Enlargement, 89
Protection, Altered, 89-90, 255
Pruritus, 90
Psychosis, 90
Pulmonary Embolism, 90
Pulse Oximetry, 90
Pulse Pressure, Increased; see Intracranial Pressure, Increased